BIOABSORBABLE POLYMERS FOR DRUG CARRIERS AND FIXATION DEVICES

BIOABSORBABLE POLYMERS FOR DRUG CARRIERS AND FIXATION DEVICES

Arbind Prasad, PhD
Sougata Jana, PhD
Editors

AAP | APPLE ACADEMIC PRESS

First edition published 2025

Apple Academic Press Inc.
1265 Goldenrod Circle, NE,
Palm Bay, FL 32905 USA

760 Laurentian Drive, Unit 19,
Burlington, ON L7N 0A4, CANADA

CRC Press
2385 NW Executive Center Drive,
Suite 320, Boca Raton FL 33431

4 Park Square, Milton Park,
Abingdon, Oxon, OX14 4RN UK

Library and Archives Canada Cataloguing in Publication

CIP data on file with Canada Library and Archives

Library of Congress Cataloging-in-Publication Data

CIP data on file with US Library of Congress

ISBN: 978-1-77491-866-1 (hbk)
ISBN: 978-1-77491-867-8 (pbk)
ISBN: 978-1-00356-981-7 (ebk)
DOI: 10.1201/9781003569817

About the Editors

Arbind Prasad, PhD
Mechanical Engineering Department, Katihar Engineering College (Under Department of Science, Technology and Technical Education, Government of Bihar), Katihar, Bihar, India

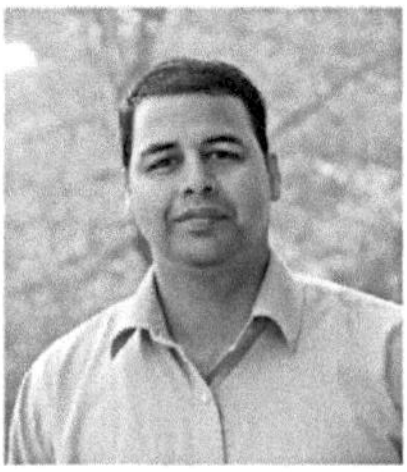

Arbind Prasad, PhD, is an Assistant Professor and Head (Mechanical Engineering) in the Department of Science, Technology and Technical Education, Government of Bihar, posted at Katihar Engineering College, Katihar, Bihar, India. He has four granted patents from his research work. He has international journal papers, book chapters, and reputed international conference papers to his credit. He has received several prestigious awards, such as a Sponsored Research Industrial Consultancy (SRIC) Award from IIT Kanpur, Best Oral Presentation from the American Chemical Society, best paper awards from IIT Guwahati during Research Conclaves. He has completed numerous projects funded by the state government. He is an Associate Editor for the *International Journal of Materials, Manufacturing and Sustainable Technologies* and early career editor for the *International Journal of Mathematical, Engineering and Management Sciences*. He is the book series editor of *Computational Intelligence and Biomedical Engineering*. He is editorial board member of various international journals and acts as active review board member of international journals. He has coordinated faculty development programs, short-term courses, symposiums, and national seminars and completed research projects sponsored under various government schemes in India. He has completed his PhD (Mechanical Engineering) from Indian Institute of Technology Guwahati, Assam, India and earned a gold medal in his MTech.

Sougata Jana, PhD
Department of Health and Family Welfare, Directorate of Health Services, Kolkata, West Bengal, India

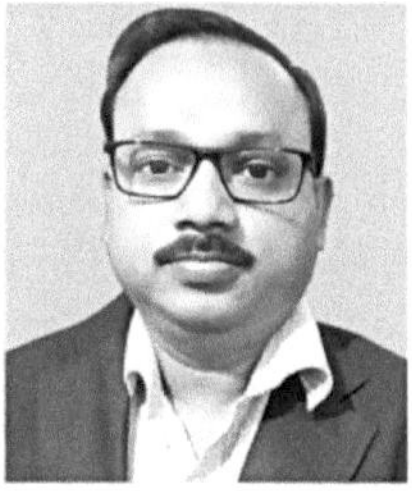

Sougata Jana, PhD, has spent 15 years in pharmacy, including teaching, research, and health services. He is affiliated with the Department of Health and Family Welfare, Directorate of Health Services, Kolkata, West Bengal. India. Dr. Jana has published over 30 research and review articles in different national and international peer-reviewed journals. He has also edited 15 books and published more than 45 book chapters in edited books by international publishers. He is a reviewer for peer-reviewed international journals. Dr. Jana is a life member of the Association of Pharmaceutical Teachers of India and holds an association with the Institution of Chemists, India. He successfully guided 17 postgraduate students in their research projects. Dr. Jana is working on drug delivery science and technology, including modification of synthetic and natural biopolymers, microparticles, nanoparticles, and semisolids and interpenetrating network (IPN) systems for controlled drug delivery. Dr. Jana completed his PhD in pharmaceutical technology at Maulana Abul Kalam Azad University of Technology (MAKAUT), West Bengal (formerly known as WBUT), India.

Contents

Contributors .... *ix*

Preface .... *xi*

1. **Introduction to Bioabsorbable Polymers: Processing and Characterization 1**
M. Francis Luther King, Arbind Prasad, and Bidyanand Mahto

2. **Bio-Absorbable Polymer-Based Scaffolds as Drug Carriers: Fabrication, Characterization, and Drug Release 31**
Gourhari Chakraborty and Pradip Das

3. **Functional Nanomaterials and their Applications in Biomedicine 61**
Nipun Jain, Ranjit Barua, and Sudipto Datta

4. **Bioactivity and Biocompatibility of Chitosan-Based Biocomposites 81**
Nancy Jaswal, Purnima Justa, Hemant Kumar, Sujeet Kumar Chaurasia, Adesh Kumar, Balaram Pani, and Pramod Kumar

5. **Degradation Studies of Bioabsorbable Polymeric Composites 105**
Atanu Kumar Paul, Gourhari Chakraborty, Shasanka Sekhar Borkotoky, and Arbind Prasad

6. **Biopolymer and Bio-Ceramics Composite for Orthopedic Applications 129**
Yusuf Olatunji Waidi, Samir Das, and Sudipto Datta

7. **Multifunctional Bio-Nanocomposite for Healthcare Application 149**
Abha Kathuria and Shruti Goel

8. **Biomechanical Studies of Biocomposites for Bone Fixation Devices 163**
Nipun Jain, Arbind Prasad, and Sudipto Datta

9. **Biocomposites in Craniofacial Fixations and Applications in Maxillofacial Fixations 181**
Hemant Kumar, Purnima Justa, Nancy Jaswal, Reenu Gangwar, Sundar Singh, Balaram Pani, and Pramod Kumar

10. **Physical and Biological Properties of Biocomposite Materials as Fixations or Sealers in Dentistry Applications 203**
V. Andal, R. Lakshmipathy, G. Jayanthi, and Arbind Prasad

11. New Frontiers of Hydrogels for Wound Healing Applications 219
Sriparna De, Madhurima Basak, Dipanjan Bhattacharjee, Arbind Prasad, and Bidyanand Mahto

12. 3D Printing of Bioabsorbable Polymeric Composites in Biomedical Applications 243
Sudipto Datta, Yusuf Olatunji Waidi, and Ranjit Barua

13. Clinical Translational Studies and Challenges of Bioabsorbable Polymeric Composites 267
Yusuf Olatunji Waidi, Nipun Jain, Ranjit Barua, and Sudipto Datta

Index 283

Contributors

V. Andal
Department of Chemistry, KCG College of Technology, Chennai, Tamil Nadu, India

Ranjit Barua
Indian Institute of Engineering Science and Technology, Howrah, West Bengal, India

Madhurima Basak
Department of Allied Health Sciences, Brainware University, Kolkata, West Bengal, India

Dipanjan Bhattacharjee
Department of Allied Health Sciences, Brainware University, Kolkata, West Bengal, India

Shasanka Sekhar Borkotoky
Department of Chemical Engineering, Assam Engineering College, Jalukbari, Guwahati, Assam, India

Gourhari Chakraborty
Department of Chemical Engineering, National Institute of Technology Tadepalligudem, West Godavari District, Andhra Pradesh, India

Sujeet Kumar Chaurasia
Center for Nanoscience and Technology, Prof. Rajendra Singh Institute of Physical Sciences for Study and Research, V.B.S. Purvanchal University, Jaunpur, Uttar Pradesh, India

Pradip Das
Spencer Laboratory, University of Delaware, Newark, USA

Samir Das
Indian Institute of Technology, Kharagpur, West Bengal, India

Sudipto Datta
Department of Materials Engineering, Indian Institute of Science, C.V. Raman Avenue, Bangalore, Karnataka, India

Sriparna De
Department of Allied Health Sciences, Brainware University, Kolkata, West Bengal, India

Reenu Gangwar
Institute of Dental Sciences, Bareilly International University, Bareilly, Uttar Pradesh, India

Shruti Goel
Department of Chemistry, IIT Roorkee, Roorkee, Uttarakhand, India

Nipun Jain
Department of Materials Engineering, Indian Institute of Science, C.V. Raman Avenue, Bangalore, Karnataka, India

Nancy Jaswal
Department of Chemistry and Chemical Science, School of Physical and Material Sciences, Central University of Himachal Pradesh, Dharamshala, Himachal Pradesh, India

G. Jayanthi
Department of Chemistry, KCG College of Technology, Chennai, Tamil Nadu, India

Purnima Justa
Department of Chemistry and Chemical Science, School of Physical and Material Sciences, Central University of Himachal Pradesh, Dharamshala, Himachal Pradesh, India

Abha Kathuria
Department of Chemistry, Ramjas College, University of Delhi, Delhi, India

M. Francis Luther King
Department of Mechanical Engineering, Swarnandhra College of Engineering and Technology (A), Narsapur, Andhra Pradesh, India

Adesh Kumar
Department of Chemistry, University of Delhi, Delhi, India

Hemant Kumar
Department of Chemistry, Ramjas College, University of Delhi, Delhi, India

Pramod Kumar
Department of Chemistry and Chemical Science, School of Physical and Material Sciences, Central University of Himachal Pradesh, Dharamshala, Himachal Pradesh, India

R. Lakshmipathy
Department of Chemistry, KCG College of Technology, Chennai, Tamil Nadu, India

Bidyanand Mahto
Government Engineering College, Vaishali (Under Department of Science, Technology, and Technical Education, Government of Bihar), Vaishali, Bihar, India

Balaram Pani
Bhaskaracharya College of Applied Sciences, Department of Chemistry, University of Delhi, Delhi, India

Atanu Kumar Paul
Department of Chemical Engineering, National Institute of Technology, Tadepalligudem, West Godavari District, Andhra Pradesh, India

Arbind Prasad
Mechanical Engineering Department, Katihar Engineering College (Under Department of Science, Technology and Technical Education, Government of Bihar), Katihar, Bihar, India

Sundar Singh
Department of Physics, Bareilly College Bareilly, Bareilly, Uttar Pradesh, India

Yusuf Olatunji Waidi
Department of Materials Engineering, Indian Institute of Science, C.V. Raman Avenue, Bangalore, Karnataka, India

Preface

There is a huge demand for bone implants and drug delivery systems, which play a significant and versatile role in various valuable applications. Advances in tissue engineering, implantable devices, drug delivery, bioimaging, scaffolds, and natural and synthetic polymeric materials have established their importance for development and utilization. Traditional procedures, implants, and other biomedical devices based on metals have many limitations, such as stress shielding, stress palpability, unmatched degradation behavior, leaching of metallic ions, and underlying bone damages. The emergence of bioresorbable composites based on naturally sourced biomaterials has a greater impact on their application. The advantages associated with bioresorbable composites, such as ease of modification of chemical, physical, surface, and biomimetic properties of polymers, have made them very appealing to researchers working in the biomedical field. Applications of biomaterials have led to the development of polymers that are biocompatible, biodegradable, and/or resorbable. A variety of research results are published almost daily on polymers and composites by enhancing their properties as biomaterials to meet the ongoing and evolving challenges in the biomedical field.

In this book, *Bioabsorbable Polymers for Drug Carriers and Fixation Devices*, deals with the latest biobased composites, processing, and characterization for drug delivery and fixation devices. There are a total of 13 chapters introduced in this book, in which Chapter 1 deals with the introduction to various bioresorbable polymers, their processing, and characterization. This will lead to an exhaustive discussion related to bioabsorbable polymers which are currently used in biomedical applications, their processing, and characterizations. Selection of the appropriate biomaterial plays a key role in the design and development of biomedical products. From the biomaterials, based on the complexity of the bone fracture, scaffolds play a vital role. Scaffolds come with various natures like they can be used for bone support, drug delivery, and other relevant roles such as multifunctional like anti-inflammatory, antimicrobial, etc. All of these are discussed in Chapter 2. The functional nanomaterials and their applications in biomedicine are explained in Chapter 3. Nowadays, emerging biomaterials are playing their effective role; such materials are chitosan and its derivatives. These materials have wide applications in biomedical implants and regenerative materials. Their bioactivity and biocompatibility have been discussed in Chapter 4. Chapter 5 provides detailed information on the degradation behavior of developing biomaterials that can create cellular response by including protein. The degradation behavior of the materials also finds fruitful applications in bioimplants and other biomedical devices. Chapter 6 relates to composite materials specifically for orthopedic applications. Various polymeric biomaterials have a lot of advantages over metallic fixation and implants. Thus, this chapter relates to biopolymers and ceramic-based composites. Chapter 7 deals with multifunctional bionanocomposites for healthcare applications. The mechanical strength always has greater significance towards the stability and durability of the bioimplants. Thus, Chapter 8 investigates the biomechanical studies of the relevant composites for bone fixation devices. The application of various biocomposites in craniofacial and maxillofacial areas is discussed in Chapter 9. Chapter 10 provides information on some of the rapidly developing groups of materials that find applications in many fields such as dentistry, medicine, and soft tissue regenerations. In this chapter, physical and biological properties have been studied, which could be useful as fixations or sealers in their areas. Chapter 11 describes various natural, synthetic, and semi-synthetic-based hydrogels for wound healing applications. These types of polymers are the most excitingly emerging class of materials and have the ability to respond to external stimuli such as temperature, pH, ionic strength, light, and electric and magnetic fields. 3D printing and clinical translation studies are described in Chapters 12 and 13, respectively. The 3D printing process of biomaterials shows remarkable growth among the bioimplants and biomaterials market. From these techniques, customized implants can be fabricated for their intended applications.

We believe that this book provides in-depth discussions and details on polymers and composites in their prospects as drug carriers and fixation devices that have applications in the biomedical field based on recent research results. Throughout the book, we have focused on recent applications with worked examples and emerging approaches to processing and characterization, which will serve the purpose of this book.

This book will prove to be a milestone for researchers, postgraduate students, industry professionals, doctors, and engineers who work in the biomedical field. We express our sincere thanks and appreciation to all the book chapter contributors from various parts of the world for contributing high-standard chapters to the book and their constant cooperation from submission to the first draft to revision and final tuning of their chapters, along with the reviews. We extend our appreciation and acknowledgment to them. Finally, we would like to thank Apple Academic Press for the opportunity, their constant support, and guidance for the successful completion of the book.

—Arbind Prasad, PhD
Mechanical Engineering Department, Katihar Engineering College, Katihar, Bihar, India
—Sougata Jana, PhD
Department of Health and Family Welfare, Directorate of Health Services, Kolkata, West Bengal, India

CHAPTER 1

Introduction to Bioabsorbable Polymers: Processing and Characterization

M. FRANCIS LUTHER KING,[1] ARBIND PRASAD,[2] and BIDYANAND MAHTO[3]

[1]*Department of Mechanical Engineering, Swarnandhra College of Engineering and Technology (A), Narsapur, Andhra Pradesh, India*

[2]*Mechanical Engineering Department, Katihar Engineering College (Under Department of Science, Technology and Technical Education, Government of Bihar), Katihar, Bihar, India*

[3]*Government Engineering College, Vaishali (Under Department of Science, Technology, and Technical Education, Government of Bihar), Vaishali, Bihar, India*

ABSTRACT

Over the course of many decades, bioresorbable polymers have been explored as promising candidates for advancing the state of the art in healthcare and biotechnology. In particular, bioresorbable polymers with a well-defined design offer significant benefits over their bulk equivalents for use in biomedical and implant devices, such as cell transport, scaffolds for tissue engineering, hydrogels, and in the pharmaceutical domains. Due to the prospective applications in artificial implant systems and biomedical devices, biocompatible implant devices based on bioresorbable materials (such as bioresorbable polymers that combine the unique characteristics of biocompatibility and simple handling) have emerged as a very active area. The innovative bio-absorbable polymers (BAPs) known as poly-hydroxy aliphatic esters have found widespread use as implantation products

Bioabsorbable Polymers for Drug Carriers and Fixation Devices. Arbind Prasad and Sougata Jana (Eds.)

(orthopedics, drug delivery, scaffolds, and sutures). Clinical applications of polylactic acid (PLA), polyglycolic acid (PGA), and polydioxanone (PDO) have been authorized by the Food and Drug Administration (FDA). Bioabsorbable polymers, their types, manufacturing, processing characteristics, and potential uses will be discussed in this chapter.

1.1 INTRODUCTION

The demand for biodegradable polymers that are biocompatible both when they are intact and as they break down is a result of increased research into ways to shorten the amount of time it takes for wounds to heal using drug delivery devices and the number of surgeries required to remove internal fixation implants. As a consequence of this, polymers that are formed of building units that exist naturally are gaining interest for use in biological applications. In addition to having excellent biocompatibility, these materials need to have a low cost throughout the synthesis, processing, as well as the purification and sterilization processes.

Medical advances pose significant difficulties for society as a whole because of the rising global population and the natural human desire to prolong one's own lifespan. The increasing incidence of bone fractures as a result of athletic and accidental injuries, as well as the aging of the population, is driving up the demand for orthopedic implants. More than 50 million fractures occur annually worldwide, and more than 8 million fracture repair procedures were performed globally in 2009 [1], according to data from the Orthopedic Industry (Report 2009–2010). Statistics reveal that the rate of fractures is not expected to decrease over the next decade due to the aging of the population. More than 7 billion people currently living on Earth will continue to work and age. Because of widespread anxiety about healthcare expenses, hospitals have begun implementing cost-cutting measures without reducing their commitment to enhancing patients' quality of life. There is a clear and present need to collaborate on developing affordable osteosynthesis implants that meet patients' needs while keeping the expenses of related medical technology, surgery, and rehabilitation to a minimum. It is possible to work with PLA in the same ways as other engineering thermoplastics. Fibers, rods, and molded pieces can all be created by melting the material. Extruding, injection molding, compression molding, solvent spinning, and casting are all viable options for working with PLA. Material that has been processed can also be machined into finished components [2].

Polymer linkages are particularly vulnerable to hydrolysis and temperature-induced depolymerization; therefore, extra caution is warranted around them [3]. If you want to keep your polymer from breaking down into water blobs during melt processing, you need to either keep it away from moisture or dry it out first. Degradation of poly(lactic acid) (PLA) is significantly influenced by processing conditions, especially temperature, shear rate, residence time, and the interactions between these variables. The loss of molecular weight caused by thermal and hydrolytic degradation directly correlates to a weakening of the material's mechanical properties. Oepen & Michaeli [4] detailed the impact of different processing parameters on the degradation of polymers during processing.

According to Oepen and Michaeli, temperature has the largest impact on the molecular weight decrease of the process factors. Above 180°C, chemical breakdown may be triggered by heat. To achieve a uniform melt during extrusion, the process temperature must be higher than the melting temperature (Tm), but it must also be kept low enough to prevent excessive loss of molecular mass. Higher processing temperatures make longer residence durations critical for effective molecular reduction [4]. As a result, polylactic acid's chain structure might undergo modifications during melt processing, either as a result of heat deterioration or hydrolysis. Temperatures exceeding 200°C cause PLA to degrade [5]. The process begins with hydrolysis, then continues on to oxidative main-chain scission and inter- or intramolecular transesterification reactions [6].

Biodegradable materials known as bioabsorbable polymers are particularly useful in short-term medical applications when the presence of a polymer implant is only briefly required. In the literature, the terms "bioabsorbable" and "bioresorbable" are often used interchangeably. By using them, it is inferred that the breakdown products of the substance are ingested by phagocytosis and then removed naturally from the biological environment. The three most common bioabsorbable polymers are poly(glycolic acid), poly(lactic acid), and poly(dioxanone). These have FDA permission for use in human clinical trials and are already widely utilized in medicine. Additional bioabsorbable polymers include polyhydroxybutyrate, polyhydroxy valerate, polycaprolactone, polyanhydrides, poly(ortho ester), poly(amino acid), and poly(ester amide) [7]. Various researchers have utilized the bioresorbable polymers for scaffold fabrication, bone regeneration, and internal fixation devices. Figure 1.1 shows the conventional drug delivery systems used for the delivery of specific drugs for their intended applications.

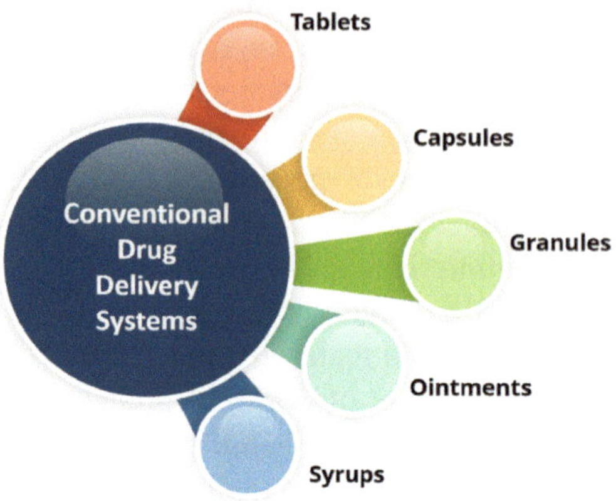

FIGURE 1.1 Conventional drug delivery systems.

Some of the limitations of the drug delivery system have been shown in Figure 1.2. It was observed that the poor adsorption of the biocomposite and the nearby sites leads to the production of infection and discourages the bone regeneration of the fractured bone. Sometimes, fluctuations in drug delivery, poor compatibility, and premature excretion create issues pertinent to bone healing.

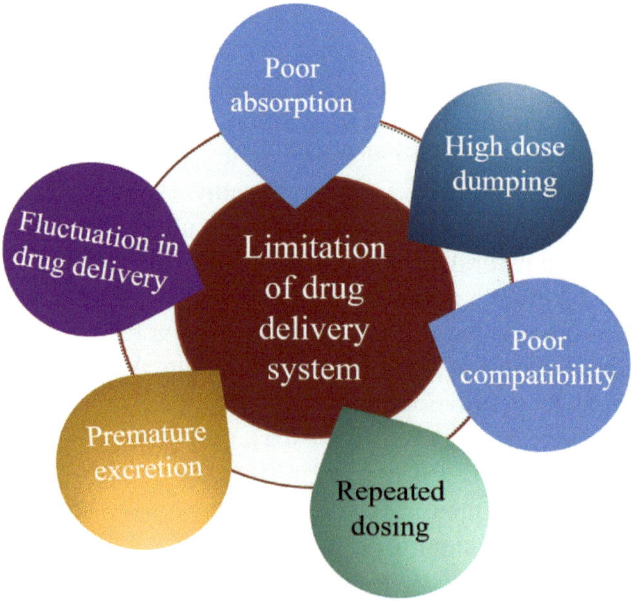

FIGURE 1.2 Limitation of the drug delivery systems.

1.2 BIOABSORBABLE POLYMERS

Bioabsorbable polymers are biodegradable materials that are beneficial in short-term medicinal applications that only need the transient presence of a polymer implant. The two words, bioabsorbable and bioresorbable, are sometimes used interchangeably in the scientific literature. To use them is to assume that the material's breakdown products are taken up by phagocytic processes and therefore eliminated from the biosphere. Poly(lactic acid), poly(glycolic acid), and poly(dioxanone) are the top three most widely used bioabsorbable polymers. They are already in widespread medical usage and have received FDA approval for human clinical trials. Polyhydroxybutyrate, polyhydroxyvalerate, polycaprolactone, polyanhydrides, poly(ortho ester)s, poly(amino acid)s, and poly(ester amide)s are some other bioabsorbable polymers [7]. Biodegradable polyesters are a popular kind of polymer, despite their often subpar thermal and mechanical qualities. Despite their high thermal and mechanical stability, polyamides are notoriously difficult to biodegrade because of their strong intermolecular bonds. Even though the amide functional groups are degradable by enzymes, the polyamide structure as a whole is resistant to biodegradation because of the high concentration of hydrogen bonds and the great regularity of its structure. Recently, numerous novel polyesteramide copolymers have been synthesized in an attempt to develop a biodegradable polymer with desirable thermal and mechanical characteristics [8]. Figure 1.3 depicts the classification of biobased polymers.

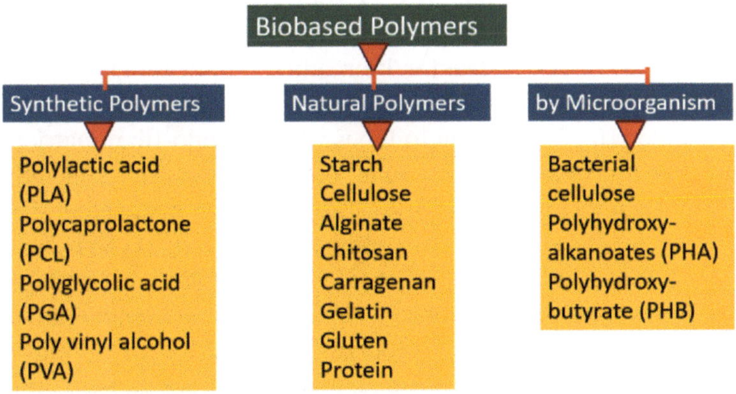

FIGURE 1.3 Classification of biobased polymers for biomedical applications.

1.2.1 NATURAL BIOABSORBABLE POLYMERS

Bioabsorbable implants have shown steady growth in clinical applications over the last few decades as a result of the extensive research done in this area. Contradictory findings regarding the absorption behavior of these materials, acquired by various groups, and the lengthy resorption time of PLA implants, which require research projects of very long duration, may have been the primary cause for the previous sluggish development. Bioabsorbable bone fixation devices have only been used clinically for the last four decades, but they have already shown to be a major improvement over metal implants for the treatment of cancellous bone fractures. There is no need for removal surgery with bioabsorbable implants, and the osteoporosis that may occur with stiff metallic implants is avoided. The healing of the bone is improved, and the financial and psychological benefits of avoiding removal treatments outweigh the costs. In surgical applications where the implant's presence is only transitory, it is certain that in the future, ultra-high strength bioabsorbable composite implants will replace conventional metallic and biostable devices.

1.2.1.1 COLLAGEN

Collagen is the most common protein in the body and plays a crucial role in the structure of skin and bones [9]. Collagen has a molecular weight (Mw) of 3,00,000 and a chain length of 300 nm, making it a polymer with repeating sequences. Collagen's innate mechanical strength and helical shape are due to the protein's repeating patterns. Despite the fact that collagen is broken down by bodily enzymes, its mechanical and biological characteristics have been thoroughly investigated for biomedical applications. Collagen functions well as a biomaterial because it is osteoconductive, biocompatible, and biodegradable [10]. In addition to tubes, sheets, nano-fiber matrices, foams, powders, and injectable viscous solutions and dispersions, it may also be treated into a number of other shapes. The mineral/organic natural composite that is mostly made up of collagen and hydroxyapatite (HA) is human bone. Therefore, composites consisting of calcium phosphate and collagen are the most biomimetic system for osseous replacement and regenerative applications [11, 12]. The biomaterial produced when collagen is combined with calcium phosphate particles may be readily molded for therapeutic purposes. Collagen coatings have been shown to enhance early cell adherence and proliferation on calcium phosphate substrates and implants [13]. As a consequence, *in vivo* implanted materials have improved osteoconduction, osteointegration, and bone-forming abilities [13]. Particle-gel mixing and powder compression procedures have been used to create composite materials that comprise calcium phosphate and collagen [14]. Dicalcium phosphate dehydrate (DCPD), commonly known as brushite, sets faster when additives like citric acid are employed, and the resultant hardened biomaterials exhibit compressive strengths that are on par with cancellous bone [15]. Citric acid increases the workability of the collagen-brushite cement paste and makes it simpler to combine the high collagen gel (3 wt.%) with the cement particles. The shorter setting time and lower viscosity achieved with citric acid improved the composite's injectability. By immersing the biomaterial in a glutaraldehyde solution (2%), we studied the impact of cross-linking into the collagen-brushite composite phase. However, studies have shown that immersing composite materials in water does not improve their compressive strength [16].

1.2.1.2 CHITOSAN

A linear polysaccharide composed of a precise ratio of glucosamine to N-acetyl glucosamine, it is a natural biopolymer derived from chitin [17]. Chitosan may range in molecular weight from 300 to 1,000 kDa, depending on where it was produced and how it was processed. Due to the protonated free amino group of glucosamine, chitosan, which is typically insoluble in aqueous solutions above pH 7, becomes soluble in dilute acids with a pH of less than 6 [18]. *In vitro* chitosan degradation has been observed for lysozyme, papain, and chitosanase. The hydrolysis of acetylated residues is catalyzed by lysozyme, which regulates the breakdown of the protein *in vivo*. Chitosan's crystallinity and acetylation affect the polymer's rate of breakdown [19]. Chitosan may be molded into scaffolds and constructions with porous micro-architecture that support osteoconduction and are biocompatible [20]. Chemical manipulations may change the rate of biodegradation and solubility, with the heavily deacetylated form showing delayed biodegradation over many months *in vivo* [19]. For this purpose, chitosan and calcium phosphate mixtures have been investigated. According to research by Seeherman et al. [20] scaffolds produced from high molecular weight chitosan have better mechanical qualities than those of scaffolds manufactured from medium molecular weight chitosan. Scaffolds constructed of chitosan plus nano-crystalline calcium phosphate have two benefits over chitosan-only scaffolds: a rough surface and "20 times greater surface area per unit mass than chitosan scaffolds alone." In the context of bone regeneration and repair, greater roughness and surface area have positive effects on protein adsorption, cell adhesion, and proliferation. Their improved mechanical capabilities are a result of calcium phosphate nano-crystals' greater association with chitosan and their more uniform distribution inside the scaffolds [21]. Chitosan was combined with collagen to produce composite micro-granules that may be used as bone replacements. This is due to the fact that the structure of the micro-granules allows for tight packing into flaws and that the linked holes between the micro-granules allow for the ingrowth of new bone and blood vessels [22]. These chitosan/collagen composite biomaterials' mechanical strength is greatly increased by the addition of filler particles like HA [23]. Chitosan/silica xerogel membranes have been demonstrated to dramatically boost new bone production when compared to pure chitosan membranes. A histomorphometric study revealed that the hybrid membrane fully repaired the defect after 3 weeks, while a chitosan membrane alone only closed 57% of the lesion. A low dose of synthetic sulfated chitosan was used to stimulate osteoblast differentiation *in vitro* and to induce ectopic bone formation *in vivo* [24]. This study examined the effects of different sulfate groups, sulfur content, and molecular weight on the bioactivity of bone morphogenetic protein 2 (BMP-2).

1.2.2 SYNTHETIC BIOABSORBABLE POLYMERS

1.2.2.1 POLY(ESTER AMIDE)S

Making polyesteramides (PEAs) from all-natural ingredients has gained traction recently since it allows for the polymer's breakdown products to be easily digested by the body. These components may be found in nature and include things like amino acids and hydroxy acids. Polyamides derived from amino acids are thought to be a good option for this purpose because of their structural similarity to real proteins. Nevertheless, working only with poly(amino acid)s has a number of drawbacks, such as high production costs, insolubility in common organic solvents, thermal deterioration during the melt process, and sluggish biodegradation rates. Even though poly(ester-amide)s have all the desirable qualities of both poly(hydroxy acid)s and poly(amino acid)s, their production is time-consuming and costly. Extreme reaction conditions are required for ring-opening melt polymerization, and as a result, poor yield and low molecular weight are commonplace, along with undesired side reactions. As a result of these unintended reactions, undesirable byproducts are produced, preventing their usage in medical settings [25].

Materials with a variety of properties can be created by incorporating polymers. By varying the ratios of three building blocks—amino acid, diol, and dicarboxylic acid—many polymers have been synthesized. A quick method to develop a wide range of properties is to combine these building blocks in different ways. Some potential applications of these polymers include vascular grafts, nerve guide tubes, bone plates, pins and screws, surgical meshes, temporary prosthetic skin, and drug delivery systems. The synthesis process occurs in three stages: (i) preparation of di-p-toluenesulfonic acid salts of bis(α-amino acid)α,ω-alkylene diesters; (ii) preparation of di-p-nitrophenyl esters of dicarboxylic acids; and (iii) solution polycondensation of the products from stages 1 and 2. Six α-amino acids were employed—L-valine, L-leucine, L-isoleucine, DL-norleucine, L- and DL-phenylalanine, and DL-methionine—along with three diols (1,3-propanediol, 1,4-butanediol, and 1,6-hexanediol) and two dicarboxylic acids (adipoyl and sebacoyl). Additional components used in the process include p-toluenesulfonic acid monohydrate, p-nitrophenol, N-dimethylacetamide, N-methyl-2-pyrrolidinone, benzene, nitrobenzene, ethyl acetate, acetone, acetonitrile, chloroform, triethylamine, N-methylmorpholine, N-tetramethyl ethylenediamine, and pyridine. The polymers were named based on the number of carbon atoms present in the dicarboxylic acid (x) and diol (y), as well as the α-amino acid (αaa) included (i.e., x-αaa-y) [25].

1.2.2.2 PLA, PGA, AND PDS

The three most typical polymers used for bioabsorbable implants include poly(lactic acid), poly(glycolic acid), and polydioxanone (PDS). PDS polymers have the highest number of clinical applications. These are alpha-polyesters or poly-(alpha hydroxy) acids. PDS was created in the early 1980s, although PLA and PGA research dates back over 50 years. Medicinal applications of PLA date back decades [26, 27]. Kulkarni and colleagues were the first to report its usage as sutures and rods for the treatment of a variety of conditions, including dog mandibular fracture repair [28].

These substances are polymers, which means they are produced through the assembly of monomers into larger molecules via covalent bonding. A polymer may be constructed from the repetition of a single monomer (a homopolymer) or from the combination of two or more different monomers (copolymer). As an added bonus, these copolymers may exhibit a disordered configuration of their monomers (random copolymer); alternatively, they might include lengthy monomer segments that alternate with blocks (block copolymer). Polymer chains may also have a chain that is linear, has branches, or is connected to other chains. In amorphous polymers, the chains of atoms are randomly arranged, whereas in crystalline polymers, the atoms are ordered in a crystalline form. Typically, these components consist of both amorphous and crystalline areas. In terms of rigidity and damping, this "semicrystalline" structure is significant. A more crystalline structure results in a more robust build because there is more microstructural organization, in addition to a reduction in chain slippage relative to nearby chains. This regression is time-dependent under pressure; the chains are constructions characterized by a viscoelastic response. Temperature has an effect on polymers, too. When heated over a certain point (glass transition temperature [Tg]), polymers soften and become pliable. It is crucial to have bioabsorbable polymers with a Tg that is above the human body's core temperature. The molecules' behavior is determined by factors such as orientation, geometric isomerism, conformity, and configuration. L-PLA (mainly amorphous) and DL-PLA (primarily crystalline) are both forms of PLA. Because of its great crystallinity, L-PLA is very resistant to hydrolysis, while due to its amorphous structure, DL-PLA is more vulnerable to hydrolysis [29]. In this sense, the PLA we use is a copolymer of the two polymers composed of isomers. There is just one kind of PGA shown in Figure 1.4. Poly(ethylene glycol) homopolymer (PGA) has superior durability compared to PLA. What we mean by "self-reinforcing PGA" is that it is substantially stiffer than any other kind of therapeutically useful biopolymer, although PGA quickly degrades. It has an acidic pH [30].

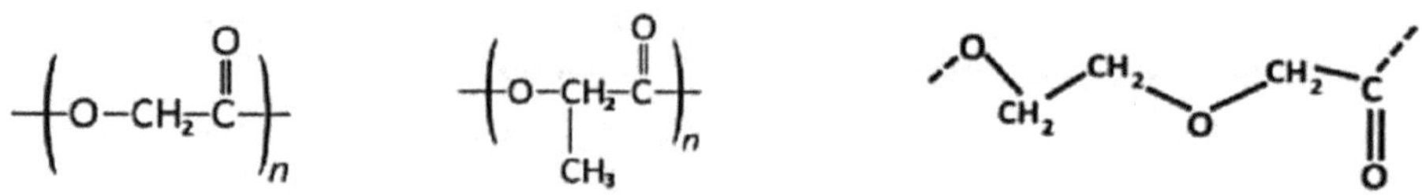

FIGURE 1.4 Structural formula for PGA, PLA, and PDS.

Source: Reproduced with permission from Maurus et al. [31]. Copyright © 2004 Elsevier Inc.

The breakdown products trigger inflammation in the neighboring tissues. Most adverse tissue reactions to bioabsorbable implants may be traced back to PGA polymers. Indeed, copolymers of PLA and PGA do exist. A good illustration of this is the suture material Vicryl (Ethicon, Somerville), which is widely used. The PGA:PLA ratio in New Jersey (NJ) is 90:10. The ratio of PGA to PLA may change the rates of degradation and mechanical properties of these materials; hence, a PGA-PLA copolymer is advantageous since it degrades faster than L-PLA but lacks the rapid degradation and acidic breakdown products that 100% PGA would have. PDS is a crystalline, colorless polymer (Figure 1.4). To facilitate manipulation, a non-toxic violet dye is added to the mix, followed by thermal processing of the polymer to provide the desired effect. Bioabsorbable implants, by definition, are designed to break down and be resorbed or expelled by the body.

First, this happens when molecules lose mass and endurance, followed by a gradual weakening as the substance deteriorates. These copolymers break apart in an untargeted way that involves ester linkages. To produce glycine, PGA must first be degraded. Glycine becomes carbon dioxide and water via the citric acid cycle or is flushed out of the body in the urine. For example, lactic acid is a breakdown product of PLA, as shown in Figure 1.5, similar to the usual human metabolic waste in that it is water and carbon dioxide after going through the citric acid cycle. PDS is either categorized as similar to PGA, where glyoxylate is broken down into glycine, carbon dioxide, and water, or expelled in the urine. Degradation takes place over a period of time that has to do with the crystalline structure, molecular weight, and pore size of the copolymer [77].

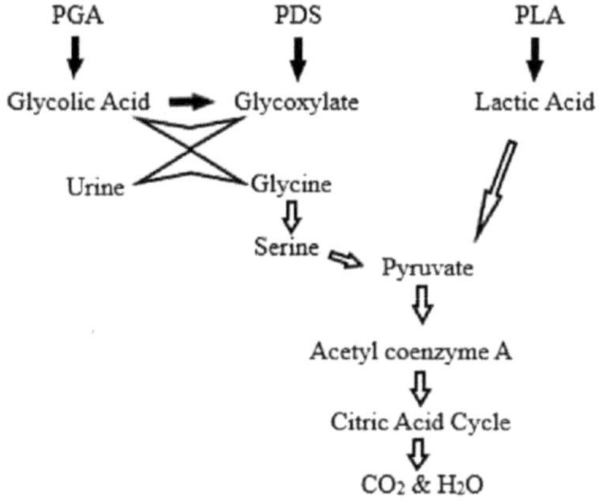

FIGURE 1.5 Breakdown of bio absorbable polymer.

Source: Reproduced with permission from Maurus et al. [31]. Copyright © 2004 Elsevier Inc.

1.3 PROPERTIES

Important BAPs have the following glass transition temperatures (T_g): PLA, 55–60°C; PGA, 35°C; and PDO, –10°C. This is a table of melting temperatures (T_m): 145–180°C for PLA and 220–230°C for PGA. Microfractures are often produced during molding due to internal tension, which negatively impacts polymer performance as a whole. After molding, annealing the material for 4 hours at 120°C may remove any residual internal tension. It seems that poly(L-lactide) lamellar crystallites are very resistant to hydrolysis [32]. In its α-form, PLA often displays a left-handed helix shape. With high molar mass PLLA, the transition to the stable β-form allows for the drawing of fibers [33–35]. PGA is more resistant to heat than PLA. Activation energies of 16.5 and 10.2 kcal/mol for PLA and PGA thermal degradation during random chain scission and 28 and 22.2 kcal/mol during selective chain end scission were measured. As PLA, PGA, and PDO are very sensitive to both moisture and heat, their thermal breakdown is rapid in the presence of moisture. Low molar mass products come from degradation mechanisms such as hydrolysis in the presence of trace amounts of water, zipper-like depolymerization owing to shearing during processing, random main chain scission by oxidation, and intermolecular transesterification [36, 37].

1.3.1 PHYSICAL CHARACTERISTICS

Of all synthetic BAPs, PLA, PGA, and PDO stand out for their superior mechanical qualities. The typical tensile strength of PGA and PLA is between 40 and 140 MPa. The moduli of elasticity are as follows: PLA = 2.7 GPa, PGA = 7.0 GPa, and PDO = 1.5 GPa. Elongation at break and tensile modulus are both greater for PGA than for PLA [38–40]. These numbers are less than the bending strength (180–195 MPa), shear strength (68 MPa), and elastic modulus (6–20 GPa) of cortical bone [41, 30]. Self-reinforcing (SR) materials produced by sintering allow for the development of BAP with high mechanical strength [42, 43]. Strength, ductility, and elastic modulus may all be greatly improved by using SR polymeric composites. The SR polymer's composite structure consists of a polymeric substance with oriented reinforcing units and a binding matrix. SR polymer implants are rigid and robust in the directed direction because both the matrix and the reinforcing components are in crystalline form and share a high degree of molecular orientation [38]. The initial bending strength of SR-PLLA pins should be 300

MPa, and the shear strength should be 220 MPa. The bending strength and initial shear strength of SR copolymers are, in descending order, 214 MPa for SR-Poly(L-DL)LA (70:30) and 121 MPa for SR-PLA/PGA (80:20) [43]. SR pins have an elastic modulus of 6–10 GPa, which is comparable to that of cortical bone [44]. Novel manufacturing processes have been developed to convert BAPs into tissue engineering scaffolds [29, 45].

1.3.2 CAPACITY TO ABSORB BIOCHEMICALS

Biodegradation, material molding history, environment (enzymatic concentration, external stress), molar mass, and crystallinity percentage are other important factors (internal stress) [36, 37, 42]. Hydrolytically unstable connections in the molecule's backbone have been used to achieve BAP; however, they have a tendency to lose molar mass after implantation. *In vivo*, materials may be degraded in a targeted or non-targeted manner [39, 40]. As PLA or PGA degrade, an acidic byproduct is created. Due to the breakdown process, PDO has transformed into a harmless byproduct. Using a chemical or enzymatic catalyst or buffering agent may have a toxic impact [40]. There is a greater rate of monomer conversion due to continuous scission. Degradation is chaotic between the surface and core sections of large, bulky implants because of the presence of surrounding tissue. A rapid rate of deterioration is produced by tissue adhesion to the surface. An improved ability to resist acid breakdown and a decreased susceptibility to hydrolysis are associated with a fine surface and/or reduced porosity [30, 41]. The pace at which a substance degrades is affected by its molecular architecture (R-group), crystallinity, and microstructure. Hydrolytic degradation occurs more rapidly in the amorphous area than in the crystalline region because of the greater quantity of water retained in the amorphous zone, owing to its larger free volume and greater segmental mobility. A crystalline region's reinforcing effects may lengthen the duration until deterioration and improve the material's mechanical characteristics. Strength and crystallinity are improved in self-reinforced PLA homopolymer [21]. Complete absorption takes over five years, but amorphous poly(D, L-lactide) may disappear in a little over a year and a half. Faster degradation is seen in the PGA-PLA copolymer than in the PLA homopolymer. PDO and PGA completely lose their molar mass after 9–12 months of degradation [46]. The water-sensitive R-group in PGA is particularly reactive. Degradation rates and the rates at which acidic breakdown products are released can be controlled by adjusting the proportions of

PLA and PGA. When PLA, PGA, or PDO are subjected to hydrolysis, lactic acid, glycolic acid, or glyoxylate are the resulting acids. Both glycolic acid and glyoxylate are eliminated from the body, with the former being filtered out by the kidneys and the latter being broken down into pyruvate and then acetyl CoA through the citric acid cycle. Glucose, which is produced from lactic acid, is broken down further to yield adenosine triphosphate (ATP) in the Cori cycle (energy cycle) [47].

1.4 PROCESSING TECHNIQUES

1.4.1 FIBER SPINNING

Melt or solution-spun processes require passing the molten polymer or solution through a barrel and forcing it through a die to create fibers. The objective is to create long, skinny filaments with a uniform cross-section. After being spun, fibers are often reinforced by a drawing process performed at a relatively high tension and low temperature, depending on the polymer being drawn. If a material can be melted without considerable degradation, then it can be spun into fibers with a relatively constant cross-section using the melt spinning technique [48]. Wet or dry solution spinning is utilized if processing the polymer in a molten state is not an option.

1.4.2 MELT SPINNING

In melt spinning, a substance is melted before being extruded through a die. After the polymer leaves the die, it rapidly cools, forming solid filaments that may be strung onto a bobbin. To reduce the diameter of the polymer filaments as they emerge from the extruder, a tensile force is often applied [49]. The screw and the die are the primary tools used in melt spinning. Melted polymer is pumped through the extruder's barrel by the screw. It helps to blend the solid polymer that is entering the extruder with the molten polymer that is circulating inside, and it regulates the extrusion rate. The die determines the extrudate's ultimate form; this shape might be single- or multifilament fibers, depending on the intended use [50].

1.4.3 SOLUTION SPINNING

For polymers that cannot form thermally stable, viscous melts, solution spinning is an alternative processing method. This is true as long as the polymer can dissolve sufficiently deeply in the right solvents. The polymer content in these solutions must range from 5% to 30% [51]. Solution wet spinning includes extruding the solution into a bath of non-solvents while using a non-volatile solvent. As the polymer travels through the bath and is finally twisted into a roll, it changes from a liquid to a solid filament. Solvent evaporates into a gaseous condition during the dry spinning process's drawdown stage.

1.4.4 COMPRESSION MOLDING

The thin film was produced using hydraulic presses. The platen heaters were set at a temperature of 140°C (284°F). A few grams of polymer, sandwiched between two sheets of Kapton (DuPont) polyimide film, were squeezed together. The platens were lowered until the top platen barely made contact with the Kapton's top layer. The platens stayed in this position for five minutes to aid in the melting of the polymer. Following the initial melting phase, the platens were compressed together for an additional five minutes at a pressure of around 1.5 tons. After the platens were separated and the polymer film had been fully squeezed, it was quenched in a water bath that was kept at room temperature. The polymer was dried under vacuum before being compacted in an oven for 8 hours at 70°C.

1.4.5 POST-EXTRUSION DRAWING

Specimens of the fibers will be sent through three sets of hot, spinning rollers. The fiber is unwound from the bobbin, drawn through the succession of rolls, and then rewound onto a take-up roll at the end of the process. Poly(ester amide) samples, for instance, were first dragged by hand over rolls 1 (56°C, 15 rpm) and 2 (52°C, 30 rpm) from bobbin 1. That was done again and again until the draw ratio was around 4x and the fiber was about 6x as drawn as it was initially. Using bobbin 3, fibers were drawn by hand again. Roll 1 was set to 48°C and 24 revolutions per minute, whereas roll 2 was set to 47°C and 40 revolutions per minute for the second drawing. The samples were easily wound off the bobbin and passed through all three sets of rollers.

1.4.6 POST-EXTRUSION ANNEALING

A vacuum oven will be used to anneal fibers at three different temperatures over the course of 1.5 hours. As a precaution against fibers catching fire from coming into contact with metal, we employed glass sample containers to keep the length of the samples consistent. Based on the DSC thermograms, the selected temperatures were determined. In the as-received polymers, they are above the Tg threshold but below the melting peak start.

1.4.7 POST-MOLDING STRETCHING

The samples of compression-molded films will be squared off to a few millimeters in size. The film was stretched at a temperature of 110°C using the T.M. Long biaxial stretcher's heaters. When the film is loaded, the samples will rest for 2 minutes to adjust to the stretching chamber's temperature. There will be both confined and unconfined circumstances for the samples.

1.5 ORIENTATION OF THE FIBER

By heating a sample fiber above its Tg and pulling it to a longer length, the polymer chains may be oriented. When polymer molecules are almost molten, applying a uniaxial tensile tension or unidirectional shear stress will force them to align in the desired direction.

When polymerization is successfully accomplished, a material that is rigid and strong along the draw direction but often slightly weak in the transverse direction is the end product. If the polymer can speed up crystallization by molecularly aligning the chains, the orientation step does so. Instead of being spherulitic, the crystalline structure is linear in these instances [50]. On a fiber sample, birefringence measurements are made to ascertain the degree of orientation. Birefringence (n) is the difference between a material's refractive indices in two orthogonal directions using linearly polarized light. The index of refraction (n) is determined by dividing the speed of light flowing through the material by the speed of light moving in a vacuum. When light travels through transparent materials, its speed decreases and it bends at the contact [52]. The amount of material bending depends on the wavelength of the light and the orientation of the substance. The refractive index changes in both directions, parallel and normal to the chain axis, as a result of differences in bonding.

If a polymer is birefringent, there will be a non-zero difference between the two refractive indices and a net orientation that results in a primary refractive index. Crystalline materials display a high degree of order and anisotropy, which makes them particularly birefringent. If a material is crystalline or semi-crystalline, birefringence measurements may show where the crystals first formed in kinetic investigations [53]. Hermann's orientation function, f, and the intrinsic birefringence, n°, are used to determine the birefringence for materials that are preferentially oriented, such as drawn fibers. The birefringence equals $\Delta n = n1 - n2 = f\Delta n°$. This orientation function measures the degree of chain orientation.

1.6 CHARACTERIZATION TECHNIQUES

The most popular technique for determining chemical composition, atomic location and size in a unit cell, and crystal structure is wide-angle X-ray scattering (WAXS) or wide-angle X-ray diffraction (WAXD). Analysis of Bragg peaks dispersed at large angles is important to this technique, which suggests that they are created by nanoscale structures. The chemical composition or phase composition of the film, as well as the crystallite size, may be determined from the resulting diffraction pattern. Using the Debye-Scherrer equation, crystallite size may be calculated from XRD data.

$$L = \frac{K\lambda}{\beta(2\theta)\mathrm{Cos}]} \tag{1}$$

Whole width at half maximum is denoted by β (2θ) in Eqn. (1), whereas the shape factor K is a function of the Miller index of the reflecting plane and the crystal's form. K is often set as 0.9 when the shape cannot be determined. Small-angle X-ray scattering (SAXS) is a technique that records the elastic scattering of X-rays induced by nanoscale features in a polymer at tiny angles, generally between 0.1° and 10°. Using this technique, data on structural units as small as 0.5 nm and as large as 1,000 nm in size may be collected using a highly refined device. Size, shape, pore size, and other characteristic features of partly ordered materials may be gleaned from the angular distribution of scattered light intensity.

As X-ray radiation may reach deep into a material, this method is not affected by the material's surface quality. Due to their limited diffracting volumes, thin films have weak diffracted intensities compared to the substrate and background, making analysis more challenging. This calls for the use of grazing incidence X-ray diffraction (GIXRD), also known as glancing angle X-ray diffraction. In order to get the most out of the signal from ultrathin layers, GIXRD measurements are taken at very small angles. A thin slit is used in the GIXRD to virtually parallelize the incident and diffracted beams. Increasing the path length of the X-ray beam through the film increases the diffracted intensity from the sample while decreasing that from the substrate, and a stationary incident beam creates a relatively tiny angle with the surface of the sample, generally 0.3–3°. X-ray diffraction (XRD) is a method used for identifying materials, analyzing textures, and establishing crystallinity, among other uses.

1.6.1 TGA AND DSC

The thermal degradation of polymers in a nitrogen environment was investigated using a Perkin Elmer Pyris 1 TGA Thermogravimetric Analyzer. The temperature range used for testing was from 25 to 500°C, with a heating rate of 20°C per minute. The original sample weight was 3–5 milligrams, and it was stored in an aluminum pan. Tg and Tm were measured using a nitrogen gas-purged Mettler Toledo Differential Scanning Calorimeter 821e. A polymer sample ranging from 3.75 mg to 5 mg was placed in aluminum dishes. The pans' lids were crimped on before three holes were pierced in the top to release nitrogen. It was programmed to heat at a rate of 10°C per minute between 25 and 160°C. To test the effect of temperature on the as-received polymer, one sample was heated to 160° Fahrenheit, cooled to 25, and then re-heated to 160°. The goal of this experiment was to determine how hot the polymer gets before it starts to crystallize. A cooling rate of 10°C per minute was utilized in this experiment. Specifically, indium was used as a reference material for the DSC instrument's calibration (H=28.45 J/g; Tm=156.61°C).

1.6.2 OPTICAL CHARACTERIZATION (BIREFRINGENCE)

A polarizing microscope equipped with a Berek compensator was used to determine the optical birefringence of the fiber samples. It was used to measure the birefringence of the film. Each configuration followed the same steps. Between the light source and the sample holder, a polarizing film was installed for better viewing. Light emission was measured by rotating the sample to find the darkest spots. After finding the "darkest places," the retardance was measured by rotating the sample 45° in both the clockwise and counterclockwise directions. To determine the birefringence, the retardance of the fiber or film was measured using a compensator, and then the measured values were adjusted.

1.6.3 CREEP TEST

The Perkin Elmer Diamond DMA was used for the creep testing. The maximum yield stress was determined at room temperature and was utilized as the constant static load in the creep experiments. The Diamond DMA was calibrated to operate at a constant strain, with a starting force amplitude of 1,000 mN and an oscillation amplitude of 5.0 m. The testing temperature was chosen based on the type of polymer to be representative of internal body temperatures. Each exam lasted for a full three hours and 10 minutes.

1.6.4 DILUTE SOLUTION VISCOMETRY

Intrinsic viscosity was measured using an Ubbelohde viscometer and a Cannon CT-1000 constant temperature bath to test for deterioration. In order to measure the polymer viscosity, it was first dissolved in dimethyl formamide (DMF). When a sample solution was well combined, 10 milliliters (mL) were pipetted into the No. 1: 420 Ubbelohde viscometer. The time required for efflux was determined using ASTM method D2857. Each trial set began with a measurement of the DMF efflux time. Each test set had five different concentrations of the 1 g PEA/150 mL DMF solution. The efflux times were taken with the viscometer floating in a 30°C water bath.

1.6.5 MELT FLOW INDEX

The melt flow rate can be calculated using a Polymer Test Systems Series 4,000 Melt Flow Indexer. The melt flow indexer was put through its paces many times, with temperatures in the barrel ranging from 120 to 230°C. Before the experiment starts, the die will be plugged while the polymer is heated to prevent any damage. Each measurement of melt flow rate will be made after 60 seconds have elapsed. There were around 4 grams of polymer utilized in each test.

1.7 APPLICATIONS OF BIOABSORBABLE POLYMERS

The use of bioabsorbable polymers as a short-term scaffold has proven very effective. Bioabsorbable polymers may be used to help in the healing of wounds, the mending of bone, and the restoration of damaged blood vessels when natural tissue is compromised due to illness, injury, or surgery. Sutures, bone anchoring devices, and vascular grafts are all examples of uses within temporary scaffolding. Temporary scaffolds are designed to deteriorate over time as the healing tissue transfers stress from the polymer.

A temporary barrier used to prevent adhesion during wound healing is another example of a product with comparable applications. When blood clots between two portions of tissue, we get adhesion. Adhesion may be a serious issue after surgery since it leads to inflammation and fibrosis. The interface between the joined tissues may cause discomfort and functional impairment if it bonds improperly, necessitating further surgery to restore the connection. In order to create a temporary barrier, a thin film or mesh is used. They facilitate more manageable wound healing by providing a barrier between adhesion-prone tissues at the time of operation. In the case of burn patients and those suffering from other skin lesion disorders, where artificial skin is an integral part of the healing process, these barriers are also employed. To gradually release medication to the appropriate site, drug delivery systems use polymeric implants that degrade over time. This is particularly prevalent when giving chemotherapy, since only the intended cells are harmed rather than the body's whole cell population. Combining medication delivery with temporary scaffolds or barriers might reduce the need for invasive operations and implants for patients who need both mechanical support and site-specific drug delivery [54].

Smart screws, smart pins (SR-LPLA-Bionx Implants), phantom soft-thread soft tissue fixation screws (LPLA-DePuy), orthosorb pins (PDO-J and J Orthopedics), biologically quiet staples (85:15/DL-PLGA-Instrument Makar), meniscal stingers (LPLA-Linvatec), and bio-anchors (LPLA-Instrument Makar) are just some of the options available (LPLA-Linvatec). A study by Denti et al. [55] looked at the effectiveness of four different bioabsorbable interference screws for bone block fixation. It has been stated that PGA screws are absorbed more rapidly than PLA screws, yet PLLA screws (Linvatec), PGA screws (Smith & Nephew), PLA-co-PGA screws (Instrument Makar), and PLA screws (Arthrex) are all commercially available.

1.7.1 THE ORTHOPEDIC USE

For the most part, bioabsorbable implants have been employed in orthopedic surgery to avoid implant removal procedures [30, 56]. Bone screws and rods made of PLA or PGA that are self-reinforced are very sturdy. Excellent mechanical properties for implantation and other uses are present in PLA (molar mass, 1,00,000). The PGA (molar mass, 20,000–1,45,000) is employed for orthopedic implants [57, 58]. Infection rates of 3–4% have been reported in association with bioabsorbable osteosynthesis devices used in orthopedic and traumatologic procedures. Scaffolds are utilized as temporary support to bodily structures to help in tissue regeneration and uniform load transformation. For the reconstruction of the finger joints, either Vicryl® (a co-polymer of 90% PGA and 10% PLLA) or Ethisorb® (a combination of PDS and a co-polymer of 90% PGA and 10% PLLA) fleeces 180 were used as scaffolds. Several biomedical applications, including tissue engineering, wound dressing, immobilized enzymes, and controlled delivery of medicines (genes), have recently shown more promise and potential using electrospun nanofiber scaffolds. Figure 1.6 shows the bone fracture healing factors. During the bone remodeling process, the biocomposites used must be biocompatible, bioactive, have interconnected pores, and also have the ability to support the fractured bone.

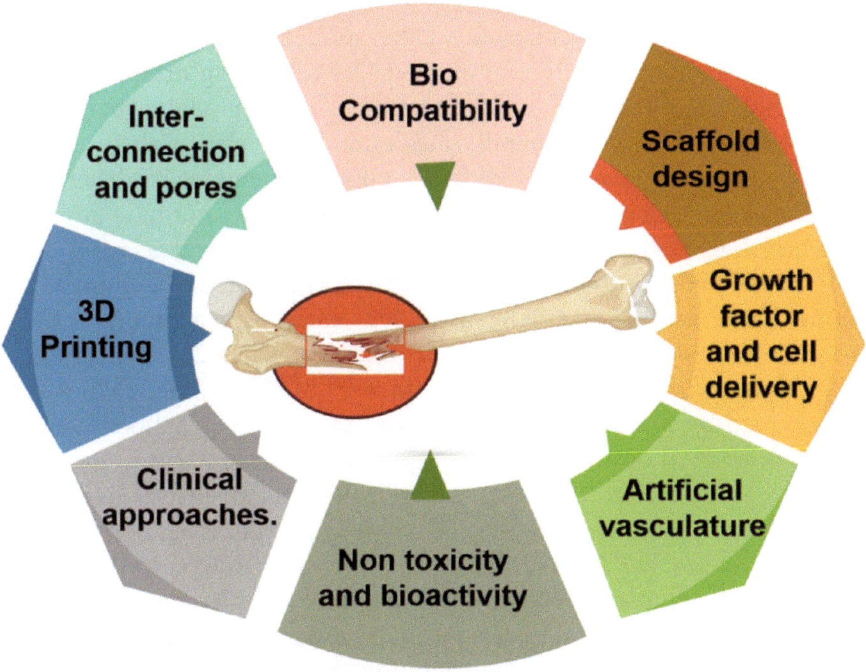

FIGURE 1.6 Factors depending on biobased composites for bone fracture healing.

1.7.2 BIOENGINEERING OF TISSUES

Compared to Vicryl (a glycolic-co-lactic acid polymer) and Dexon, PDO scaffolds performed better in tissue engineering thanks to their high flexibility, delayed degradation, increased strength retention, and decreased inflammatory response rates (polyglycolic acid). After 3 weeks, the breaking strength of monofilament sutures generally drops by half [59, 60]. The half-life of copolymer PLA-PGA scaffolds varies with the ratio of monomers present. Optimal pore sizes for bone regeneration, skin regeneration, and cell proliferation are 100–150 microns, 20–125 microns, and 20–60 microns, respectively. The bioactivity of electrospun scaffolds may be improved by modifying their surfaces with particular bioactive compounds for use in a variety of medicinal applications. Nanoparticle-polylactic acid (PLA) composites have been identified as a biocompatible conducting material with potential use as a biosensor in tissue engineering [61]. Studies *in vivo* revealed that polyheterocycles would be renally cleared slowly [62].

1.7.3 MANAGED DRUG DELIVERY SYSTEMS

Desorption of the drug attached to the surface and/or diffusion through the nanoparticle matrix are two methods for regulating drug release. After the completion of the active agent release, biodegradable polymers are designed to break down naturally inside the body. Hence, there will be no need to remove any unwanted materials once the medicine has been released [63–65]. Adjusting polymer properties, such as copolymer ratio and crystallinity, enables BAPs to be tailored for controlled drug release and disease-specific localization [66–68]. Several PLGA (Poly(lactic-co-glycolic acid)) formulations are commercially available, each with a unique molecular weight (10–100 kDa) and copolymer ratio (50:50, 75:25, and 85:15). The breakdown process and the release profile of the entrapped medication are affected by the molecular weight and the copolymer molar ratios [46, 69]. The creation of microchannels and a large surface area in the polymer matrix may be facilitated by highly crystalline nanoparticles, allowing for simple drug release. Sterilization and storage procedures such as γ-radiation, ethylene oxide (EtO), or plasma etching are all effective ways to sterilize bioabsorbable implants before they are used in humans, and all three methods are recommended before clinical usage, as outlined in references [4, 70]. Sterilization and storage conditions have an effect on the molecular weight, mechanical properties, and performance of polymers. Toxicity from EtO sterilization residue disfavors its usage for bioimplants. A low dosage of 250 kGy γ-radiation improves chain scission in the polymer, whereas a greater dose introduces crosslinks between linear chains, making 215 kGy γ-radiation the preferred approach for bioimplants. Biodegradable materials are kept in a cool, dry place with low humidity [75, 76]. Figure 1.7 shows the drug delivery systems in various forms. These forms are nowadays widely used not only for drug delivery but also to provide multifunctional properties to the composites for their efficient applications [71–74].

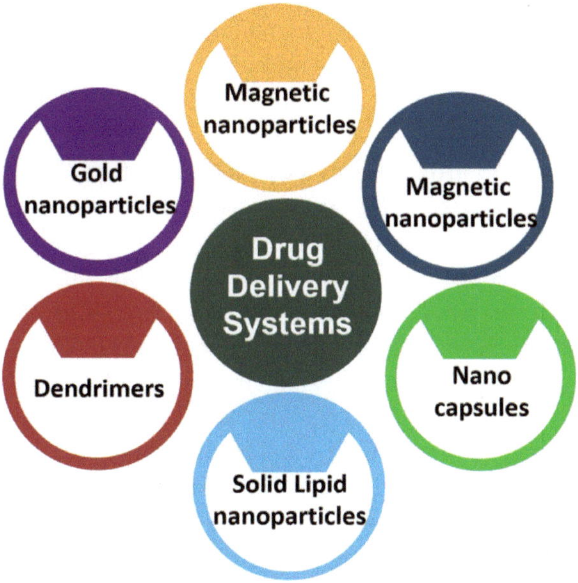

FIGURE 1.7 Various materials used as drug delivery systems.

1.8 CONCLUSION

Bioabsorbable materials are now routinely used in orthopedic procedures. Especially in the realm of sports medicine, these instruments have broadened the surgeon's toolkit. Bioabsorbable implants are often used for anterior cruciate ligament reconstruction, shoulder surgery, meniscal repair, and fracture treatment, and include interference screws, suture anchors, meniscal repair devices, and simple fracture fixation devices. In solid form, PLA may be either amorphous or semicrystalline, depending on the stereochemistry and thermal history. Tg and Tm are significantly impacted by factors such as molecular weight, thermal history, fundamental structure, and overall optical makeup. Combinations of L and D monomers may alter the morphologies of PLA. Increasing the D concentration makes PLA more amorphous, whereas increasing the L content makes PLA more (semi)crystalline. The glass transition temperature at infinite molecular weight is greater when there is a larger proportion of the L-stereoisomer.

Both aerobic and anaerobic composting environments are capable of breaking down PLA-made products. The advantages of ultra-high strength bioresorbable polymeric composites go well beyond their amazing mechanical capabilities, which make structural disintegration increasingly difficult as crystallinity rises. By using physiologically active ingredients that hasten or promote healing, or make up components of healing tissues, they may further improve their osteogenic potential. Future developments in tissue engineering, which combines material science, biotechnology, and medicine to produce artificial devices that can be transformed into living, functional tissues or organs like bone, cartilage, connective tissue, tendons, and ligaments, will be made possible thanks to biodegradable implants. For certain uses, PGA is preferable to PLA because of its high thermal distortion temperature, strong mechanical qualities, high degradability, and good gas barrier properties. Several methods exist for fusing PGA and PLA together, including co-polymerization, physical mixing, and multilayer lamination. Earlier studies found that adding PGA to PLA greatly enhanced both its biodegradability and mechanical characteristics. There has been a lot of research on adding PGA to PLA, mostly for use in medical settings. The biggest problem with mass-producing PGA is that it is more expensive than competing biodegradable polymers.

KEYWORDS

- **artificial devices**
- **biodegradable polymers**
- **bioresorbable polymers**
- **fabrication**
- **thermal distortion**
- **tissue engineering**

REFERENCES

1. Wright, S. (1999). *Global Orthopedic Markets–Bridging the Divide*. Great Britain.
2. Middleton, J. C., & Tipton, A. J. (2000). Synthetic biodegradable polymers as orthopedic devices. *Biomaterials, 21*(23), 2335–2346.
3. Auras, R. A., Lim, L. T., Selke, S. E., & Tsuji, H. (2011). *Poly(lactic acid): Synthesis, Structures, Properties, Processing, and Applications* (Vol. 10). John Wiley & Sons.
4. Michaeli, W., & Oepen, R. V. (1993). Processing of degradable polymers. In *Technical Papers of the Annual Technical Conference–Society of Plastics Engineers Incorporated* (pp. 796). Society of Plastics Engineers Inc.
5. Södergård, A., & Näsman, J. H. (1994). Stabilization of poly (L-lactide) in the melt. *Polymer Degradation and Stability, 46*(1), 25–30.
6. Fan, Y., Nishida, H., Shirai, Y., Tokiwa, Y., & Endo, T. (2004). Thermal degradation behavior of poly (lactic acid) stereo complex. *Polymer Degradation and Stability, 86*(2), 197–208.
7. Alexander, H., Brunski, J. B., Cooper, S. L., Hench, L. L., Hergenrother, R. W., Hoffman, A. S., & Yannas, I. V. (1996). Classes of materials used in medicine. In *Biomaterials Science* (pp. 37–130). Academic Press.
8. He, Y., Qian, Z., Zhang, H., & Liu, X. (2004). Alkaline degradation behavior of polyester amide fibers: Surface erosion. *Colloid and Polymer Science, 282*, 972–978.
9. Prasad, A., Ravi Sankar, M., & Katiyar, V. (2017). State of art on solvent casting particulate leaching method for orthopedic scaffolds fabrication. *Materials Today: Proceedings, 4*(2), 898–907.
10. Altman, G. H., Diaz, F., Jakuba, C., Calabro, T., Horan, R. L., Chen, J., & Kaplan, D. L. (2003). Silk-based biomaterials. *Biomaterials, 24*(3), 401–416.
11. Gupta, A., Patel, S., Prajapati, R., Katiyar, P., Biswas, S., & Katiyar, V. (2017). Multifunctional nanohydroxyapatite-promoted toughened high-molecular-weight stereo complex poly (lactic acid)-based bio nanocomposite for both 3D-printed orthopedic implants and high-temperature engineering applications. *ACS Omega, 2*(7), 4039–4052.
12. Roveri, N., Falini, G., Sidoti, M. C., Tampieri, A., Landi, E., Sandri, M., & Parma, B. (2003). Biologically inspired growth of hydroxyapatite nanocrystals inside self-assembled collagen fibers. *Materials Science and Engineering: C, 23*(3), 441–446.
13. Brodie, J. C., Goldie, E., Connel, G., Merry, J., & Grant, M. H. (2005). Osteoblast interactions with calcium phosphate ceramics modified by coating with type I collagen. *Journal of Biomedical Materials Research Part A: An Official Journal of The Society for Biomaterials, The Japanese Society for Biomaterials, and The Australian Society for Biomaterials and the Korean Society for Biomaterials, 73*(4), 409–421.
14. Schneiders, W., Reinstorf, A., Pompe, W., Grass, R., Biewener, A., Holch, M., & Rammelt, S. (2007). Effect of modification of hydroxyapatite/collagen composites with sodium citrate, phosphoserine, phosphoserine/RGD-peptide and calcium carbonate on bone remodeling. *Bone, 40*(4), 1048–1059.
15. Armentano, I., Dottori, M., Fortunati, E., Mattioli, S., & Kenny, J. M. (2010). Biodegradable polymer matrix nanocomposites for tissue engineering: A review. *Polymer Degradation and Stability, 95*(11), 2126–2146.
16. Tamimi, F., Sheikh, Z., & Barralet, J. (2012). Dicalcium phosphate cements: Brushite and monetite. *Acta Biomaterialia, 8*(2), 474–487.

17. Kumar, M. N. R. (2000). A review of chitin and chitosan applications. *Reactive and Functional Polymers, 46*(1), 1–27.
18. Dornish, M., Kaplan, D., & Skaugrud, Ø. (2001). Standards and guidelines for biopolymers in tissue-engineered medical products: ASTM alginate and chitosan standard guides. *Annals of the New York Academy of Sciences, 944*(1), 388–397.
19. Shi, C., Zhu, Y., Ran, X., Wang, M., Su, Y., & Cheng, T. (2006). Therapeutic potential of chitosan and its derivatives in regenerative medicine. *Journal of Surgical Research, 133*(2), 185–192.
20. Seeherman, H., Li, R., & Wozney, J. (2003). A review of preclinical program development for evaluating injectable carriers for osteogenic factors. *JBJS, 85*(suppl_3), 96–108.
21. Chesnutt, B. M., Viano, A. M., Yuan, Y., Yang, Y., Guda, T., Appleford, M. R., & Bumgardner, J. D. (2009). Design and characterization of a novel chitosan/nanocrystalline calcium phosphate composite scaffold for bone regeneration. *Journal of Biomedical Materials Research Part A: An Official Journal of The Society for Biomaterials, The Japanese Society for Biomaterials, and The Australian Society for Biomaterials and the Korean Society for Biomaterials, 88*(2), 491–502.
22. Prasad, A., Devendar, B., Ravi Sankar, M., & Robi, P. S. (2015). Micro-scratch based tribological characterization of hydroxyapatite (HAp) fabricated through fish scales. *Materials Today: Proceedings, 2*(4–5), 1216–1224.
23. Prasad, A., Bhasney, S., Katiyar, V., & Ravi Sankar, M. (2017). Biowastes processed hydroxyapatite filled poly (lactic acid) bio-composite for open reduction internal fixation of small bones. *Materials Today: Proceedings, 4*(9), 10153–10157.
24. Zhou, H., Qian, J., Wang, J., Yao, W., Liu, C., Chen, J., & Cao, X. (2009). Enhanced bioactivity of bone morphogenetic protein-2 with low dose of 2-N, 6-O-sulfated chitosan in vitro and in vivo. *Biomaterials, 30*(9), 1715–1724.
25. Katsarava, R., Beridze, V., Arabuli, N., Kharadze, D., Chu, C. C., & Won, C. Y. (1999). Amino acid-based bio analogous polymers. Synthesis, and study of regular poly (ester amide) s based on bis (α-amino acid) α, ω-alkylene diesters, and aliphatic dicarboxylic acids. *Journal of Polymer Science Part A: Polymer Chemistry, 37*(4), 391–407.
26. Ray, J. A., Doddi, N., Regula, D., Williams, J. A., & Melveger, A. (1981). Polydioxanone (PDS), a novel monofilament synthetic absorbable suture. *Surgery, Gynecology & Obstetrics, 153*(4), 497–507.
27. Lowe, C. E. (1955). Patent 2,668,162, 1954. (b) Schneider. AK US Patent, 2.
28. Prasad, A. (2021). State of art review on bioabsorbable polymeric scaffolds for bone tissue engineering. *Materials Today: Proceedings, 44*, 1391–1400.
29. Daniels, A. U., Chang, M. K., Andriano, K. P., & Heller, J. (1990). Mechanical properties of biodegradable polymers and composites proposed for internal fixation of bone. *Journal of Applied Biomaterials, 1*(1), 57–78.
30. Törmälä, P. (1992). Biodegradable self-reinforced composite materials; manufacturing structure and mechanical properties. *Clinical Materials, 10*(1–2), 29–34.
31. Maurus, P. B., & Kaeding, C. C. (2004). Bioabsorbable implant material review. *Operative Techniques in Sports Medicine, 12*(3), 158–160.
32. Weir, N. A., Buchanan, F. J., Orr, J. F., Farrar, D. F., & Boyd, A. (2004). Processing, annealing and sterilisation of poly-L-lactide. *Biomaterials, 25*(18), 3939–3949.
33. De Santis, P., & Kovacs, A. (1968). Molecular conformation of poly (S-lactic acid). *Biopolymers: Original Research on Biomolecules, 6*(3), 299–306.

34. Cartier, L., Okihara, T., Ikada, Y., Tsuji, H., Puiggali, J., & Lotz, B. (2000). Epitaxial crystallization and crystalline polymorphism of polylactides. *Polymer, 41*(25), 8909–8919.
35. Eling, B., Gogolewski, S., & Pennings, A. J. (1982). Biodegradable materials of poly (l-lactic acid): 1. Melt-spun and solution-spun fibers. *Polymer, 23*(11), 1587–1593.
36. Dawes, E., & Rushton, N. (1997). Response of macrophages to poly (L-lactide) particulates which have undergone various degrees of artificial degradation. *Biomaterials, 18*(24), 1615–1623.
37. Hurrell, S., Milroy, G. E., & Cameron, R. E. (2003). The degradation of polyglycolide in water and deuterium oxide. Part I: The effect of reaction rate. *Polymer, 44*(5), 1421–1424.
38. Prasad, A. (2021). Bioabsorbable polymeric materials for biofilms and other biomedical applications: Recent and future trends. *Materials Today: Proceedings, 44*, 2447–2453.
39. Pietrzak, W. S., Sarver, D. R., & Verstynen, M. L. (1997). Bioabsorbable polymer science for the practicing surgeon. *The Journal of Craniofacial Surgery, 8*(2), 87–91.
40. Koelling, A. S., Ballintyn, N. J., Salehi, A., Darden, D. J., Taylor, M. E., Varnavas, J., & Melton, D. R. (1997). In vitro real-time aging and characterization of poly (L/D-lactic acid). In *Proceedings of the 1997 16th Southern Biomedical Engineering Conference* (pp. 197–201). IEEE.
41. Reilly, D. T., & Burstein, A. H. (1975). The elastic and ultimate properties of compact bone tissue. *Journal of Biomechanics, 8*(6), 393–405.
42. Tormala, P., Paasimaa, S., Lehto, M., & Lehtimaki, M. (2000). U.S. Patent No. 6,113,640. Washington, DC: U.S. Patent and Trademark Office.
43. Joukainen, A., Pihlajamäki, H., Mäkelä, E. A., Ashammakhi, N., Viljanen, J., Pätiälä, H., & Rokkanen, P. (2000). Strength retention of self-reinforced drawn poly-L/DL-lactide 70/30 (SR-PLA70) rods and fixation properties of distal femoral osteotomies with these rods. An experimental study on rats. *Journal of Biomaterials Science, Polymer Edition, 11*(12), 1411–1428.
44. Miller, R. A., Brady, J. M., & Cutright, D. E. (1977). Degradation rates of oral resorbable implants (polylactates and polyglycolates): Rate modification with changes in PLA/PGA copolymer ratios. *Journal of Biomedical Materials Research, 11*(5), 711–719.
45. Bhatia, S., Shalaby, S. W., Powers, D. L., Lancaster, R. L., & Ferguson, R. L. (1995). The effect of site of implantation and animal age on properties of polydioxanone pins. *Journal of Biomaterials Science, Polymer Edition, 6*(5), 435–446.
46. Prasad, A., Chakraborty, G., & Kumar, A. (2022). Bio-based environmentally benign polymeric resorbable materials for orthopedic fixation applications. In *Advanced Materials for Biomedical Applications* (pp. 251–266). CRC Press.
47. Blasier, R. D., Bucholz, R., Cole, W., Johnson, L. L., & Mäkelä, E. A. (1997). Bioresorbable implants: Applications in orthopedic surgery. *Instructional Course Lectures, 46*, 531–546.
48. Pearson, J. R. A. (1985). *Mechanics of Polymer Processing*. Elsevier.
49. Spruiell, J. E. (2001). Structure formation during melt spinning. In *Structure Formation in Polymeric Fibers* (pp. 6–26). Springer.
50. Powell, P. C., & Housz, A. I. (1998). *Engineering with Polymers*. CRC Press.
51. Ziabicki, A. (1976). *Fundamentals of Fiber Formation*. Wiley.
52. Peacock, A. (2000). Characterization and testing. In *Handbook of Polyethylene: Structures, Properties, and Applications* (pp. 350–351). CRC Press.

53. Cambridge Polymer Group. (2004). The theory of birefringence. Retrieved from: www.campoly.com (accessed on 8 August 2024).
54. Coury, A. J., Levy, R. J., Mcmillin, C. R., Pathak, Y., Ratner, B. D., Schoen, F. J., & Williams, R. L. (1996). Degradation of materials in the biological environment. In *Biomaterials Science* (pp. 243–281). Academic Press.
55. Denti, M., Randelli, P., Lo Vetere, D., Moioli, M., & Tagliabue, M. (2004). Bioabsorbable interference screws for bone-patellar tendon-bone anterior cruciate ligament reconstruction: Clinical and computerized tomography results of four different models. A prospective study. *Journal of Orthopedics and Traumatology, 5*, 151–155.
56. Hurrell, S., & Cameron, R. E. (2002). The effect of initial polymer morphology on the degradation and drug release from polyglycolide. *Biomaterials, 23*(11), 2401–2409.
57. Ge, H., Hu, Y., Yang, S., Jiang, X., & Yang, C. (2000). Preparation, characterization, and drug release behaviors of drug-loaded ε-caprolactone/l-lactide copolymer nanoparticles. *Journal of Applied Polymer Science, 75*(7), 874–882.
58. Izumikawa, S., Yoshioka, S., Aso, Y., & Takeda, Y. (1991). Preparation of poly(l-lactide) microspheres of different crystalline morphology and effect of crystalline morphology on drug release rate. *Journal of Controlled Release, 15*(2), 133–140.
59. Lehman, W. B., Strongwater, A. B., Tune, D., Kummer, F., Atar, D., Grant, A. D., & Rohovsky, M. W. (1994). Internal fixation with biodegradable plate and screws in dogs. *Journal of Pediatric Orthopedics B, 3*(2), 190–193.
60. Boland, E. D., Coleman, B. D., Barnes, C. P., Simpson, D. G., Wnek, G. E., & Bowlin, G. L. (2005). Electrospinning polydioxanone for biomedical applications. *Acta Biomaterialia, 1*(1), 115–123.
61. Wang, Z., Roberge, C., Wan, Y., Dao, L. H., Guidoin, R., & Zhang, Z. (2003). A biodegradable electrical Bioconductor made of polypyrene nanoparticle/poly (d, l-lactide) composite: A preliminary in vitro biostability study. *Journal of Biomedical Materials Research Part A: An Official Journal of The Society for Biomaterials, The Japanese Society for Biomaterials, and The Australian Society for Biomaterials and the Korean Society for Biomaterials, 66*(4), 738–746.
62. Wang, Z., Roberge, C., Dao, L. H., Wan, Y., Shi, G., Rouabhia, M., & Zhang, Z. (2004). In vivo evaluation of a novel electrically conductive polypyrene/poly (d, l-lactide) composite and polypyrene-coated poly (d, l-lactide-co-glycolide) membranes. *Journal of Biomedical Materials Research Part A: An Official Journal of The Society for Biomaterials, The Japanese Society for Biomaterials, and The Australian Society for Biomaterials and the Korean Society for Biomaterials, 70*(1), 28–38.
63. Prego, C., Fabre, M., Torres, D., & Alonso, M. J. (2006). Efficacy and mechanism of action of chitosan nano capsules for oral peptide delivery. *Pharmaceutical Research, 23*, 549–556.
64. Higuchi, T. (1963). Mechanism of sustained-action medication. Theoretical analysis of rate of release of solid drugs dispersed in solid matrices. *Journal of Pharmaceutical Sciences, 52*(12), 1145–1149.
65. Jenquin, M. R., & McGinity, J. W. (1994). Characterization of acrylic resin matrix films and mechanisms of drug-polymer interactions. *International Journal of Pharmaceutics, 101*(1–2), 23–34.
66. Bala, I., Hariharan, S., & Kumar, M. R. (2004). PLGA nanoparticles in drug delivery: The state of the art. *Critical Reviews™ in Therapeutic Drug Carrier Systems, 21*(5).

67. Panyam, J., & Labhasetwar, V. (2003). Biodegradable nanoparticles for drug and gene delivery to cells and tissue. *Advanced Drug Delivery Reviews, 55*(3), 329–347.
68. Ghosh, S. (2004). Recent research and development in synthetic polymer-based drug delivery systems. *Journal of Chemical Research, 2004*(4), 241–246.
69. Avgoustakis, K. (2004). Pegylated poly (lactide) and poly (lactide-co-glycolide) nanoparticles: Preparation, properties and possible applications in drug delivery. *Current Drug Delivery, 1*(4), 321–333.
70. Zislis, T., Martin, S. A., Cerbas, E., Heath 3rd, J. R., Mansfield, J. L., & Hollinger, J. O. (1989). A scanning electron microscopic study of in vitro toxicity of ethylene-oxide-sterilized bone repair materials. *The Journal of Oral Implantology, 15*(1), 41–46.
71. Prasad, A., Bhasney, S. M., Prasannavenkadesan, V., et al. (2023). Polylactic acid reinforced with nano-hydroxyapatite bioabsorbable cortical screws for bone fracture treatment. *Journal of Polymer Research, 30*, 177. https://doi.org/10.1007/s10965-023-03542-8.
72. Sarkar, K., Dutta, K., Chatterjee, A., Sarkar, J., Das, D., Prasad, A., Chattopadhyay, D., Acharya, K., Das, M., Verma, S. K., & De, S. (2023). Nanotherapeutic potential of antibacterial folic acid-functionalized nanoceria for wound-healing applications. *Nanomedicine, 18*(2). https://doi.org/10.2217/nnm-2022-0233.
73. Katiyar, V., Prasad, A., Sankar, M. R., & Bhasney, S. M. (2022). Process for the preparation of polymer composite based cancellous screw and pins (Indian Patent No. 401811).
74. Prasad, A. (2022). Biomaterial-Based Nanofibers Scaffolds in Tissue Engineering Application. In *Functional Biomaterials* (pp. 245–264). Springer, Singapore.
75. Babanalbandi, A., Hill, D. J. T., & Whittaker, A. K. (1997). Volatile products and new polymer structures formed on 60Co γ-radiolysis of poly (lactic acid) and poly (glycolic acid). *Polymer Degradation and Stability, 58*(1–2), 203–214.
76. Gupta, M. C., & Deshmukh, V. G. (1983). Radiation effects on poly (lactic acid). *Polymer, 24*(7), 827–830.
77. Athanasiou, K. A., Liu, G. T., Lavery, L. A., Lanctot, D. R., & Schenck, R. C. Jr., (1998). Biomechanical Topography of Human Articular Cartilage in the First Metatarsophalangeal Joint. *Clinical Orthopaedics and Related Research, 348*, 269–281.

CHAPTER 2

Bio-Absorbable Polymer-Based Scaffolds as Drug Carriers: Fabrication, Characterization, and Drug Release

GOURHARI CHAKRABORTY[1] and PRADIP DAS[2]

[1]*Department of Chemical Engineering, National Institute of Technology, Tadepalligudem, Andhra Pradesh, India*

[2]*Spencer Laboratory, University of Delaware, Newark, USA*

ABSTRACT

Bio-degradable polymers have flourished as raw materials for biomedical applications in current times because of their inherent properties such as biocompatibility and resorbability. Sustained release of the drug via a suitable carrier can improve the overall effectiveness of the drug and minimize the loss of costly materials. Bio-absorbable polymers can also be exploited as drug carriers using different techniques like sol-gel, 3D printing, electrospinning, and cross-linking. The loading extent and release nature of the drugs can be varied based on chemical linking or physical interaction with the polymer. In some cases, external coating or pore-filling (electrospun bandage) techniques are also adopted. Hence, it can be inferred that the nature of the polymer and the fabrication technique of bio-absorbable polymer-based scaffolds have a remarkable impact on sustained drug delivery. Additionally, the applicability of scaffolds also depends on their mechanical properties, bioactivity, hydrophilicity, swelling nature, etc. Proper characterization of scaffolds determining their structure and properties is important prior to application. This chapter elucidates the emerging upgrades in the fabrication routes, characterization techniques, and nature of the release of drug-loaded

Bioabsorbable Polymers for Drug Carriers and Fixation Devices. Arbind Prasad and Sougata Jana (Eds.)

bioabsorbable scaffolds. The various scaffold-manufacturing technologies, drug-loading techniques, polymers, and active medicinal components used to manufacture drug-loaded scaffolds are discussed. Furthermore, existing kinetics of drug release, modes of action of drug delivery, and loading techniques of bioactive substances are explored in order to produce drug-loaded fibrous structures with the requisite morphological and physicochemical features. Finally, contemporary drug-releasing fiber system applications in wound healing, tissue engineering, and *in vivo* drug administration are presented. Future trends and opportunities for extensive research are explored in relation to scaffold-based drug delivery systems.

2.1 INTRODUCTION

Bio-absorbable polymers have applicability in almost all dimensions because of their processability, superior properties, and bio-based nature. Polylactic acid (PLA), polyhydroxyalkanoates (PHAs), chitosan, silk, collagen, polycaprolactone (PCL), poly(butylene succinate) (PBS), and different block copolymers are emerging as precursors for product development on various occasions [1–6]. Biomedical applications of biodegradable polymeric materials and composites extend to tissue culture, orthopedics, drug delivery, nerve regeneration, and 3D printing applications. Drug release at the affected site in the human body is one of the predominant issues in medical science because of the complexity of release kinetics [7]. Designed or injectable polymeric platforms or structures often assist in the treatment of various diseases. These constructs are called scaffolds, and on many occasions, biodegradable polymeric scaffolds are emerging as a fascinating subject for biomedical applications like drug delivery. Scaffolds are classified as injectable, implant, and 3D printed, depending on the nature of the fabrication and application. Natural polymers like proteins and polysaccharides were utilized as scaffold ingredients alongside synthetic polymers [8]. Scaffold properties are intensely dependent on polymer properties and fabrication techniques. Nano drug-delivery systems are emerging in the medical sector because of their flexibility in formulation, efficient material utilization, and control of the release [9]. Scaffolds are the pillars of tissue culture-based biomedical applications, with improved cell adhesion, cell proliferation, and cell differentiation information. Conventional and non-conventional routes of scaffold fabrication techniques determine the nature of applications in the forms of sponges, foams, fibers, etc. [10]. Biodegradable scaffolds are more efficient than conventional ones because of their mechanical stability and biocompatibility properties inside the body [11]. In the case of complex bone diseases, the implantation of scaffolds in association with signaling molecules stimulates bone formation. In the formation of autologous bone, the polymer scaffold gets degraded, and regenerated bone replaces the defect site. Chitosan, PCL, HA, etc., have been observed to have significant applicability in scaffold making for bone defect applications [12]. Wound healing was observed to improve with the use of drug-loaded scaffolds. Drug delivery systems were observed to be responsive based on the precursor polymer, scaffold fabrication routes, and application types. In order to control the release kinetics, different stimuli-responsive materials/composites are emerging, which impact precise control over the sustained release of drugs [13].

In this present chapter, the implementation of absorbable polymers for drug-loaded scaffolds is discussed elaborately (Figure 2.1). In view of the impact of the origin of the scaffold, one section is added emphasizing prime scaffold fabrication techniques. Scaffold efficiency depends on polymer properties and scaffold properties. The properties of scaffolds are elaborately discussed and incorporated, accounting for major structural and application-oriented features of scaffolds. The employment of absorbable polymer-based scaffolds for drug release cases, along with modifications in recent research applications, is thoroughly discussed in corroboration with current literature. Finally, the outlook and summary section of the chapter is appended at the end, prior to acknowledgment and citations.

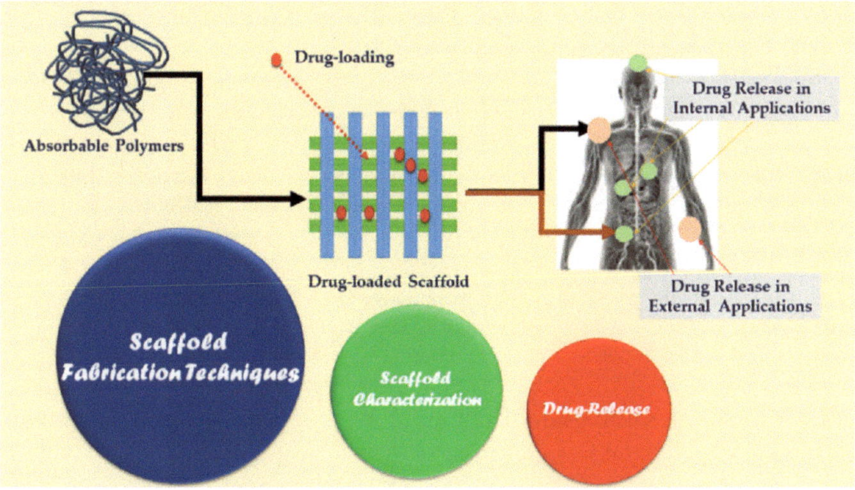

FIGURE 2.1 Bio-absorbable polymer-based scaffolds as drug carrier.

2.2 BIO-ABSORBABLE POLYMERS FOR DRUG DELIVERY APPLICATIONS

Degradable polymers, because of their resorbable nature, eliminate the need for further operation of the affected site after the healing of defects (Figure 2.2 and Table 2.1). Transport phenomena and reaction kinetics determine the route of the degradation of the samples. Bulk degradation and surface degradation are the two major physically observed phenomena for biodegradable polymeric items. Alongside other factors like pH, crystallinity, geometry, additives, processing, etc., polymer type turns out to be primarily responsible for the resorbability kinetics of the polymeric items [14]. Bio-absorbable polymers were utilized for the casting of scaffolds for drug delivery applications as follows.

TABLE 2.1 Major Bio-Absorbable Polymers for Scaffold Fabrication

Polymer	Properties	Source	Nature of Application	References
Alginate	Anionic, polysaccharides	Brown algae and bacteria	Drug delivery, gene therapy, nano-remediation	[16]
Chitosan	Polysaccharides, water-soluble	Available in chitin form in insect's cuticles, crabs, etc.	Antimicrobial, drug delivery, biocatalysis	[20]
HA	Anionic, linear glycosaminoglycan	Hyaluronan synthases in the inner cell membrane	Drug delivery, cartilage repair, tissue engineering	[26]
Collagen	Three helix polypeptide chain, opaque, viscoelastic	Bovine, fish scale, bird's feet, frog skin	Scaffold, drug delivery	[31, 32]
PGA	Semicrystalline, aliphatic polyester, T_g-35 to 45°C, T_{m-}220–233°C	Polycondensation of glycolic acid	Fracture fixation, suture, scaffolds	[40, 41]
PLA	Aliphatic, polyester, $T_g \sim 60$°C, T_m- 180–200°C	Polycondensation of lactic acid, ROP of lactide	Implant, scaffold, fixation element, suture, drug delivery	[40, 43, 44]
PCL	Polyester, biodegradable, $T_g \sim -60$°C, $T_m \sim$ 64°C	ROP of ε-caprolactone	Suture, scaffold	[48, 49]

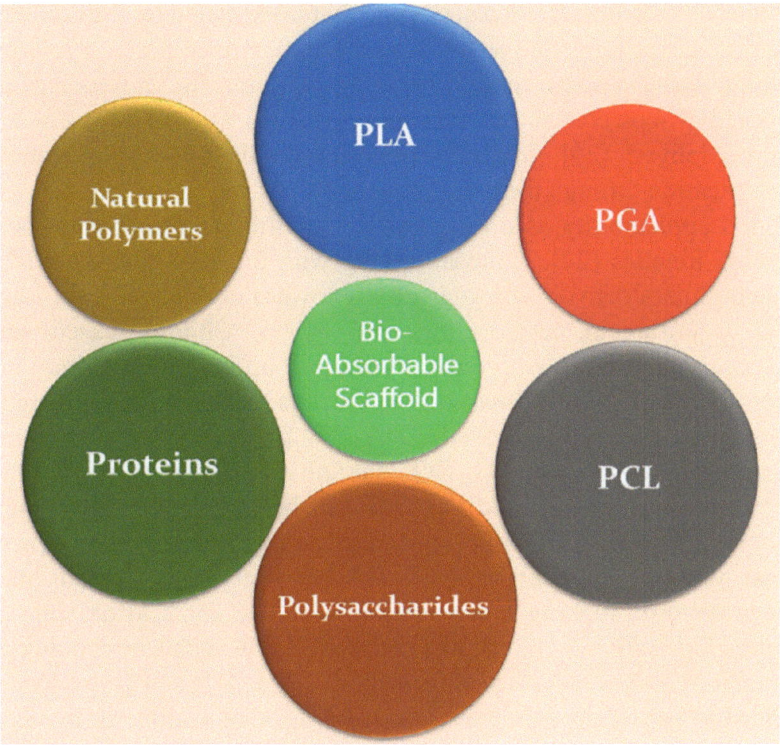

FIGURE 2.2 Polymers utilized for fabrication of scaffolds as drug carrier.

2.2.1 NATURAL POLYMERS

Natural polymers are derived polymers directly from living systems. These polymers are hydrophilic in nature and less toxic in medical applications. The excellent biocompatibility of these polymers makes them suitable for applications in the biomedical field. Alginates, chitosan, hyaluronic acid (HA), proteins, and collagen are major naturally occurring polymers that are in use for scaffold preparation [8, 15]. Alginate is a biopolymer with hydroxyl and carboxylate moieties, and it possesses good biodegradability, biocompatibility, and solubility in water. It is gathered from the brown algae cell walls and purified according to conditions. Alginate-based scaffolds were fabricated using techniques like electrospinning, electrospraying, thermally induced phase separation, and complexation, etc. [16]. Different alginate-based composite scaffolds were observed to have potential applicability in fields like extracellular matrix for tissue culture and drug delivery, 3D printed scaffolds for cancer treatment, diabetic wound healing, etc. [17–19].

Chitosan is the β-linked polysaccharide that is extracted by the deacetylation of chitin and contains amine functional group substitutions. It is present in the chitin form in some fungi, crabs, shrimp, etc. The presence of surface functional groups creates the possibility of application in biomedical fields like drug delivery [20]. Solubility of chitosan aids in its application in scaffold fabrication through the membrane and hydrogel form [21]. Chitosan has profound applicability as a drug carrier in different forms with variations in release kinetics [22]. Chitosan, along with different materials like folic acid and glutaraldehyde, showed activity toward drug carriers for Paclitaxel (PTX), doxorubicin, tetracycline, and others. Chitosan-based scaffolds were observed to be effective for myocardial infarction [24]. Similarly, for cancer treatment, chitosan-based drug carriers were successfully studied by researchers [25]. Hyaluronic acid (HA) is a glycosaminoglycan compound without a sulfate group ($C_{14}H_{21}NO_{11}$ subunit structure) and is present in the body. Diverse chemical modifications can be made because of the availability of alcohol, carboxylic acid, and amine functional groups, which endorse versatile applicability [26]. HA has superior biocompatibility and biodegradability, making it an automatic choice for scaffold ingredients. Different fabrication methods, like phase inversion and electrospinning, were adopted for HA-based scaffold fabrication [27]. HA-based drug carriers were observed to be effective for the release of drugs like insulin, α-chymotrypsin, IgG, and nimodipine, with various release kinetics [28]. In wound dressing, sponges, fibers, cloths, foams, colloids, and bandages are used in most cases. The employment of HA was found to be promising in wound dressing [29]. In many cases, shortcomings of HA, such as low viscosity, less mechanical stability, and rapid *in vivo* degradability, were addressed by using modifications like crosslinking and reinforcement, etc. [26, 30]. Collagen is one of the most abundant proteins present in mammals, with the capability to support cell growth. A wide range of collagens is available (28 categories), which can be categorized into three major types: skin, bone, and tendon-based (Type I); cartilage-based (Type II); and skin, vasculature-based (Type III). Collagen has a fibril triple helix structure, and its properties are dependent on the source and processing [31, 32]. Mineralization of collagen promotes interest in the material in view of bone regeneration and scaffold-based applications [33]. Collagen-based scaffolds fabricated by various methods have been observed to be effective in bone research [34]. In accordance with that, it has applicability in making scaffolds that can be utilized for drug delivery. Fish-based collagens have been observed to have superior applicability in drug delivery. Drug delivery is also dependent on diffusion, the presence of solvents, the presence of external stimuli, etc. [35]. In current research findings, it was observed that collagen has substantial applicability for cardiovascular medicine preparation [36].

2.2.2 POLYESTERS

This type of polymer contains a hetero backbone structure, i.e., –COO. The synthesis routes of this type of polymer are mostly microbial synthesis and condensation polymerization, excluding naturally occurring polyesters. The naturally occurring polyester shellac, which contains fatty acid as the main chain backbone, is used as a coating material for medicines [15]. Polyhydroxyalkanoates are produced by microorganisms through different mechanisms like glycolysis, β-oxidation, etc. PHA is a category of polymers with excellent biocompatibility and biodegradability, which extends its application in biomedical fields [37]. Poly-3-hydroxybutyrate (PHB), poly-(3-hydroxybutyrate-co-3-hydroxyvalerate) (PHBV), and poly(3-hydroxybutyrate-co-3-hydroxyvalerate-co-3-hydroxyhexanoate) (PHBVHHx) have substantial bioactivity for bone scaffold applications [38]. Electrospun scaffolds of PHAs were observed to have adequate applicability as scaffolds, including drug-loaded scaffolds [39]. Poly(glycolic acid) (PGA) is a biodegradable polymer that was first utilized as a suture in 1962 and manufactured by Dexon. Its semicrystalline nature, low glass transition temperature, processable melting temperature, along with its absorbable nature, convert PGA into a commercially attractive precursor for biomedical item production [40]. It can be produced through ring-opening polymerization of glycolide, polycondensation of glycolic acid, and other catalytic routes. PGA-based blends and copolymers (PLGA, PGC) are also observed to have similar applicability in various fields [41]. In the case of short-term tissue engineering scaffolds, PGA is utilized. In similar studies, PGA-based copolymers and blends were observed to have more controlled drug release behavior [41, 42]. Poly(lactic acid) (PLA) is a leading biodegradable aliphatic polyester with thermoplastic properties. The processability of PLA through melt or solution pathways makes it a versatile material with sustainable product development capabilities [1–4]. Scaffolds can be prepared through electrospinning, freeze-drying, casting, leaching, etc., involving PLA [43–45]. PLA-based scaffolds were investigated for musculoskeletal, nervous, cardiovascular, and other tissue engineering applications [45]. PLA was observed to be a potential material as a carrier for cells and drugs. PLA-based materials were found to be effective in delivering drugs to the liver or kidney [46]. PLA-based electrospun scaffolds containing

Doxorubicin were found to be excellent drug-releasing carriers. It was also noted that the impact on the healing of tumors was dependent on the release properties. The release property was observed to be dependent on the loading, and Dox-loaded PLA turned out to be an effective implantable scaffold [47]. Polycaprolactone (PCL) has higher stability compared to PLA because of its structure. Even though it has comparatively less biocompatibility, it is still used for the fabrication of scaffolds [48]. The high permeability of drugs and slow biodegradation of PCL are factors that imply superior applicability in drug delivery [49]. Alongside tissue engineering, PCL-based components are also impressive for the release of therapeutic agents [50]. Zein-incorporated PCL was observed to have a porous structure with 89% porosity. Tetracycline hydrochloride release was observed to be sustained in nature [51]. Polydioxanone (PDS) is a colorless degradable polymer that has profound applicability in the biomedical domain. Where prolonged degradation of the material is required, PDS-based biomaterials can be employed. PDO is used for making sutures and films for medical applications [52, 53]. PDO-based tubular electrospun structures were observed to have significant antimicrobial activity when loaded with antibiotics (Sigma), namely MET, CIP, and MINO [54]. In some cases, drug-loaded nanomaterials are also incorporated into the polymer matrix for the preparation of scaffolds. Composites reduce shortcomings such as mechanical property, brittleness, and fast degradability of this class of polymers.

2.2.3 OTHER POLYMERS

Other than the above-mentioned polymers, some other polymers are also in the developing stage for bio-absorbable product development. Bacterial cellulose (BC), which is produced by microorganisms, has superior solubility, which opens up its applicability as a bio-absorbable material and as a drug deliverable scaffold [55]. Silk is another promising protein that can be applied for scaffold fabrication for delivering therapeutics [56]. Some other polymers, like poly(ortho esters), polyphosphazene, polyanhydrides, poly(amino acids), etc., due to their superior bio-absorbability, show prospects as drug carriers [15].

2.3 SCAFFOLD FABRICATION TECHNIQUES

Cells and tissues are arranged into a 3D architecture in the body. In order to build this functional tissue and organs, scaffolds that allow cell distribution and direct their growth in all directions must be created employing a variety of fabrication processes. Here, the primary fabrication methods for scaffolds are discussed (Figure 2.3). Scaffold properties like mechanical strength, porosity, surface texture, etc., are dependent on the scaffold fabrication route. Preparing the scaffolds via solvent casting is relatively quick, straightforward, and cheap. It relies entirely on a solvent's evaporation to create platforms using one of the two methods; it does not require any significant equipment. One method involves immersing the mold in a polymeric solution and letting it evaporate for a sufficient amount of time to produce a layer of polymeric membrane. Another technique consists of pouring the polymeric solution into a mold and giving it enough time to evaporate the solvent, forming a polymeric membrane layer that adheres to the mold.

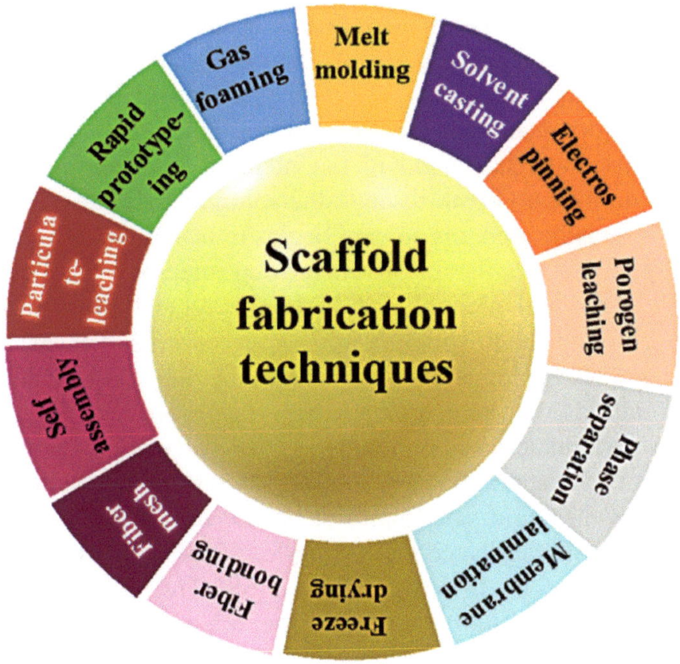

FIGURE 2.3 Scaffold fabrication techniques.

One of the well-liked methods that is frequently utilized to create scaffolds for tissue engineering applications is particulate leaching. The porous structures are made using substances known as porogens, such as salt, wax, or sugar. Here, salt is pulverized into tiny particles of the desired size, and those particles are then added to a mold and filled with a porogen. The mold containing the salt is subsequently filled with a polymer solution. The salt crystals are washed away with water to create the scaffold's pores after the solvent has evaporated. This method makes very porous scaffolds by using high-pressure carbon dioxide gas. The content of gas dissolved in the polymer holds the key to the porosity and porous structure of the scaffolds. This procedure includes saturating a highly porous polymer with carbon dioxide gas at a high pressure (800 psi). In this situation, the polymer will phase split as the dissolved carbon dioxide becomes unstable. To reduce the free energy, the carbon dioxide molecules cluster, leading to the formation of pores. These pores result in a considerable drop in polymer density and an increase in polymer volume. Following the foaming process, a three-dimensional porous structure (scaffolds) is created. The electrospinning method for constructing scaffolds makes use of electrostatic force to produce polymeric fibers with sizes ranging from nano to micro. High-intensity electric fields between two electrodes with electrical charges of opposite polarity govern this process. Two electrodes are used: one in a polymer solution and the other in a collector. Typically, a drop of solution is formed by pumping a polymer solution. After that, an electric field is created with the intention of generating a force, which allows the droplets to break through the solution's surface tension. When a jet of polymer is formed, the solvent begins to evaporate as a result, and this process continues once the nanofibers are deposited on the collector, forming the fibers. Polyvinyl alcohol and hydroxyethyl cellulose-based scaffolds fabricated through electrospinning were observed to have a tensile strength of 2.5 MPa and 200% elongation [57]. One of the most popular techniques for creating scaffolds with regulated porosity is porogen leaching. The foundation of the particulate leaching method is the dispersion of porogen through the processes of evaporation, cross-linking, or other reaction liquids that may solidify, either in liquid particulates or powdered materials. In the case of a PLA/CNF scaffold fabricated via casting-leaching using sodium chloride as a porogen, a porosity of ~76% was observed [58]. The fiber mesh technique for making scaffolds uses individual fibers that are either woven or interwoven into three-dimensional patterns with a range of pore sizes. As a synthetic suture thread, PGA is the first biocompatible and biodegradable polymer to be spun into fiber. It is made by first coating a nonwoven mesh made of another polymer with a polymer solution, then evaporating the mixture. Synthetic polymer (PLLA) was dissolved in chloroform as part of the fiber bonding procedure for scaffold creation, and non-woven mesh containing PGA fiber was then added. After the solvent was eventually evaporated, a composite material made of non-bonded PGA fiber inserted in a PLLA matrix was created. Self-assembly is the molecule's natural organization into a clearly defined, ordered structure needed for a particular function. Nanofibers are tiny fibers created by the self-assembly of natural or synthetic molecules. Rapid prototyping (RP) is referred to as a strong free-form method. This method of fabricating scaffolds is more sophisticated. It is a fabrication technology that is computer-controlled. By adopting the layer manufacturing process, 3D objects can be produced quickly. There are several different methods for making scaffolds that are mentioned. In order to manage the pore interconnectivity and shape, which are crucial for the transfer of nutrients and waste from one pore to another, these scaffold construction techniques were devised. In melt modeling, the Teflon mold is filled with PLGA powder and gelatin microspheres of a particular diameter, and then the mold is heated above the PLGA's glass transition temperature while applying pressure to the mixture. Pressure-assisted microsyringe-based 3D printing was employed for scaffold preparation from bio-absorbable polymers like chitosan, gelatin, and alginate, etc. [59]. Another SFF-like method for creating three-dimensional, anatomically accurate biodegradable polymeric foam scaffolds is membrane lamination. The fabrication process involves layer-by-layer introduction of peptides and proteins, solvent casting, particle leaching, and membrane lamination. To create porous scaffolds, the freeze-drying method is used. The sublimation theory serves as the foundation for this procedure. To create a solution with the correct concentration, the polymer must first be dissolved in a solvent. Under a high vacuum, the solution is frozen, and the solvent is extracted to create a scaffold with high porosity and interconnectivity. Poly(ethylene glycol) diacrylate and silk fibroin-based scaffolds were fabricated with the aid of lyophilization for transdermal drug delivery. The porosity of the scaffold was observed to be dependent on the concentration, with a maximum value reported as ~92% [60].

2.4 CHARACTERIZATION OF SCAFFOLDS AND DRUG RELEASE

These architectural characteristics would include strut thickness, cross-sectional area, anisotropy, interconnectivity, surface area-to-volume ratio, porosity, pore size, and permeability [61]. These factors affect the mechanical strength and biofunctionality of the scaffold. They can be assessed using various methods, such as theoretical evaluation, scanning electron microscopy (SEM) analysis, flow and mercury porosimetry, gas pycnometry, and adsorption.

The expansion and diffusion of the vasculature are necessary for molecular transport in tissue-engineered structures. Vasculature serves as the primary means of transport at the implantation sites, whereas diffusion is the only method used for *in vitro* culture. The porous links need to be improved in order to ease molecular transport and ensure the viability of the cells. Porosity is one of the crucial characteristics that has garnered a lot of attention in the research. The scaffold's mechanical strength, diffusion, and cell seeding effectiveness would all depend on its porosity. To achieve homogeneous cell delivery, cellular attachment, and neotissue formation, a material must have significant porosity and a large surface area-to-volume ratio [62, 63]. In addition to porosity, focus on scaffold design has shown that pore interconnectivity and permeability also have an impact on molecular transport. The diffusion efficiency may be reduced by very porous scaffolds with non-interconnected pores. Chondrocytes were cultivated by Suh et al. on scaffolds with similar porosity but varied levels of interconnectivity. In scaffolds with increased interconnected pores, they observed superior cell attachment and proliferation [64]. There are two major groups that comprise scaffold design. Regular honeycombed scaffolds and woven textile meshes belong to this category of the first design, which features a strict geometrical layout. The second type of scaffold design entails the uneven production and deposition of scaffold struts or walls. Numerous properties, including those in Table 2.2, would be interesting due to the limited consistency and control.

TABLE 2.2 Scaffolds Main Structural Characteristics

Characteristics	Elaboration
Porosity	Porosity is defined as the sum of the volume of the pores and the scaffold material times 100%.
Pore size	The pores' average diameter.
Wall thickness	Typical scaffold strut diameter or typical scaffold wall thickness.
Cross section area	A calculation of the scaffold's surface area in a certain sectional plane.
Permiability	A measurement of how easily fluid flows through the pores of the scaffold.

Scanning electron microscopy (SEM) analysis is a potent investigative technique that creates intricate, high-magnification images of the surface topography of a subject using a focused electron beam. *Energy-dispersive X-ray spectroscopy, or EDX analysis*, allows our experts to delve further into the specifics of the material after a region of interest on the sample has been located and examined using SEM. SEM examination offers direct measurements of pore size and strut/wall thickness, complementing these theoretical estimations of porosity [65, 66]. The following equation was used to calculate the scaffold's porosity percentage, A_p and A_T, respectively, the total area of each cross-section's pores and the total area of each cross-section.

$$Porosity(\%) = \frac{A_p}{A_T} \times 100$$

It is also possible to estimate anisotropy, cross-sectional area, and interconnectedness visually. However, physical sectioning of the scaffold is required to examine its interior, and this would cause unnecessary compression and edge effects that would undermine the accuracy of the findings. Due to layer fusion, variable strut diameter, and complex architectures, the surface area to volume ratio cannot be quantitatively calculated using the theoretical and SEM approaches.

With the exception of the fact that it uses electrons rather than photons or light, transmission electron microscopy (TEM) is a microscopy technique that is similar to light microscopy in many ways. However, because electrons have a much higher resolution than light due to the readily accessible small de Broglie wavelengths, it also exhibits some minor functional differences [67]. The best thickness for examined samples, however, is in the low nm range, making it inappropriate for many scaffolds and limited to the examination of individual fibers [66]. Individual fibers have been treated with it, particularly those that contain nanomaterial.

A well-known and well-established technique for examining porous materials is mercury porosimetry. This method makes use of mercury, a non-wetting liquid that doesn't enter pore spaces unless there is adequate pressure [67]. Using this method, the sample is placed inside a penetrometer and subjected to gas evacuation while mercury is allowed to flow. The sample is under atmospheric pressure, and mercury surrounds it. The bulk volume of the sample is calculated from the mercury volume readings. The scaffolding material and pore spaces make up the bulk volume, which is the same as the apparent volume. In order to encourage mercury infiltration, maximum pressure is gradually built up. Measurement of the total volume of the mercury intruded at maximum pressure enables the determination of the total open pore volume and porosity. An intrusion curve tracks the cumulative volume of the intruded mercury at each pressure step as it happens. Then the Washburn equation is used to calculate the distribution of pore volume by pore size and pore sizes which is as follows [68, 69], $DP = 4\gamma\text{Cos}\theta$

Where the pore diameter is denoted by D, γ denotes the surface tension of mercury, P is the applied pressure, and θ is the contact angle between the pore wall and mercury.

In addition to the structural analysis, mechanical property evaluation is also important for the application of the scaffold. Tensile properties like ultimate tensile strength (UTS), elongation (EB), and elastic modulus determine the load-bearing capacity of the scaffold. In some cases, scaffold activity can be checked by determining UTS at different time intervals under *in vitro* exposure. Thermal stability of the scaffold is sometimes important in order to place it for application. This can be examined using a thermogravimetric analyzer (TGA), which provides information about the degradation profile. In addition to these, other investigations like crystal nature using *differential scanning calorimetry (DSC),* surface hydrophilicity using *contact angle measurement (goniometer),* and material identity using *X-ray diffraction analyzer (XRD)* can be incorporated to extract an overall idea about the scaffold system.

Release behavior measurements in *in vitro* or *in vivo* conditions are also equally important to examine the effectiveness of the scaffold. Different solvent systems and buffer solutions are used as *in vitro* media for release studies. *UV spectroscopy* and *fluorescence spectroscopy* help with the quantification of the released drug. Kinetic analysis and mechanism determination are carried out on the basis of these findings.

2.5 RECENT ADVANCEMENT OF DRUG DELIVERY APPLICATIONS

Bio-absorbable polymer-based scaffolds are utilized to a large extent in drug delivery in association with or along with tissue engineering applications. In many cases, drug-loaded bandages are employed solely for wound healing. Sponges, patches, bandages, mats, cloth, fibers, and films are some of the forms of scaffolds applied over different kinds of affected areas. Bio-absorbable polymeric drug carriers are employed in external wounds for skin as well as for internal damages like bone regeneration and cancer treatment, etc. (Table 2.3). Dodero et al. [70] fabricated sodium alginate (SA), ZnO nanoparticle, and PCL-based electrospun patches for skin wound healing applications. ZnO was synthesized using a green route in order to implement it for antimicrobial purposes. Sr^{2+} modification was conducted on the surface of the patches without altering the biocompatibility of PCL. Cationic and anionic model drugs were observed to be promising in surface adsorption and desorption of the electrospun patches [70]. Monterrubio et al. [71] fabricated a PLA-based drug delivery system for the delivery of the anti-cancer drug SN-38 in the case of tumor control in pediatric oncology. Nanofibers were fabricated through electrospinning, and *in vivo* analysis indicated that the drug can penetrate up to 2 mm into the tumor and resist growth [71]. Similarly, collagen-based scaffolds were introduced for spinal cord injury, and it was noticed that amino acid-based scaffolds have a significant effect on the promotion of the migration of neural stem cells (NSCs) [72]. Scaffold application in bone repair is increasing in recent times. Drug-loaded scaffolds can improve the growth of bone and effectively cure the fracture.

TABLE 2.3 Representative Drug Releasing Scaffolds

Scaffold	Type	Application	Observation	References
Alginate-PCL	Electrospun	Skin wound patches	Controllable between burst and controlled.	[70]
PLA	Electrospun	Pediatric solid tumors	SN-38 penetrates upto 2 mm inside tumor and resists the growth.	[71]
PLA-collagen	3D-printed	Bone regeneration and antimicrobial	Burst release within first 1 h and continuous release up to 24 h for Minocycline hydrochloride (MH).	[75]
PLA-cellulose acetate	Electrospun	Wound dressing patch	Thymoquinone (TQ) release was 17.7–55.9% depending upon the formulation of the scaffolds.	[78]
PCL-PVA	Electrospun (Core-cell)	Colon cancer	Paclitaxel (PTX) release was 18% within 150 h at pH 4.	[84]
Hydroxypropyl guar-graft-poly(N-vinyl caprolactam)	Thermoresponsive hydrogel	Injectable scaffold for antimicrobial drug release (Bone)	Sustained release pattern was observed	[88]
PLGA-PLA	Hot melt extruded scaffold	Implantable scaffold	Brust release less for high drug loaded scaffolds.	[97]
Alginate	IPN-hydrogel	Oral applications	Diclofenac sodium release is pH specific	[105]
PLGA	Scaffold and microsphere	Antimicrobial	Cumulative release was observed to be ~40% for the scaffold after 9 days	[107]

Quinlan et al. [73] investigated the impact of drug-loaded alginate-collagen-based freeze-dried scaffolds on bone repair. Vascular endothelial growth factor (VEGF) release was observed to be increasing within 4 days, and protein release dropped after 7 days. Burst release of >160 ng VEGF was recorded for the 10% protein-loaded scaffold [73]. Alginate-PVA incorporated silk-based scaffolds fabricated through 3D printing were observed to have the capacity to mimic the bone extracellular matrix. An extrusion-based 3D printing strategy was adopted for the work, with $CaCl_2$ leaching for porous scaffold fabrication. The scaffolds were observed to be microporous and showed remarkable cell proliferation up to 7 days [74]. Fused deposition modeling (FDM) was also adopted for scaffold fabrication for antimicrobial and bone regeneration applications. Minocycline hydrochloride (MH) and citrate-hydroxyapatite nanoparticles (cHA) were coated on the surface of the 3D printed scaffolds after alkali treatment of the scaffolds. Collagen was used for the effective deposition of the MH and cHA on the surface of the scaffolds. A highest compressive strength of the scaffold was noted as ~ 13.6 MPa, and surface hydrophilicity was observed to be improved with the introduction of collagen-based coating. Cumulative release study of MH indicated the presence of burst release within the first hour and continuous release up to 24 hours. Effective antibacterial activity was observed towards *S. aureus* with biofilm production. cHA-coated scaffolds were observed to have significant cell proliferation towards mesenchymal stromal cell cultures [75]. 3D-printed scaffolds are user-specific and have the liberty of design alteration. PCL-based 3D-printed scaffolds were observed to have a microporous structure with pore sizes of 20–70 μm, where pores were created by porogen leaching. Scaffolds were observed to be efficient in loading model drugs doxorubicin (DOX), paclitaxel (PTX), and cefazolin (CEF). Sustained release of drugs was noticed within 150–500 hours, depending upon the drug [76]. Electrospun scaffolds are also in use for many cases of tissue engineering involving drug delivery. A PLA/PCL blend with a 50/50 weight ratio was electrospun over an aluminum collector for bovine serum albumin (BSA) release study. Release behavior was examined in phosphate-buffered saline (PBS) solution and was observed to be effective because of its porous fibrous nature [77]. Wound dressing is one of the areas where drug-loaded mats and bandages are employed to a substantially large extent. Gomaa et al. [78] utilized polylactic acid/cellulose acetate-based nanofibrous mats for wound dressing. The representative antimicrobial drug thymoquinone (TQ) was loaded in the scaffold for the study. The release behavior of the TQ-loaded electrospun mats was carried out in PBS solution containing 1%

SDS at 37°C. *In vitro* drug release studies showed that loading efficiency was within 79.5%–90.5%. Release within the initial 24 hours was observed to be between 17.7% and 55.9%, depending upon the formulation of the scaffolds. After 9 days, the maximum cumulative release was recorded to be 79.1%. The presence of cellulose acetate promoted the burst-release nature of the scaffold [78]. Similarly, core/shell electrospun fiber-based scaffolds were observed to be effective in the release of dexpanthenol for wound dressing. Satisfactory results were obtained for cell proliferation and viability, which implied the effectiveness of the scaffolds for wound dressing [79]. In some cases, in order to improve the activity of the scaffold, aniline-agarose systems were utilized for drug release [80]. Hydrophilic molecule encapsulation in hydrophobic systems like PLA was conducted using a probe sonicator, and a release study was conducted in order to formulate different carrier drug systems with long release periods [81]. Mg-based alloys were utilized as bioresorbable drug-release materials in association with biodegradable polymers like PCL, PLA, etc. [82]. Song et al. [83] utilized PEG-PCL-based micelles for the delivery of curcumin. Drug loading was observed at approximately 12.83%, and entrapment efficiency was noted as 98.53%. Linolenic acid modification improved the release of curcumin from 20 days to 50 days [83]. Tumors are one of the main causes of cancerous cell development. Effective control of the release of anti-cancer drugs can provide suitable alternatives to radiation therapy for cancer treatment. PLA/PCL electrospun with coaxial nature was observed to be impressive in the anticancer drug paclitaxel (PTX) release study. There was no release of the drug at pH 7.4, whereas release was approximately 18% within 150 hours at pH 4. This indicates the pH-dependent release behavior of the scaffold, making it a possible candidate for colon cancer treatment [84]. Drug release studies are increasing in the field of injectable scaffolds for drug delivery. Drug delivery in the central nervous system (CNS) faces barriers such as the blood-brain barrier (BBB), blood-cerebrospinal fluid barrier, and blood-brain tumor barrier (BBTB). Common CNS disorders include brain tumors, brain and spinal cord injuries, and neurodegenerative diseases like Alzheimer's disease (AD) and Parkinson's disease (PD). A thermoresponsive hydrogel with a sol-gel transformation temperature of approximately 32°C was employed for CNS disorder treatment. Ellagic acid, BMSC, NT-3, EPO, etc., were loaded in chitosan, collagen, and hyaluronan-methylcellulose gel systems and examined successfully as injectable gels for various disorder cases [85]. Thermoresponsive hydrogels were also studied for cancer treatment through chemotherapy, photothermal therapy, photodynamic therapy, gene therapy, etc. [86]. Similarly, hydrophobic polymer-based gels were also studied as injectable gels for drug delivery in many cases [87]. Parameswaran-Thankam et al. [88] used guar-gum-based thermoresponsive hydrogel as an injectable scaffold for drug delivery. Hydroxypropyl guar (HPG)-poly(N-vinyl caprolactam) (PNVCL) graft polymer was synthesized as a thermoresponsive gel with a gel point temperature of approximately 34°C. Time-dependent structural information was obtained after the incorporation of the gel. Ciprofloxacin, a model drug, was used to gather information about the release mechanism, and a sustained release pattern was noticed [88]. Cellulose nanocrystal (CNC) and polyamidoamine (PAMAM) dendrimer were two nano-carriers (NCs) introduced inside the gelatin system for the synthesis of an injectable scaffold for inflammatory drug release studies. Betamethasone sodium phosphate (BSP) release behavior was observed to be dependent on the compositions of the cryogels [89]. mPEG-PELG copolymer was used for the synthesis of an injectable drug-loaded scaffold. Mouse NGF release was observed to be dependent on loading and release conditions [90]. Chitosan-based injectable hydrogel was utilized for the treatment of Parkinson's disease [91], and gelatin-based self-healing gel was employed for drug delivery [92].

Implantable scaffolds for drug delivery are another area where affected tissue can be cured using implantable scaffolds. Different reinforcement additions can improve the various properties of scaffolds. Spray-dried HA (sd HA) was loaded into the PLA matrix through the FDM method. Porosity was noted to be higher (55%) in comparison to the PLA scaffold. Thus, the made scaffold proved to be promising for bone regeneration applications [93]. In the case of localized drug delivery for cancer treatment, PLGA-PEG and PLGA-PEG-based degradable scaffolds were utilized. Prodigiosin (PG) or paclitaxel (PTX), anti-cancer drugs, were loaded into the polymer solution, and scaffolds were fabricated using freeze-drying. *In vitro,* drug release behavior in PBS solution was observed to be temperature-dependent. A cell viability study was carried out using triple-negative breast cancer (TNBC) cells (MDA-MB-231). After 48 hours, burst release was 39.5% at 44°C for PLGA-PEG_PTX [94]. Hyaluronic acid-based sponge-type scaffolds were observed to be effective for hepatocarcinoma cells. Scaffold degradation rates were observed to be dependent on exposure conditions [95]. Yang et al. [96] constructed a PLGA-based scaffold through extrusion printing. Five-Fluorouracil, which is a breast cancer drug, was loaded for the release study. Uniform distribution of the drug was observed through mapping. *In vitro* release studies indicated burst release within the first week, followed by sustained release for up to 30 days [96]. Melt-extruded implants were also found to be promising for drug release applications. PLGA/PLA-based melt-drawn fiber was created incorporating the drug dexamethasone. *In vitro*, drug release studies were investigated at pH 7.4 and 37°C. Melt-extruded fibers were observed to have a diameter of 1.2 to 1.4 mm and a length of 5.8 to 5.9 mm, depending on the drug loading. Burst release was found to be less for higher loading of drug in PLGA [97]. HA-Bio-Streptavidin-Alginate (HBSA)-based hydrogel was synthesized for bioprinting of scaffolds for adipose tissue growth. Double-crosslinked hydrogel was observed to be effective for chondrogenic formation [98]. Implantable scaffolds were also subjected to cancer immunotherapy [99]. In some cases, bioabsorbable polymers were employed as coating materials for glass or metallic implantable scaffolds. This improves the biocompatibility of the scaffolds [100]. Different advanced technologies are emerging for improved scaffold fabrication, like cryoprinting based on extrusion 3D printing [101]. It was observed that bioabsorbable polymer-based scaffolds are emerging as implantable scaffolds for spinal cord injuries and were observed to be effective for the regeneration of neuronal cells [102]. Calcium carbonate ($CaCO_3$) and alginate-based scaffolds were investigated for various types of drug delivery because of their pH stability, flexibility, porosity, and water-soluble nature, etc. [103].

Stimuli-responsive scaffold system is also becoming the need in proper control and selective release of drugs. This can help in the optimum dosage of the drug, local drug delivery and less chance of adverse side effects. Nanoparticle inclusion in the polymeric system can introduce responsive features in the scaffold. Magnetic nanoparticles, conductive materials, and shape memory materials are some of the elements utilized in the fabrication of scaffolds. In some cases, near-infrared (NIR), ultrasound-sensitive (US), X-ray, alternating magnetic field (AMF), static magnetic field (SMF), and electroporation (EP) responsive scaffolds are emerging as effective releasing carriers [104]. Alginate-based scaffolds were observed to have pH sensitivity in releasing drugs. Model drugs like amoxicillin (AMX), trimethoprim (TMP), etc., were incorporated in IPN-hydrogels for release studies for oral applications. The release of diclofenac sodium was observed to be 4.5% at pH 1.2 and 95% at pH 7 [105]. Hyaluronic acid-based drug-eluting systems were studied successfully with stimuli-responsive nature [106]. The impact of shape memory on drug delivery was studied by Du et al. in 2017 [107] using a PLGA system. Vancomycin release profile was examined using PBS solution, and cumulative release was observed to be ~40% for the scaffold after 9 days, whereas for the drug-loaded microsphere, the release was around 70% [107].

Scaffold research is prevailing in all aspects of disease control and treatment. Depending on the need for the application, polymers are modified with nanomaterials, or fabrication techniques are tuned to achieve improved product development (Figure 2.4).

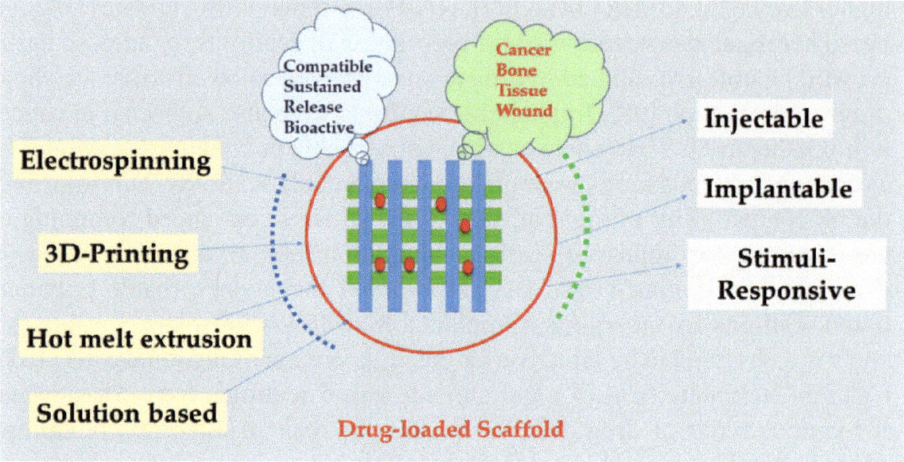

FIGURE 2.4 Recent trends of drug loaded scaffolds.

2.6 OUTLOOK AND SUMMARY

In this chapter, discussions are made covering various aspects of bio-absorbable polymeric scaffolds employed for drug delivery. Bio-absorbable polymers, with their properties and possibilities in scaffold fabrication use, are thoroughly enlightened in corroboration with recent research. The scaffold fabrication technique, which is one of the prime factors to control the porosity and morphology of scaffolds, is incorporated along with basic characterization techniques for structure-property evaluation of the scaffolds. The major focus of the chapter is on the emerging works in the area of drug delivery using bio-absorbable polymers, which are also thoroughly discussed from the aspects of application, emerging fabrication techniques, materials, and advanced features. In the future, more development will come for the upgradation of drug-loaded scaffolds applicable for CNS damages, cardiac recoveries, cancer treatment, etc. Stimuli-responsive scaffolds, which can make the applicability one step ahead, need to be addressed in the future. Bio-degradation, bio-absorption, and bio-resorbability need to be studied more in association with release studies to reduce the toxic effect or side effects.

In vivo studies in the human system need to be focused on more to make more commercially useful systems.

ACKNOWLEDGMENT

Authors are thankful to the National Institute of Technology Andhra Pradesh for providing the necessary facilities to prepare this book chapter.

KEYWORDS

- **alternating magnetic field**
- **bio-absorption**
- **bio-degradation**
- **fabrication**
- ***in vivo* studies**
- **polymers**
- **scaffolds**
- **static magnetic field**

REFERENCES

1. Chakraborty, G., Valapa, R. B., Pugazhenthi, G., & Katiyar, V. (2018). Investigating the properties of poly (lactic acid)/exfoliated graphene-based nanocomposites fabricated by versatile coating approach. *International Journal of Biological Macromolecules, 113*, 1080–1091. https://doi.org/10.1016/j.ijbiomac.2018.03.050.
2. Chakraborty, G., Pugazhenthi, G., & Katiyar, V. (2019). Exfoliated graphene-dispersed poly (lactic acid)-based nanocomposite sensors for ethanol detection. *Polymer Bulletin, 76*(5), 2367–2386. https://doi.org/10.1007/s00289-018-2536-8.
3. Chakraborty, G., Katiyar, V., & Pugazhenthi, G. (2021). Improvisation of polylactic acid (PLA)/exfoliated graphene (GR) nanocomposite for detection of metal ions (Cu2+). *Composites Science and Technology, 213*, 108877. https://doi.org/10.1016/j.compscitech.2021.108877.
4. Chakraborty, G., Bhattacharjee, S., Katiyar, V., & Pugazhenthi, G. (2023). Melt rheology analysis through experimental and constitutional mechanical models of exfoliated graphene based polylactic acid (PLA) nanocomposites. *Journal of Polymer Research, 30*(1), 10. https://doi.org/10.1007/s10965-023-03006-2.

5. Sringari, S. S., Chakraborty, G., & Prasad, A. (2021). Biodegradable and biocompatible polymeric nanocomposites for tissue engineering applications. In A. Prasad (Ed.), *Nanomanufacturing and Nanomaterials Design* (pp. 205–225). CRC Press. https://doi.org/10.1201/9780429298327-12.
6. Prasad, A., Chakraborty, G., & Kumar, A. (2022). Bio-based environmentally benign polymeric resorbable materials for orthopedic fixation applications. In A. Kumar & S. K. Nayak (Eds.), *Advanced Materials for Biomedical Applications* (pp. 251–266). CRC Press. https://doi.org/10.1201/9781003137597-16.
7. Prajapati, S. K., Jain, A., Jain, A., & Jain, S. (2019). Biodegradable polymers and constructs: A novel approach in drug delivery. *European Polymer Journal, 120*, 109191. https://doi.org/10.1016/j.eurpolymj.2019.109191.
8. Calori, I. R., Braga, G., de Jesus, P. D. C. C., Bi, H., & Tedesco, A. C. (2020). Polymer scaffolds as drug delivery systems. *European Polymer Journal, 129*, 109621. https://doi.org/10.1016/j.eurpolymj.2020.109621.
9. Guenday, C., Anand, S., Gencer, H. B., Munafo, S., Moroni, L., Fusco, A., & Danti, S. (2020). Ciprofloxacin-loaded polymeric nanoparticles incorporated electrospun fibers for drug delivery in tissue engineering applications. *Drug Delivery and Translational Research, 10*, 706–720. https://doi.org/10.1007/s13346-020-00719-7.
10. Nayak, A. K., Mohanta, B. C., Hasnain, M. S., Hoda, M. N., & Tripathi, G. (2020). Alginate-based scaffolds for drug delivery in tissue engineering. In A. K. Nayak & M. S. Hasnain (Eds.), *Alginates in Drug Delivery* (pp. 359–386). Academic Press. https://doi.org/10.1016/B978-0-12-817640-3.00012-9.
11. Dorati, R., DeTrizio, A., Modena, T., Conti, B., Benazzo, F., Gastaldi, G., & Genta, I. (2017). Biodegradable scaffolds for bone regeneration combined with drug-delivery systems in osteomyelitis therapy. *Pharmaceuticals, 10*(4), 96. https://doi.org/10.3390/ph10040096.
12. Aoki, K., & Saito, N. (2020). Biodegradable polymers as drug delivery systems for bone regeneration. *Pharmaceutics, 12*(2), 95. https://doi.org/10.3390/pharmaceutics12020095.
13. Castillo-Henríquez, L., Castro-Alpízar, J., Lopretti-Correa, M., & Vega-Baudrit, J. (2021). Exploration of bioengineered scaffolds composed of thermo-responsive polymers for drug delivery in wound healing. *International Journal of Molecular Sciences, 22*(3), 1408. https://doi.org/10.3390/ijms22031408.
14. Casalini, T. (2017). Bioresorbability of polymers: Chemistry, mechanisms, and modeling. In A. B. Kohn (Ed.), *Bioresorbable Polymers for Biomedical Applications* (pp. 65–83). Woodhead Publishing. https://doi.org/10.1016/B978-0-08-100262-9.00004-6.
15. Pertici, G. (2017). Introduction to bioresorbable polymers for biomedical applications. In A. B. Kohn (Ed.), *Bioresorbable Polymers for Biomedical Applications* (pp. 3–29). Woodhead Publishing. https://doi.org/10.1016/B978-0-08-100262-9.00001-0.
16. Fernando, I. P. S., Lee, W., Han, E. J., & Ahn, G. (2020). Alginate-based nanomaterials: Fabrication techniques, properties, and applications. *Chemical Engineering Journal, 391*, 123823. https://doi.org/10.1016/j.cej.2019.123823.
17. De Silva, R. T., Dissanayake, R. K., Mantilaka, M. P. G., Wijesinghe, W. S. L., Kaleel, S. S., Premachandra, T. N., & de Silva, K. N. (2018). Drug-loaded halloysite nanotube-reinforced electrospun alginate-based nanofibrous scaffolds with sustained antimicrobial protection. *ACS Applied Materials & Interfaces, 10*(40), 33913–33922. https://doi.org/10.1021/acsami.8b13736.

18. Abasalizadeh, F., Moghaddam, S. V., Alizadeh, E., Akbari, E., Kashani, E., Fazljou, S. M. B., & Akbarzadeh, A. (2020). Alginate-based hydrogels as drug delivery vehicles in cancer treatment and their applications in wound dressing and 3D bioprinting. *Journal of Biological Engineering, 14*(1), 1–22. https://doi.org/10.1186/s13036-020-00266-1.
19. Shah, S. A., Sohail, M., Khan, S. A., & Kousar, M. (2021). Improved drug delivery and accelerated diabetic wound healing by chondroitin sulfate grafted alginate-based thermoreversible hydrogels. *Materials Science and Engineering: C, 126*, 112169. https://doi.org/10.1016/j.msec.2021.112169.
20. Aranaz, I., Alcántara, A. R., Civera, M. C., Arias, C., Elorza, B., Heras Caballero, A., & Acosta, N. (2021). Chitosan: An overview of its properties and applications. *Polymers, 13*(19), 3256. https://doi.org/10.3390/polym13193256.
21. Hossain, M. R., Mallik, A. K., & Rahman, M. M. (2020). Fundamentals of chitosan for biomedical applications. In M. K. Shukla, S. Thomas, & Z. T. Jiang (Eds.), *Handbook of Chitin and Chitosan* (pp. 199–230). Elsevier. https://doi.org/10.1016/B978-0-12-817970-1.00008-2.
22. Kurakula, M., & Naveen, N. R. (2021). Electro spraying: A facile technology unfolding the chitosan-based drug delivery and biomedical applications. *European Polymer Journal, 147*, 110326. https://doi.org/10.1016/j.eurpolymj.2020.110326.
23. Ahmad, A., Mubarak, N. M., Naseem, K., Tabassum, H., Rizwan, M., Najda, A., & Hussain, S. (2020). Recent advancement and development of chitin and chitosan-based nanocomposite for drug delivery: Critical approach to clinical research. *Arabian Journal of Chemistry, 13*(12), 8935–8964. https://doi.org/10.1016/j.arabjc.2020.09.002.
24. Beleño Acosta, B., Advincula, R. C., & Grande-Tovar, C. D. (2023). Chitosan-based scaffolds for the treatment of myocardial infarction: A systematic review. *Molecules, 28*(4), 1920. https://doi.org/10.3390/molecules28041920.
25. Shanmuganathan, R., Edison, T. N. J. I., LewisOscar, F., Kumar, P., Shanmugam, S., & Pugazhendhi, A. (2019). Chitosan nano polymers: An overview of drug delivery against cancer. *International Journal of Biological Macromolecules, 130*, 727–736. https://doi.org/10.1016/j.ijbiomac.2019.02.151.
26. Dovedytis, M., Liu, Z. J., & Bartlett, S. (2020). Hyaluronic acid and its biomedical applications: A review. *Engineered Regeneration, 1*, 102–113. https://doi.org/10.1016/j.engreg.2020.10.001.
27. Chircov, C., Grumezescu, A. M., & Bejenaru, L. E. (2018). Hyaluronic acid-based scaffolds for tissue engineering. *Romanian Journal of Morphology and Embryology, 59*(1), 71–76.
28. Huang, G., & Huang, H. (2018). Application of hyaluronic acid as carriers in drug delivery. *Drug Delivery, 25*(1), 766–772. https://doi.org/10.1080/10717544.2018.1461950.
29. Alven, S., & Aderibigbe, B. A. (2021). Hyaluronic acid-based scaffolds as potential bioactive wound dressings. *Polymers, 13*(13), 2102. https://doi.org/10.3390/polym13132102.
30. Séon-Lutz, M., Couffin, A. C., Vignoud, S., Schlatter, G., & Hébraud, A. (2019). Electrospinning in water and *in situ* crosslinking of hyaluronic acid/cyclodextrin nanofibers: Towards wound dressing with controlled drug release. *Carbohydrate Polymers, 207*, 276–287. https://doi.org/10.1016/j.carbpol.2018.11.074.

31. Sionkowska, A., Skrzyński, S., Śmiechowski, K., & Kołodziejczak, A. (2017). The review of versatile application of collagen. *Polymers for Advanced Technologies, 28*(1), 4–9. https://doi.org/10.1002/pat.3866.
32. Avila Rodríguez, M. I., Rodríguez Barroso, L. G., & Sánchez, M. L. (2018). Collagen: A review on its sources and potential cosmetic applications. *Journal of Cosmetic Dermatology, 17*(1), 20–26. https://doi.org/10.1111/jocd.12450.
33. Oosterlaken, B. M., Vena, M. P., & de With, G. (2021). *In vitro* mineralization of collagen. *Advanced Materials, 33*(16), 2004418. https://doi.org/10.1002/adma.202004418.
34. Zhang, D., Wu, X., Chen, J., & Lin, K. (2018). The development of collagen-based composite scaffolds for bone regeneration. *Bioactive Materials, 3*(1), 129–138. https://doi.org/10.1016/j.bioactmat.2017.08.004.
35. Furtado, M., Chen, L., Chen, Z., Chen, A., & Cui, W. (2022). Development of fish collagen in tissue regeneration and drug delivery. *Engineered Regeneration, 3*, 217–231. https://doi.org/10.1016/j.engreg.2022.05.004.
36. Copes, F., Pien, N., Van Vlierberghe, S., Boccafoschi, F., & Mantovani, D. (2019). Collagen-based tissue engineering strategies for vascular medicine. *Frontiers in Bioengineering and Biotechnology, 7*, 166. https://doi.org/10.3389/fbioe.2019.00166.
37. Sharma, V., Sehgal, R., & Gupta, R. (2021). Polyhydroxyalkanoate (PHA): Properties and modifications. *Polymer, 212*, 123161. https://doi.org/10.1016/j.polymer.2020.123161.
38. Lim, J., You, M., Li, J., & Li, Z. (2017). Emerging bone tissue engineering via Polyhydroxyalkanoate (PHA)-based scaffolds. *Materials Science and Engineering: C, 79*, 917–929. https://doi.org/10.1016/j.msec.2017.05.124.
39. Sanhueza, C., Acevedo, F., Rocha, S., Villegas, P., Seeger, M., & Navia, R. (2019). Polyhydroxyalkanoates as biomaterial for electrospun scaffolds. *International Journal of Biological Macromolecules, 124*, 102–110. https://doi.org/10.1016/j.ijbiomac.2018.11.116.
40. Low, Y. J., Andriyana, A., Ang, B. C., & Zainal Abidin, N. I. (2020). Bioresorbable and degradable behaviors of PGA: Current state and future prospects. *Polymer Engineering & Science, 60*(11), 2657–2675. https://doi.org/10.1002/pen.25449.
41. Samantaray, P. K., Little, A., Haddleton, D. M., McNally, T., Tan, B., Sun, Z., & Wan, C. (2020). Poly (glycolic acid) (PGA): A versatile building block expanding high performance and sustainable bioplastic applications. *Green Chemistry, 22*(13), 4055–4081. https://doi.org/10.1039/D0GC01394A.
42. García, M. C. (2018). Drug delivery systems based on nonimmunogenic biopolymers. In K. N. Parikh (Ed.), *Engineering of Biomaterials for Drug Delivery Systems* (pp. 317–344). Woodhead Publishing. https://doi.org/10.1016/B978-0-08-101750-0.00010-5.
43. Maghsoudi, S., Taghavi Shahraki, B., Rabiee, N., Fatahi, Y., Dinarvand, R., Tavakolizadeh, M., & Tayebi, L. (2020). Burgeoning polymer nano blends for improved controlled drug release: A review. *International Journal of Nanomedicine, 15*, 4363–4392. https://doi.org/10.2147/IJN.S252170.
44. Avérous, L. (2008). Polylactic acid: Synthesis, properties, and applications. In M. N. Belgacem & A. Gandini (Eds.), *Monomers, Polymers and Composites from Renewable Resources* (pp. 433–450). Elsevier. https://doi.org/10.1016/B978-008045316-3.00021-1.
45. Cheng, Y., Deng, S., Chen, P., & Ruan, R. (2009). Polylactic acid (PLA) synthesis and modifications: A review. *Frontiers of Chemistry in China, 4*(3), 259–264. https://doi.org/10.1007/s11458-009-0056-8.

46. Tyler, B., Gullotti, D., Mangraviti, A., Utsuki, T., & Brem, H. (2016). Polylactic acid (PLA) controlled delivery carriers for biomedical applications. *Advanced Drug Delivery Reviews, 107*, 163–175. https://doi.org/10.1016/j.addr.2016.06.018.
47. Dai, J., Jin, J., Yang, S., & Li, G. (2017). Doxorubicin-loaded PLA/pearl electrospun nanofibrous scaffold for drug delivery and tumor cell treatment. *Materials Research Express, 4*(7), 075403. https://doi.org/10.1088/2053-1591/aa7e96.
48. Malikmammadov, E., Tanir, T. E., Kiziltay, A., Hasirci, V., & Hasirci, N. (2018). PCL and PCL-based materials in biomedical applications. *Journal of Biomaterials Science, Polymer Edition, 29*(7–9), 863–893. https://doi.org/10.1080/09205063.2017.1394711.
49. Mohamed, R. M., & Yusoh, K. (2016). A review on the recent research of polycaprolactone (PCL). *Advanced Materials Research, 1134*, 249–255. https://doi.org/10.4028/www.scientific.net/AMR.1134.249.
50. Mondal, D., Griffith, M., & Venkatraman, S. S. (2016). Polycaprolactone-based biomaterials for tissue engineering and drug delivery: Current scenario and challenges. *International Journal of Polymeric Materials and Polymeric Biomaterials, 65*(5), 255–265. https://doi.org/10.1080/00914037.2015.1103241.
51. Fereshteh, Z., Fathi, M., Bagri, A., & Boccaccini, A. R. (2016). Preparation and characterization of aligned porous PCL/zein scaffolds as drug delivery systems via improved unidirectional freeze-drying method. *Materials Science and Engineering: C, 68*, 613–622. https://doi.org/10.1016/j.msec.2016.06.013.
52. Martins, J. A., Lach, A. A., Morris, H. L., Carr, A. J., & Mouthuy, P. A. (2020). Polydioxanone implants: A systematic review on safety and performance in patients. *Journal of Biomaterials Applications, 34*(7), 902–916. https://doi.org/10.1177/0885328219880272.
53. Lee, H., Yoon, K., & Lee, M. (2018). Outcome of facial rejuvenation with polydioxanone thread for Asians. *Journal of Cosmetic and Laser Therapy, 20*(3), 189–192. https://doi.org/10.1080/14764172.2018.1463901.
54. Bottino, M. C., Albuquerque, M. T., Azabi, A., Münchow, E. A., Spolnik, K. J., Nör, J. E., & Edwards, P. C. (2019). A novel patient-specific three-dimensional drug delivery construct for regenerative endodontics. *Journal of Biomedical Materials Research Part B: Applied Biomaterials, 107*(5), 1576–1586. https://doi.org/10.1002/jbm.b.34242.
55. Badshah, M., Ullah, H., Khan, A. R., Khan, S., Park, J. K., & Khan, T. (2018). Surface modification and evaluation of bacterial cellulose for drug delivery. *International Journal of Biological Macromolecules, 113*, 526–533. https://doi.org/10.1016/j.ijbiomac.2018.02.131.
56. Pandey, V., Haider, T., Jain, P., Gupta, P. N., & Soni, V. (2020). Silk as a leading-edge biological macromolecule for improved drug delivery. *Journal of Drug Delivery Science and Technology, 55*, 101294. https://doi.org/10.1016/j.jddst.2019.101294.
57. El Fawal, G., Hong, H., Song, X., Wu, J., Sun, M., Zhang, L., & Wang, H. (2020). Polyvinyl alcohol/hydroxyethyl cellulose containing ethosomes as a scaffold for transdermal drug delivery applications. *Applied Biochemistry and Biotechnology, 191*(4), 1624–1637. https://doi.org/10.1007/s12010-020-03314-y.
58. Radakisnin, R., Abdul Majid, M. S., Mohd Jamir, M. R., Mat Tahir, M. F., Meng, C. E., & Al Alshahrani, H. (2021). Physical, thermal, and mechanical properties of highly porous polylactic acid/cellulose nanofiber scaffolds prepared by salt leaching technique. *Nanotechnology Reviews, 10*(1), 1469–1483. https://doi.org/10.1515/ntrev-2021-0107.

59. Aguilar-de-Leyva, Á., Linares, V., Casas, M., & Caraballo, I. (2020). 3D printed drug delivery systems based on natural products. *Pharmaceutics, 12*(7), 620. https://doi.org/10.3390/pharmaceutics12070620.
60. Gao, Y., Hou, M., Yang, R., Zhang, L., Xu, Z., Kang, Y., & Xue, P. (2019). Highly porous silk fibroin scaffold packed in PEGDA/sucrose microneedles for controllable transdermal drug delivery. *Biomacromolecules, 20*(3), 1334–1345. https://doi.org/10.1021/acs.biomac.8b01612.
61. Lin, A. S., Barrows, T. H., Cartmell, S. H., & Guldberg, R. E. (2003). Microarchitectural and mechanical characterization of oriented porous polymer scaffolds. *Biomaterials, 24*(3), 481–489. https://doi.org/10.1016/S0142-9612(02)00381-6.
62. Zein, I., Hutmacher, D. W., Tan, K. C., & Teoh, S. H. (2002). Fused deposition modeling of novel scaffold architectures for tissue engineering applications. *Biomaterials, 23*(4), 1169–1185. https://doi.org/10.1016/S0142-9612(01)00232-0.
63. Schantz, J. T., Hutmacher, D. W., Chim, H., Ng, K. W., Lim, T. C., & Teoh, S. H. (2002). Induction of ectopic bone formation by using human periosteal cells in combination with a novel scaffold technology. *Cell Transplantation, 11*(2), 125–138. https://doi.org/10.3727/000000002783986014.
64. Suh, S. W., Shin, J. Y., Kim, J., Kim, J., Beak, C. H., Kim, D. I., & Choo, I. W. (2002). Effect of different particles on cell proliferation in polymer scaffolds using a solvent-casting and particulate leaching technique. *ASAIO Journal, 48*(5), 460–464. https://doi.org/10.1097/00002480-200209000-00022.
65. Holland, T. A., & Mikos, A. G. (2006). Biodegradable polymeric scaffolds. Improvements in bone tissue engineering through controlled drug delivery. In A. G. Mikos & P. Ducheyne (Eds.), *Tissue Engineering I* (pp. 161–185). Springer. https://doi.org/10.1007/3-540-28181-6_7.
66. Walsh, D., Furuzono, T., & Tanaka, J. (2001). Preparation of porous composite implant materials by *in situ* polymerization of porous apatite containing ε-caprolactone or methyl methacrylate. *Biomaterials, 22*(11), 1205–1212. https://doi.org/10.1016/S0142-9612(00)00321-4.
67. Lopez Marquez, A., Gareis, I. E., Dias, F. J., Gerhard, C., & Lezcano, M. F. (2022). Methods to characterize electrospun scaffold morphology: A critical review. *Polymers, 14*(3), 467. https://doi.org/10.3390/polym14030467.
68. Ho, S. T., & Hutmacher, D. W. (2006). A comparison of micro-CT with other techniques used in the characterization of scaffolds. *Biomaterials, 27*(8), 1362–1376. https://doi.org/10.1016/j.biomaterials.2005.08.035.
69. Webb, P. A. (2001). An introduction to the physical characterization of materials by mercury intrusion porosimeter with emphasis on reduction and presentation of experimental data. Micromeritics Instrument Corp, Norcross, Georgia.
70. Dodero, A., Alloisio, M., Castellano, M., & Vicini, S. (2020). Multilayer alginate–polycaprolactone electrospun membranes as skin wound patches with drug delivery abilities. *ACS Applied Materials & Interfaces, 12*(28), 31162–31171. https://doi.org/10.1021/acsami.0c07301.
71. Monterrubio, C., Pascual-Pasto, G., Cano, F., Vila-Ubach, M., Manzanares, A., Schaiquevich, P., & Carcaboso, A. M. (2016). SN-38-loaded nanofiber matrices for local control of pediatric solid tumors after subtotal resection surgery. *Biomaterials, 79*, 69–78. https://doi.org/10.1016/j.biomaterials.2015.11.050.

72. Zhang, L., Fan, C., Hao, W., Zhuang, Y., Liu, X., Zhao, Y., & Dai, J. (2021). NSCs migration promoted and drug delivered exosomes-collagen scaffold via a bio-specific peptide for one-step spinal cord injury repair. *Advanced Healthcare Materials, 10*(8), 2001896. https://doi.org/10.1002/adhm.202001896.
73. Quinlan, E., López-Noriega, A., Thompson, E. M., Hibbitts, A., Cryan, S. A., & O'Brien, F. J. (2017). Controlled release of vascular endothelial growth factor from spray-dried alginate microparticles in collagen–hydroxyapatite scaffolds for promoting vascularization and bone repair. *Journal of Tissue Engineering and Regenerative Medicine, 11*(4), 1097–1109. https://doi.org/10.1002/term.2028.
74. Sangkert, S., Kamolmatyakul, S., Gelinsky, M., & Meesane, J. (2021). 3D printed scaffolds of alginate/polyvinylalcohol with silk fibroin based on mimicked extracellular matrix for bone tissue engineering in maxillofacial surgery. *Materials Today Communications, 26*, 102140. https://doi.org/10.1016/j.mtcomm.2020.102140.
75. Martin, V., Ribeiro, I. A., Alves, M. M., Gonçalves, L., Claudio, R. A., Grenho, L., & Bettencourt, A. F. (2019). Engineering a multifunctional 3D-printed PLA-collagen-minocycline-nanoHydroxyapatite scaffold with combined antimicrobial and osteogenic effects for bone regeneration. *Materials Science and Engineering: C, 101*, 15–26. https://doi.org/10.1016/j.msec.2019.03.060.
76. Dang, H. P., Shabab, T., Shafiee, A., Peiffer, Q. C., Fox, K., Tran, N., & Tran, P. A. (2019). 3D printed dual macro-, microscale porous network as a tissue engineering scaffold with drug delivering function. *Biofabrication, 11*(3), 035014. https://doi.org/10.1088/1758-5090/ab0d57.
77. Herrero-Herrero, M., Gómez-Tejedor, J. A., & Vallés-Lluch, A. (2018). PLA/PCL electrospun membranes of tailored fibers diameter as drug delivery systems. *European Polymer Journal, 99*, 445–455. https://doi.org/10.1016/j.eurpolymj.2017.12.008.
78. Gomaa, S. F., Madkour, T. M., Moghannem, S., & El-Sherbiny, I. M. (2017). New polylactic acid/cellulose acetate-based antimicrobial interactive single dose nanofibrous wound dressing mats. *International Journal of Biological Macromolecules, 105*, 1148–1160. https://doi.org/10.1016/j.ijbiomac.2017.07.109.
79. Najafiasl, M., Osfouri, S., Azin, R., & Zaeri, S. (2020). Alginate-based electrospun core/shell nanofibers containing dexpanthenol: A good candidate for wound dressing. *Journal of Drug Delivery Science and Technology, 57*, 101708. https://doi.org/10.1016/j.jddst.2020.101708.
80. Atoufi, Z., Zarrintaj, P., Motlagh, G. H., Amiri, A., Bagher, Z., & Kamrava, S. K. (2017). A novel bio electro active alginate-aniline tetramer/agarose scaffold for tissue engineering: Synthesis, characterization, drug release and cell culture study. *Journal of Biomaterials Science, Polymer Edition, 28*(15), 1617–1638. https://doi.org/10.1080/09205063.2017.1352086.
81. Gai, M., Frueh, J., Tao, T., Petrov, A. V., Petrov, V. V., Shesterikov, E. V., & Sukhorukov, G. B. (2017). Polylactic acid nano-and microchamber arrays for encapsulation of small hydrophilic molecules featuring drug release via high intensity focused ultrasound. *Nanoscale, 9*(21), 7063–7070.
82. Xu, W., Yagoshi, K., Koga, Y., Sasaki, M., & Niidome, T. (2018). Optimized polymer coating for magnesium alloy-based bioresorbable scaffolds for long-lasting drug release and corrosion resistance. *Colloids and Surfaces B: Biointerfaces, 163*, 100–106.
83. Song, Z., Zhu, W., Liu, N., Yang, F., & Feng, R. (2014). Linolenic acid-modified PEG-PCL micelles for curcumin delivery. *International Journal of Pharmaceutics, 471*(1–2), 312–321.

84. Yan, E., Jiang, J., Ren, X., Gao, J., Zhang, X., Li, S., & Li, Y. (2021). Polycaprolactone/polyvinyl alcohol core-shell nanofibers as a pH-responsive drug carrier for the potential application in chemotherapy against colon cancer. *Materials Letters, 291*, 129516.
85. Bellotti, E., Schilling, A. L., Little, S. R., & Decuzzi, P. (2021). Injectable thermoresponsive hydrogels as drug delivery system for the treatment of central nervous system disorders: A review. *Journal of Controlled Release, 329*, 16–35.
86. Xiao, Y., Gu, Y., Qin, L., Chen, L., Chen, X., Cui, W., & He, X. (2021). Injectable thermosensitive hydrogel-based drug delivery system for local cancer therapy. *Colloids and Surfaces B: Bio Interfaces, 200*, 111581.
87. Arun, Y., Ghosh, R., & Domb, A. J. (2021). Biodegradable hydrophobic injectable polymers for drug delivery and regenerative medicine. *Advanced Functional Materials, 31*(44), 2010284.
88. Parameswaran-Thankam, A., Parnell, C. M., Watanabe, F., RanguMagar, A. B., Chhetri, B. P., Szwedo, P. K., & Ghosh, A. (2018). Guar-based injectable thermoresponsive hydrogel as a scaffold for bone cell growth and controlled drug delivery. *ACS Omega, 3*(11), 15158–15167.
89. Goodarzi, K., Shariatzadeh, F. J., Solouk, A., Akbari, S., & Mirzadeh, H. (2020). Injectable drug-loaded gelatin-based scaffolds as minimally invasive approach for drug delivery system: CNC/PAMAM nanoparticles. *European Polymer Journal, 139*, 109992.
90. Liu, Y., Yu, S., Gu, X., Cao, R., & Cui, S. (2019). Tissue-engineered nerve grafts using a scaffold-independent and injectable drug delivery system: A novel design with translational advantages. *Journal of Neural Engineering, 16*(3), 036030.
91. Ren, Y., Zhao, X., Liang, X., Ma, P. X., & Guo, B. (2017). Injectable hydrogel based on quaternized chitosan, gelatin and dopamine as localized drug delivery system to treat Parkinson's disease. *International Journal of Biological Macromolecules, 105*, 1079–1087.
92. Wang, L., Deng, F., Wang, W., Li, A., Lu, C., Chen, H., & Li, L. (2018). Construction of injectable self-healing macroporous hydrogels via a template-free method for tissue engineering and drug delivery. *ACS Applied Materials & Interfaces, 10*(43), 36721–36732.
93. Corcione, C. E., Gervaso, F., Scalera, F., Padmanabhan, S. K., Madaghiele, M., Montagna, F., & Maffezzoli, A. (2019). Highly loaded hydroxyapatite microsphere/PLA porous scaffolds obtained by fused deposition modelling. *Ceramics International, 45*(2), 2803–2810.
94. Obayemi, J. D., Jusu, S. M., Salifu, A. A., Ghahremani, S., Tadesse, M., Uzonwanne, V. O., & Soboyejo, W. O. (2020). Degradable porous drug-loaded polymer scaffolds for localized cancer drug delivery and breast cell/tissue growth. *Materials Science and Engineering: C, 112*, 110794.
95. Turtoi, M., Anghelache, M., Bucatariu, S. M., Deleanu, M., Voicu, G., Safciuc, F., & Calin, M. (2021). A novel platform for drug testing: Biomimetic three-dimensional hyaluronic acid-based scaffold seeded with human hepatocarcinoma cells. *International Journal of Biological Macromolecules, 185*, 604–619.
96. Yang, Y., Qiao, X., Huang, R., Chen, H., Shi, X., Wang, J., & Tan, Z. (2020). E-jet 3D printed drug delivery implants to inhibit growth and metastasis of orthotopic breast cancer. *Biomaterials, 230*, 119618.

97. Bode, C., Kranz, H., Fivez, A., Siepmann, F., & Siepmann, J. (2019). Often neglected: PLGA/PLA swelling orchestrates drug release: HME implants. *Journal of Controlled Release, 306*, 97–107.
98. Nedunchezian, S., Banerjee, P., Lee, C. Y., Lee, S. S., Lin, C. W., Wu, C. W., & Wang, C. K. (2021). Generating adipose stem cell-laden hyaluronic acid-based scaffolds using 3D bioprinting via the double crosslinked strategy for chondrogenesis. *Materials Science and Engineering: C, 124*, 112072.
99. Yang, C., Blum, N. T., Lin, J., Qu, J., & Huang, P. (2020). Biomaterial scaffold-based local drug delivery systems for cancer immunotherapy. *Science Bulletin, 65*(17), 1489–1504.
100. Hum, J., & Boccaccini, A. R. (2018). Collagen as coating material for 45S5 bioactive glass-based scaffolds for bone tissue engineering. *International Journal of Molecular Sciences, 19*(6), 1807.
101. Remaggi, G., Catanzano, O., Quaglia, F., & Elviri, L. (2022). Alginate Self-Crosslinking Ink for 3D Extrusion-Based Cryoprinting and Application for Epirubicin-HCl Delivery on MCF-7 Cells. *Molecules, 27*(3), 882.
102. Faccendini, A., Vigani, B., Rossi, S., Sandri, G., Bonferoni, M. C., Caramella, C. M., & Ferrari, F. (2017). Nanofiber scaffolds as drug delivery systems to bridge spinal cord injury. *Pharmaceuticals, 10*(3), 63.
103. Huang, Y., Cao, L., Parakhonskiy, B. V., & Skirtach, A. G. (2022). Hard, soft, and hard-and-soft drug delivery carriers based on CaCO3 and alginate biomaterials: Synthesis, properties, pharmaceutical applications. *Pharmaceutics, 14*(5), 909.
104. Mertz, D., Harlepp, S., Goetz, J., Bégin, D., Schlatter, G., Bégin-Colin, S., & Hébraud, A. (2020). Nanocomposite polymer scaffolds responding under external stimuli for drug delivery and tissue engineering applications. *Advanced Therapeutics, 3*(2), 1900143.
105. Ilgin, P., Ozay, H., & Ozay, O. (2020). Synthesis and characterization of pH responsive alginate based-hydrogels as oral drug delivery carrier. *Journal of Polymer Research, 27*, 1–11.
106. Choi, K. Y., Han, H. S., Lee, E. S., Shin, J. M., Almquist, B. D., Lee, D. S., & Park, J. H. (2019). Hyaluronic acid–based activatable nanomaterials for stimuli-responsive imaging and therapeutics: Beyond CD44-mediated drug delivery. *Advanced Materials, 31*(34), 1803549.
107. Du, L., Yang, S., Li, W., Li, H., Feng, S., Zeng, R., & Tu, M. (2017). Scaffold composed of porous vancomycin-loaded poly (lactide-co-glycolide) microspheres: A controlled-release drug delivery system with shape-memory effect. *Materials Science and Engineering: C, 78*, 1172–1178.

CHAPTER 3

Functional Nanomaterials and their Applications in Biomedicine

NIPUN JAIN,[1] RANJIT BARUA,[2] and SUDIPTO DATTA[1]

[1]*Department of Materials Engineering, Indian Institute of Science, C.V. Raman Avenue, Bangalore, Karnataka, India*

[2]*Indian Institute of Engineering Science and Technology, Howrah, West Bengal, India*

ABSTRACT

Nanomaterials, which are materials having units bearing size between 1 and 100 nanometers, have lately become the subject of much interest as they are known to hold a lot of promise in fields such as pharmacy and biomedicine due to their unique physicochemical properties attributed to their elevated surface area and size. The engineering of the nanostructures, by adapting right surface or bulk modification, makes them multipurpose and open up new avenues in the biomedical applications like biosensing, drug delivery, imaging, medical implantation, carcinogenic treatment, and tissue engineering. This chapter focuses on the current state of developments in functionalization of nanomaterials for use in Biomedical fields. An overview of the classification of the nanomaterials and the methods of surface functionalization is presented. Further, the application of nanomaterial in diagnostic imaging, drug/gene delivery, tissue engineering and regeneration, cancer therapy, and implantology is discussed. Lastly, another section that gives conclusions and future perspectives is presented.

Bioabsorbable Polymers for Drug Carriers and Fixation Devices. Arbind Prasad and Sougata Jana (Eds.)

3.1 INTRODUCTION

Recently, nanomaterials have received quite a bit of recognition due to their unusual physical and chemical characteristics caused by their large surface area and small dimensions. Thus, they offer plenty of applications for use in various fields, especially in biomedicine, cancer therapy, [1] targeted delivery of pharmaceutical agents, [2] regenerative medicine, [3] organ mimic implants, [4] imaging, [5], etc. Additionally, numerous nanomaterial designs, such as in the form of plates, tubes, particles, and wires, possess particular qualities that offer a wide range of potential biological applications [6]. However, it is necessary to evaluate their future cytotoxic effects, which can be controlled by the structural characteristics and chemical composition. [7] Additionally, the colloidal stability of the nanomaterials must be preserved within physiological settings, preferably over a broad pH scale. It is crucial to consider these factors to fulfill the specific requirements of nanomaterials. Their interactions with biological molecules must be governed to change and functionalize the nanomaterial surface. The creation, manipulation, and targeted deployment of functionalized nanoparticles (FNP) present an innovative and intriguing potential for the fabrication of multifunctional biological systems [9]. Likewise, specific functional groups make the nanoparticles compatible with one another and prevent aggregation in later phases. As a result, FNPs have improved pharmacokinetic properties *in vivo* and can travel more effectively following systemic administration. FNPs can penetrate the tissues easily by using fine capillaries and gaps in the epithelial covering, thus delivering the agent of choice to the desired site [10]. Furthermore, FNPs' excellent physicochemical properties, such as dissolution, diffusion, immunogenicity, and targeted delivery with minimal loss to their surroundings, are enhanced due to their very small size [11]. Different approaches can be used to develop and modify the interface. These are labeled as either replacement, non-covalent, or covalent interactions according to the fundamental idea of the major linkage being used [12]. The replacement technique includes ligand addition and exchange between molecules and nanoparticles to modify the interface [13]. Weak non-covalent forces like electrostatic attraction for ionic molecules, Van der Waals forces, or more complicated interactions like host-guest [14]. For the goal of biomedical applications, covalent interaction-based approaches have been more common. This gives the nanoparticles more functionality as it directly changes the exterior environment [15]. Despite the reports of several studies on nanoparticle manufacturing, their interface modification for use in medicine and nanotechnology is not well reported [1, 2, 16].

This article aims to summarize and review various functionalization techniques categorized by functional groupings and specific benefits. On top of that, the versatility of these functionalized compounds with particular uses will be covered through specific examples. Different NP functionalization strategies have been devised, and their varied applications have garnered much attention. NPs have undergone extensive research due to their advantageous qualities, such as controlled biodegradation and biological compatibility in physiological pathways, vast availability, suitability for targeted treatment, and a broad spectrum of possible synthesis processes. The present article provides fresh perspectives on NP modification, emphasizing its potential cytotoxicity and curative, diagnostic, targeted agent delivery, and tissue engineering purposes.

3.2 CHARACTERISTICS OF FUNCTIONALIZED NANOMATERIALS IN PHARMACEUTICS

NPs are used in diverse medical applications involving imaging, drug delivery, gene therapy, molecular compound monitoring, hyperthermia, magnetic resonance imaging, and emission tomography [17]. It must be understood that biomolecular linkages rely largely on the nanoparticle surface's chemical constitution. As a result, numerous target molecular ligands, consisting of peptides [18], aptamers [19], and antibodies [20], have been developed that can be easily placed on the nanoparticle surface. Such targeted moiety components can enable the incorporation and uptake of nanoparticles into various tissues governed by specific receptor interactions. The NP's surface can be modified with specific ligands, making it easier to target membrane-surface receptors actively. This increases cellular internalization and selective absorption [21]. Finding novel biomarkers and their suitable ligands for targeted delivery is of special interest to investigators worldwide. For imaging purposes, the signal of nanoparticles can be increased by binding to analytes and biomarkers, thus making detection simpler. Functionalization occurs when the nanoparticle's surface is embellished with "biologically responsive cues" that engage the cell to trigger a particular response [22]. Various ligands have been found that can attach to nanoparticle surfaces, making it possible to use them for intracellular delivery, disease diagnosis, biomolecule, and cell sensing. Due to the simplicity of such a technique, researchers can readily create the appropriate functionalities for use in the clinic [23]. Small-sized ligands are frequently chosen for functionalizing purposes because their moieties make attaching to surfaces covalently straightforward. Polymeric particles, capsules, micelles, dendrimers, liposomes, nanospheres, and nanogels are just a few examples of the various surface-modified NPs that have been created as multipurpose agents for use in pharmaceutical applications [24]. Both drug adsorption at the surface and drug encapsulation are possible, and they can also make nanoparticles biocompatible and shield them from aggregation [25]. Enhancing the nanoparticle's physical, chemical, and mechanical properties leads to synergistic effects [26]. For instance, Hirayama et al. characterized the loading and discharge of the malarial drug quinine using silica nanoparticles. It improves drug adsorption capacity by interacting with NPs and silane agents [27]. A barrier such as polymers (small hydrodynamic radius) is used to avoid a head-on connection between the particle core and cell surface receptors. Therefore, when imparting features of macromolecular systems, coated polymers surpass small molecule interactions. Coating with polymers like polyethylene glycol (PEG) enhances the permeability and retention (EPR) impact, thus enabling passive tumor targeting. This theory explains why circulating particles tend to concentrate significantly more in tumor tissues than in normal ones. PEG coating prolongs circulation time, encourages tumor tissue absorption, and reduces serum protein adsorption [28]. Certain features of biomolecule-functionalized nanoparticles, such as material distribution and low toxicity, are impractical to attain by utilizing artificial compounds. The earliest nanotechnology examples involve creating oligonucleotide-AuNP conjugates by synthesizing gold-thiol linkages [28]. In order to create a hydrophilic and stable coating, Kleinfeldt and coworkers [29] stacked cationic and anionic layers of polyallylamine and acrylic acid. Makvandi et al. [30] examined the advantages of different polymer functionalization groups (glycan clusters, dendrimers, and polymers) and various nanomaterials in water treatment, food containers, textiles, and pharmaceutical treatments. Despite significant advancements in nanotechnology and its medicinal applications, various challenges have been identified. By manipulating FNPs, new paths are opened for developing undiscovered multipurpose equipment for medicinal and nanobiotechnology applications [31]. Since the late 1980s, there has been much curiosity about utilizing nano-sized particles [32]. With the help of multiple examples, different techniques for nanoparticle functionalization are explained below. A recent review [33] discussed the uses of functionalized gold nanoparticles in the biomedical field. This goal was accomplished by carefully examining the manufacturing process, thus understanding AuNP structure pathways and utilizing their applications in oncology, electrochemistry, and biology. Multi-functionalization allows for the simultaneous achievement of multiple qualities. Multifunctional AuNPs have been shown to be useful in transporting cancer medications and antibiotics by enhancing the effects of photothermal therapy [34]. Figure 3.1 highlights ways polymers might functionalize gold nanoparticles as sensing materials [35].

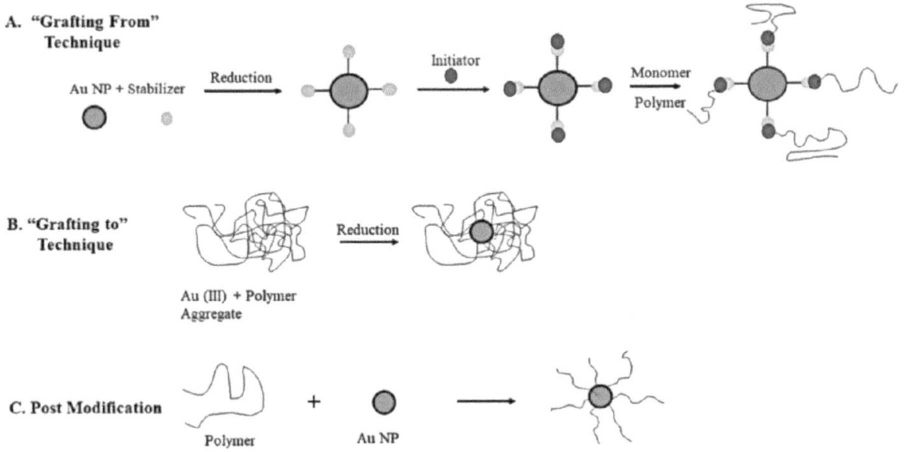

FIGURE 3.1 AuNPs functionalization (a); "grafting to;" (b) "post modification;" and (c) techniques.

Source: Adapted from Ref. [35, 60]

The covalent binding of polymeric fragments to the nanoparticle surface can be executed using the "grafting to/grafting from" approach. The foremost approach is to create a reformed polymer capable of interacting with functional groups on the nanoparticle surface. Because of the poor reactions and high steric hindrance, this approach has the drawback of restricting the quantity of polymer that may be grafted. This approach has the benefits of being simple (one-pot synthesis) and having access to various polymers [36]. In the "grafting from" approach, monomer-based polymerization is used to build the polymer from the nanoparticle surface. This strategy works well because it enables the insertion of polymer fragments, thus creating high-density compounds, and provides control over the molecular weight of the formed species. The post-modification strategy is majorly popular and a straightforward technique for creating gold nanocomposites since merging the two as-prepared materials can eliminate undesirable elements. Low polymer introduction effectiveness caused by conjugated polymers' steric barriers and unintentional adsorption via the polymers' functional groups are the downsides of this strategy. For example, covalently bound nanocomposites are created when polymers containing SH-terminated groups are combined with AuNPs. Additionally, using carbodiimide as a coupling agent, the gold nanoparticle's surface was modified with anionic and cationic layers of polyacrylic acid and allylamine. This was accomplished by forming an amide connection between the amine groups of papain and the carboxyl groups of altered nanoparticles. Bioanalysis and biopharmaceutical analysis have both used the produced molecule [37]. Carbon nanotubes (CNTs) provide a unique mixture of mechanical and electrical qualities and have encouraged research into using them in various biomedical applications [38]. They are an allotropic form of carbon that Iijima originally described in 1991. They were created in various styles, including chemical vapor deposition (CVD), laser ablation, and electric arc discharge [39]. They may be considered a single layer of graphene that has been rolled up and is occasionally sealed off at the ends. An important characteristic that affects a CNT's numerous qualities is the number of concentric walls that make up the structure. Since more imperfections increase the number of layers, changing and functionalizing them is easier, usually at the expense of losing some of their physical attributes. CNT uses in the biomedical field present some difficulties that must be overcome. A major issue is based on safety concerns, which result in the continuous use of highly pure tubes to prevent the discharge of harmful molecules. However, large-scale use of these is practically impossible because of their high cost, thus requiring a sacrifice of quality for quantity. The ability to obtain excellent CNT dispersions in solvents and aqueous solutions is another challenge. CNTs are extremely hydrophobic, making them challenging to stabilize in suspension and disseminate in a solvent. They can be stabilized by adding a dispersion agent, surfactant, or through surface functionalization [40]. In electrochemical sensors, several scientists have considered utilizing functionalized CNTs [41]. Additionally, they can serve as contrasting mediators in certain imaging techniques [42]. When functionalized with different markers, they can accurately pinpoint the location and presence of specific cells. CNT-based cancer treatments have also been described [43]. For instance, tumor clearance and improved survival were achieved in mice by injecting MWCNT at the tumor site accompanied by laser treatment [43a]. After that, Wang et al. [43b] delineated how the intravenous delivery of SWCNT produced an immunological response and showed a synergistic effect with cytotoxic killing and photothermal treatment, significantly eradicating the persistent lesions. It has also been noted that combining imaging techniques with PTT can expedite the discovery of linked lymph nodes and treat main tumors [43c]. As photothermal conversion has recently improved, MWCNT/AuNS hybrids have made it possible to shorten the duration of laser stimulation during therapy [43d]. B16-F10 melanoma cells were cultivated with various concentrations of MWCNTs/AuNS for 24 hours to examine the blended material's potential for increased removal of cancer cells. The cells were then exposed to various laser exposure periods and power densities, and the ideal parameters were determined. Compared to the AuNSs alone, the hybrids had higher photothermal efficiency, which caused most of the cancer cells to separate from substrates. Additionally, utilizing molecular delivery and PTT widens the scope of cancer treatment. However, the tissue's laser penetration depth limits CNT-assisted PTT, and it must still demonstrate its effectiveness for thicker samples. Because of its biocompatibility and minimal inflammatory reactions, hydrogels are frequently used in the biomedical industry. Tissue engineering has recently utilized CNT-based hydrogels [44]. The mechanical and electrical conductivity are improved when CNTs are added to these gels. Their orientation within the hydrogel may be changed, allowing for precise adjustment of the tailored scaffolds' features. For example, adding CNTs to gelatin methacrylate (GelMA) hydrogels efficiently strengthens them without compromising their porosity or cell proliferation [44a]; Figure 3.2 shows various NPs surface-modified by molecules/ligands.

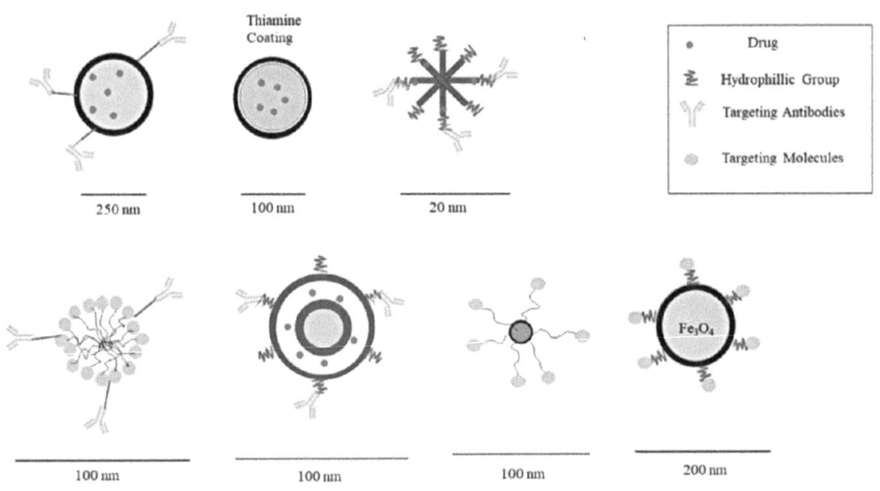

FIGURE 3.2 Various NPs surface-modified by molecules/ligands for active directing [35, 60].
Source: Adapted from Ref. [35, 60]

3.3 CYTOTOXIC EFFECTS OF FUNCTIONALIZED NANOMATERIALS

Several factors, such as size, shape, constituents, concentration, crystallinity, and chemical groups on the surface, substantially influence nanoparticle cytotoxicity and ingestion [45]. The chemical composition can cause oxidative stress and regulate its binding with cells, cellular ingestion, and intracellular transport. For example, CNTs cause greater lung damage than solid carbon or silica NPs, but TiO_2 and Fe_2O_3 are thought to be less poisonous than asbestos. Silver nanoparticles are more virulent than asbestos [45]. The crystalline structure also governs the degree of toxicity. While anatase NPs do not cause any toxic effect, rutile particles (200 nm) produce oxidative stress without UV light [46]. The NP size is another component that significantly affects toxicity. Smaller particles can access cells through phagocytosis, pinocytosis, and endocytosis because they can easily pass the physiological barriers [45c]. Weak, non-covalent interactions control how well the particles can enter. NPs with large surface areas aggregate in liquids, bind with different component molecules, and induce oxidative stress [45a]. Moreover, the shape (aspect ratio) influences cellular ingestion effectiveness and impacts cell viability [45b]. Additionally, surface functionalization influences how they are distributed and regulated in living cells. For example, functionalizing Au nanoparticles is essential for enhancing absorption and delivery potential, as well as maximizing their delivery within the body. The prospective toxic reactions of various polymeric coatings, such as polyethylene glycol (PEG) and polyethyleneimine (PEI), have been studied. Their toxicity and the impact of oxidative factors on DNA damage have also been examined [45c]. All nanoparticles considerably raised intracellular ROS levels, but neither AuNPs nor AuNPs/PEG changed the oxidant/antioxidant parameters.

3.4 APPLICATIONS OF FUNCTIONAL NANOMATERIALS IN BIOMEDICINE

Nanotechnology has updated and impacted the fields of diagnostic medicine, healthcare services, vaccinations, and immunization procedures [46]. Biological agents are combined with different NPs through chemical and physical functionalization. There are various categories into which the biomedical uses of NPs can be divided, which are discussed briefly in the following subsections.

3.4.1 DIAGNOSTIC APPLICATIONS

Magnetic resonance imaging and optical coherence tomography are the two most common techniques that frequently include nanomaterials. They are increasingly necessary to create high-resolution, high-contrast pictures for precision diagnoses and can provide pertinent data in preclinical and clinical settings. Semiconductor nanocrystals called QDs are frequently used in optics [47]. Lead-based QDs have been utilized to noninvasively scan animals with septic encephalopathy, indicating that these nanomaterials may be employed to image various circulatory systems [47a]. Magnetic hybrid nanomaterials (MHNs), on the other hand, are nanoparticles that incorporate magnetic components. These are biocompatible and may be used as contrast mediums for multimodal imaging probes, which have recently sparked much attention [47b]. They combine magnetic properties with useful components like noble metals to exhibit superparamagnetism and novel properties that can be applied in positron emission tomography, single-photon emission computed tomography, computed tomography contrast modalities, magnetic resonance imaging, and other imaging techniques [47c]. The synergistic effects of combining several nanomaterials make higher sensitivity and spatial resolution possible. Magnetic nanoparticles called porous iron oxide nano agents (PIONs) can be used for photoacoustic imaging (PAI). A magnetic field can direct them toward cancer tissues and be used as a foundation for imaging when combined with a plasmid vector.

3.4.2 THERAPEUTIC APPLICATIONS

Due to their beneficial therapeutic qualities, functionalized nanomaterials such as up- and down-conversion lanthanide NPs, AuNPs, QDs, and superparamagnetic iron oxide nanoparticles (SPIONs) have revolutionized the biomedical industry in recent years [48]. They have been utilized to improve previously effective illness therapeutic techniques. They can stimulate the expansion of finer strategies to improve therapies for serious human diseases like cancer and associated disorders. SPIONs can make photodynamic therapy drugs and associated tumor-specific ligands under their remarkable reactivity to the applied magnetic field in photodynamic therapy, where drug administration should be avoided to prevent any harm to surrounding active cells. Additionally, functionalization can enhance their PDT-related qualities [48a]. For instance, under the action of magnetic fields, water-soluble surface-capped SPIONs have increased heat transfer efficiency, eliminating tumors. It has been observed that a variety of biocompatible polymers, including dextran, PEG, PVP, dendrimers, proteins, and functionalized gold nanoparticles, may stabilize SPIONs in an aqueous solution [48c]. The most common methods for changing a SPION's surface are ligand exchange or directly providing a coating agent after creation in the latter, a hydrophobic ligand from the surface is switched out for a hydrophilic ligand. PDT's applicability is limited by its light-related toxicity. A focused platform has been created that includes SPIONS, PC4, a cancer-targeting ligand, and a second-generation PDT medication to reduce toxicity [48b]. Fibronectin-mimetic peptide (Fmp) was initially coupled with carboxyl-functionalized SPIONs. Then, to create Fmp-IO-Pc4, the PDT drug PC4 was incorporated within the ligand-bonded SPIONs. More effectively than free Pc4, IO-Pc4 and Fmp-IO-Pc4 decreased the dimensions of xenograft tumors. As a result, they can lower PDT medication dosage and improve therapy effectiveness. The directed IO-Pc4 NPs have excellent power to function as a PDT medication and an MRI agent in the clinic.

3.4.3 DRUG DELIVERY APPROACHES USING FUNCTIONALIZED NANOPARTICLES

The capability to insert medicines or genetic material such as plasmid DNA and siRNA with functionalized nanoparticles that generate no negative side effects has ushered in a new age of treatments for selective drug or gene delivery to cells [49]. It is envisaged that applying nanoengineering to treat diseases minimizes systemic adverse reactions. Innovative treatments for age-related neurodegenerative illnesses, enhanced controlled release of drugs, and sustainable delivery in solid tumors can be created using nanotechnology. People have considered using CNTs as unusual delivery transporters for therapeutics as they possess unique properties, such as high aspect ratio, improved conductivity, toughness, and cellular compatibility [49a]. Different mechanisms are used by various cell types to absorb CNTs. Therapeutics targeting inflammation, dexamethasone steroids for osteogenesis, gemcitabine, methotrexate, docetaxel, paclitaxel, and other anticancer compounds can be efficiently delivered *via* CNTs. Furthermore, the straightforward functionalized surfaces of these carbon nanotubes have promoted their application for the delivery of genes with plasmid DNA (pDNA), miRNA, and siRNA for various diseases. The primary objectives of CNT functionalization are to support their biocompatibility and enhance their physical properties, such as solubility and dispersibility. They accumulate and disperse poorly throughout the body, increasing their cytotoxicity [49b]. Their surfaces can be functionalized to increase drug delivery efficiency while reducing cytotoxicity [49c]. SWCNTs and human serum albumin (HSA) have been linked to facilitate the intracellular transport of PTX [50], enhancing PTX's ability to fight cancer cells. When connected to lipids and naturally occurring dendrimers made of amino acids, SWCNTs are used for effective nucleic acid transport [51]. Additionally, SWNTs' functional groups on the surface carry away siRNA for gene-based therapy. When subjected to negatively charged siRNA, cationic SWNTs with noncovalently functionalized 1,2-dioleoyl-3-trimethylammonium-propane dramatically decreased the proliferation of prostate cancer [52]. Although there may be other problems, CNT-based toxicity and its implications for the environment are currently the most important, primarily due to their non-biodegradable nature [53].

3.4.4 FUNCTIONALIZED NANOMATERIALS USE IN REGENERATIVE MEDICINE

Regenerative therapy attempts to reconstruct damaged tissues injured by a certain disease, trauma, or congenital disability instead of the conventional approach, which primarily aims to cure the symptoms. Techniques such as tissue engineering, cellular therapy, medical equipment, and synthetic organs accomplish these goals [54]. Collagen and inorganic hydroxyapatite comprise bone with a pecking order from nanometers to micrometers. Nanomaterials present some unique strategies for bone regeneration, considering the severe limitations of conventional therapy. Nanostructured scaffolds govern cell division, transport, and differentiation, leading to active tissue creation. They provide a more practical architectural foundation for the cells, similar to native bone structures. Several groups [55] have attempted to imitate the inherent composite design of bone by manipulating the mechanical characteristics (stiffness, strength, and toughness). This is achieved by constructing structures in the form of nanoparticles or nanofibers within the polymer scaffolds. For example, blends of chitosan and hydroxyapatite assist the growth of mesenchymal stem cells. The genetic basis of these stem cells' proliferation has been studied *in vitro* [55a]. Additionally, some other polymeric substances like PEG, PCL, and PLGA can be combined with nanohydroxyapatite to improve the effects on bone regeneration and repair [56]. The following summarizes some representative functionalized nanomaterials used in regenerative medicine. Overall, regenerating or restoring injured tissue depends on using nanomaterials in tissue engineering. Researchers have been employing various combinations of nanomaterials to create new biomaterials during the past few years. These nanoparticles are employed as substitutes in tissue engineering or repair of malfunctioning organs. Care must be taken to consider factors like the sensitivity of implanted materials, the resulting immunological reactions, the possibility of toxic effects, the effect on reproduction, the effect on fetal growth, etc.

3.4.5 FUNCTIONALIZED NANOMATERIALS USED IN CANCER TREATMENT

Multifunctional nanoparticles are developed for directing cancer treatment by adjusting physiochemical characteristics. These must be transported to the designated site and triggered by stimuli for accurate therapy. Stimuli-responsive nanomaterials can improve and achieve beneficial tumor targeting by using smart nanosystems that respond to internal and external stimuli such as a change in pH, enzyme concentration, redox potential, and ROS. These external stimuli include light, magnetic fields, ultrasound, and electric fields. H^+ ion concentration change is frequently employed, especially those that utilize either the slightly acidic (endosomal and lysosomal pH = 5.5–6.0) or the slightly alkaline extracellular environment (pH 6.8) of solid tumor tissue. Charge-charge interactions led to the development of negatively charged NPs made of positively charged DOX and HA polypyrrole (PPy) [57]. After internalization by cancer cells, HA loses some of the negative charges, and these interactions with protons change the acidic pH environment. This causes the medicines to be released from the NPs and their optical characteristics to turn on spontaneously. Through numerous interactions with indomethacin and DTX, PEI conjugated by PEG through Schiff base (PEG-s-PEI) creates pH-based nanoassembly structures [58]. They were more pH-sensitive at the extracellular pH of the tumor microenvironment than in normal tissues, which allowed them to circulate longer in the blood but be heavily phagocytosed by tumor cells. Due to the EPR effect, functionalized nanoparticles cause selective infiltration in the tumor-growing region. In contrast to normal tissue, tumors have different chemicals that aid in increased targeting, such as VEGF and basic FGF. They also have a more permeable vascular system and a poorly defined lymphatic system. NPs are used in cancer immunotherapies and can monitor important immune cells during metastasis.

3.5 CONCLUSION

The evolution of functionalized nanoparticles for imaging, regenerative medicine, drug delivery, and cancer therapy has been examined extensively. Several nanoparticles, both organic (CNTs, graphene, and QDs) and inorganic (silica, Fe_3O_4, TiO_2, ZnO), have been made possible by the special properties exhibited by them, such as miniature size, increased surface area, compliant design, remarkable optical/mechanical properties, high cellular compatibility, and facile functionalized surfaces. According to preliminary clinical studies, due to certain characteristics (focused targeting in cancer and easy internalization), nanoparticles with particular surface components resulted in better potency and minimal toxicity. Because of their prolonged body retention times, the principal drawback of functionalized nanoparticles when used in clinical trials is their potential for adverse side effects. For further clinical translation, it is crucial to quantitatively analyze the harmful impacts of the surface-modified nanoparticles, considering factors like their localization in various organs and their metabolic pathways. Firstly, various animal models should be used to assess their biodistribution and toxicity. If the outcomes are positive, clinical studies should be conducted to analyze them further. The creation of degradable nanoparticles will also benefit future formal applications. Small nano-sized particles can be quickly eliminated from the body through urine. Their biodegradability is yet another important issue. Some inorganic nanoparticles, such as MnO_2, $CaCO_3$, $Ca_3(PO_4)_2$, and transition-metal-based salts, can be degraded into effective ions [59]. Functional nanoparticles can have their biodegradability customized by being doped with inorganic elements or by adding biodegradable polymers. However, much work still needs to be done to escalate the aggregation of desired nanoparticles in the damaged organs. The local injection may substitute systemic medication administration for some conditions. In conclusion, functional nanomaterials have enormous promise for enhancing how different diseases are treated. However, the possibility of their adverse effects has prevented their rational application. Most of the nanoparticles discussed in this article are still in the early stages. Thus, additional study is required to determine their chronic exposure and rate of biodegradation. As a result, the FDA has only cleared a small number of nanomaterial-based nanomedicines for marketing.

KEYWORDS

- **biodegradation**
- **cellular compatibility**
- **chronic exposure**
- **immune cells**
- **inorganic nanoparticles**
- **nanomaterials**
- **nanomedicines**
- **nanoparticles**

REFERENCES

1. (a) Hong, E. J., Choi, D. G., & Shim, M. S. (2016). *Acta Pharmaceutica Sinica B, 6*, 297–307. doi: 10.1016/j.apsb.2016.02.001. (b) Rahdar, A., Hajinezhad, M. R., Hamishekar, H., Ghamkhari, A., & Kyzas, G. Z. (2021). *Polymer Bulletin, 78*, 4877–4898. doi: 10.1007/s00289-021-03668-8.
2. (a) Patra, J. K., Das, G., Fraceto, L. F., Campos, E. V. R., Rodriguez-Torres, M. del P., Acosta-Torres, L. S., & Sharma, S. (2018). *Journal of Nanobiotechnology, 16*, 1–33. doi: 10.1186/s12951-018-0396-8. (b) Bilal, M., Qindeel, M., Raza, A., Mehmood, S., & Rahdar, A. (2021). *Journal of Drug Delivery Science and Technology, 66*, 102916. doi: 10.1016/j.jddst.2021.102916. (c) Er, S., Laraib, U., Arshad, R., Sargazi, S., Rahdar, A., Pandey, S., & Díez-Pascual, A. M. (2021). *Nanomaterials, 11*, 3002. doi: 10.3390/nano11113002.
3. (a) Díez-Pascual, A. M., & Diez-Vicente, A. L. (2016). *ACS Applied Materials & Interfaces, 8*, 17902–17914. doi: 10.1021/acsami.6b04909. (b) Díez-Pascual, A. M., & Diez-Vicente, A. L. (2014). *ACS Applied Materials & Interfaces, 6*, 17277–17288. doi: 10.1021/am5043285.
4. (a) Giubilato, E., Cazzagon, V., Amorim, M. J., Blosi, M., Bouillard, J., Bouwmeester, H., & Fadeel, B. (2020). *Materials, 13*, 4532. doi: 10.3390/ma13104532. (b) Díez-Pascual, A. M., & Rahdar, A. (2022). *Nanomaterials, 12*, 949. doi: 10.3390/nano12060949.
5. Wang, G., Li, Z., Luo, X., Yue, R., Shen, Y., & Ma, N. (2018). *Nanoscale, 10*, 16508–16520. doi: 10.1039/C8NR04066H.

6. (a) Qiu, Z., & Tang, D. (2020). *Journal of Materials Chemistry B, 8*, 2541–2561. doi: 10.1039/C9TB02648A. (b) Shu, J., & Tang, D. (2017). *Chemistry–An Asian Journal, 12*, 2780–2789. doi: 10.1002/asia.201701197. (c) Lloyd, J. R., Byrne, J. M., & Coker, V. S. (2011). *Current Opinion in Biotechnology, 22*, 509–515. doi: 10.1016/j.copbio.2011.04.005. (d) Diez-Pascual, A. M. (2021). *Macromolecular, 1*, 173–176. doi: 10.1021/acs.macromol.1c00173.
7. Kobayashi, K., Wei, J., Iida, R., Ijiro, K., & Niikura, K. (2014). *Polymer Journal, 46*, 460–468. doi: 10.1038/pj.2014.37.
8. Sanità, G., Carrese, B., & Lamberti, A. (2020). *Frontiers in Molecular Biosciences, 7*, 587012. doi: 10.3389/fmolb.2020.587012.
9. Schultz, A. G., Boyle, D., Chamot, D., Ong, K. J., Wilkinson, K. J., McGeer, J. C., & Goss, G. G. (2014). *Environmental Chemistry, 11*, 207–226. doi: 10.1071/EN14035.
10. Zhou, Q., Lin, Y., Zhang, K., Li, M., & Tang, D. (2018). *Biosensors and Bioelectronics, 101*, 146–152. doi: 10.1016/j.bios.2017.10.038.
11. Sonju, J. J., Dahal, A., Singh, S. S., & Jois, S. D. (2021). *Journal of Controlled Release, 329*, 624–644. doi: 10.1016/j.jconrel.2020.11.041.
12. (a) Yu, Z., Gong, H., Xu, J., Li, Y., Zhen, Y., Liu, X., & Tang, D. (2022). *Analytical Chemistry, 94*, 3418–3426. doi: 10.1021/acs.analchem.1c04827. (b) Yu, Z., Xu, J., Gong, H., Li, Y., Li, L., Wei, Q., & Tang, D. (2022). *ACS Applied Materials & Interfaces, 14*, 5101–5111. doi: 10.1021/acsami.1c21656. (c) Huang, L., Zeng, Y., Liu, X., & Tang, D. (2021). *ACS Applied Materials & Interfaces, 13*, 46440–46450. doi: 10.1021/acsami.1c12217.
13. Li, H., Wang, Q., & Liang, G. (2021). *ACS Applied Nano Materials, 4*, 2621–2633. doi: 10.1021/acsanm.1c00095.
14. Krishnadevi, K., RatnaKumari, S., Prasanna, D., Prasanna, H. B. N., & Anuradha, V. (2022). *Journal of Colloid and Interface Science, 607*, 1776–1785. doi: 10.1016/j.jcis.2021.09.106.
15. (a) Mahmoudpour, M., Ding, S., Lyu, Z., Ebrahimi, G., Du, D., Dolatabadi, J. E. N., & Torbati, M. (2021). *Nano Today, 39*, 101177. doi: 10.1016/j.nantod.2021.101177. (b) Mahmoudpour, M., Karimzadeh, Z., Ebrahimi, G., Hasanzadeh, M., & Dolatabadi, J. E. N. (2021). *Critical Reviews in Analytical Chemistry*. doi: 10.1080/10408347.2021.1919987.
16. Theus, A. S., Ning, L., Jin, L., Roeder, R. K., Zhang, J., & Serpooshan, V. (2021). *Essays in Biochemistry, 65*, 429–439. doi: 10.1042/EBC20210040.
17. (a) Tang, D., Cui, Y., & Chen, G. (2013). *Analyst, 138*, 981–990. doi: 10.1039/C2AN36259B. (b) Pei, X., Zhang, B., Tang, J., Liu, B., Lai, W., & Tang, D. (2013). *Analytica Chimica Acta, 758*, 1–18. doi: 10.1016/j.aca.2012.10.018. (c) Su, J., & Tang, D. (2020). *Analytical Chemistry, 92*, 363–377. doi: 10.1021/acs.analchem.9b04518.
18. Rong, L., Qin, S. Y., Zhang, C., Cheng, Y. J., Feng, J., Wang, S. B., & Zhang, X. Z. (2018). *Materials Today Chemistry, 9*, 91–102. doi: 10.1016/j.mtchem.2018.06.004.
19. Xie, S., Ai, L., Cui, C., Fu, T., Cheng, X., Qu, F., & Tan, W. (2021). *ACS Applied Materials & Interfaces, 13*, 9542–9560. doi: 10.1021/acsami.0c20728.
20. Farahavar, G., Abolmaali, S. S., Gholijani, N., & Nejatollahi, F. (2019). *Biomaterials Science, 7*, 4000–4016. doi: 10.1039/C9BM00488H.
21. Azevedo, C., Macedo, M. H., & Sarmento, B. (2018). *Drug Discovery Today, 23*, 944–959. doi: 10.1016/j.drudis.2018.01.028.
22. Gravely, M., Safaee, M. M., & Roxbury, D. (2019). *Nano Letters, 19*, 6203–6212. doi: 10.1021/acs.nanolett.9b02398.

23. (a) Yu, Z., Gong, H., Li, Y., Xu, J., Zhang, Y., Zhen, Y., Liu, X., & Tang, D. (2021). *Analytical Chemistry, 93*, 13389–13397. doi: 10.1021/acs.analchem.1c02923. (b) Yu, Z., Cai, G., Liu, X., & Tang, D. (2021). *Analytical Chemistry, 93*, 2916–2925. doi: 10.1021/acs.analchem.0c05186. (c) Zeng, R., Wang, W., Chen, M., Wan, Q., Wang, C., Knopp, D., & Tang, D. (2021). *Nano Energy, 82*, 105711. doi: 10.1016/j.nanoen.2021.105711.
24. Muthu, M. S., & Sanjay, S. (2009). *Nanomedicine, 4*, 105–118. doi: 10.2217/nnm.08.14.
25. (a) Gole, B., Sanyal, U., Banerjee, R., & Mukherjee, P. S. (2016). *Inorganic Chemistry, 55*, 2345–2354. doi: 10.1021/acs.inorgchem.5b02870. (b) Rawat, D., Kumari, A., & Singh, R. R. (2022). *Functionalized Nanomaterials for Catalytic Application.* doi: 10.1002/9781119809036.ch13.
26. (a) Charoensri, K., Rodwihok, C., Wongratanaphisan, D., Ko, J. A., Chung, J. S., & Park, H. J. (2021). *Polymer, 13*, 425. doi: 10.3390/polym13030425. (b) Nemati, F., Rezaie, M., Tabesh, H., Eid, K. A. M., Xu, G., Ganjali, M. R., Hosseini, M., Karaman, C., Erk, N., & Show, P. L. (2022). *Environmental Research, 208*, 112685. doi: 10.1016/j.envres.2021.112685. (c) Díez-Pascual, A. M., & Diez-Vicente, A. L. (2014). *ACS Applied Materials & Interfaces, 6*, 10132–10145. doi: 10.1021/am501919a. (d) Díez-Pascual, A. M., & Diez-Vicente, A. L. (2014). *ACS Applied Materials & Interfaces, 6*, 17277–17288. doi: 10.1021/am5043285. (e) Díez-Pascual, A. M., & Diez-Vicente, A. L. (2015). *ACS Applied Materials & Interfaces, 7*, 5561–5573. doi: 10.1021/am507469b.
27. Hirayama, H., Amolegbe, M. A., Islam, M. S., Rahman, M. A., Goto, N., Sekine, Y., & Hayami, S. (2021). *Journal of Materials Chemistry, 9*, 5043–5046. doi: 10.1039/D1TB00642C.
28. Mout, R., Moyano, D. F., Rana, S., & Rotello, V. M. (2012). *Chemical Society Reviews, 41*, 2539–2544. doi: 10.1039/C2CS15362B.
29. Kleinfeldt, L., Gädke, J., Biedendieck, R., Krull, R., & Garnweitner, G. (2019). *ACS Omega, 4*, 16300–16308. doi: 10.1021/acsomega.9b02000.
30. Makvandi, P., Wang, C. Y., Zare, E. N., Borzacchiello, A., Niu, L. N., & Tay, F. R. (2020). *Advanced Functional Materials, 30*, 1910021. doi: 10.1002/adfm.201910021.
31. (a) Huang, L., Chen, J., Yu, Z., & Tang, D. (2020). *Anal. Chem., 92*, 2809–2814. https://doi.org/10.1021/acs.analchem.9b04658. (b) Zhang, K., Lv, S., Zhou, Q., & Tang, D. (2020). *Sens. Actuators B Chem., 307*, 127631. https://doi.org/10.1016/j.snb.2019.127631. (c) Lv, S., Zhang, K., Lv, S., Zhu, L., & Tang, D. (2020). *Anal. Chem., 92*, 1470–1476. https://doi.org/10.1021/acs.analchem.9b03743.
32. Li, X., Wei, J., Aifantis, K. E., Fan, Y., Feng, Q., Cui, F. Z., & Watari, F. (2016). *J. Biomed. Mater. Res. Part A, 104,* 1285–1296. https://doi.org/10.1002/jbm.a.35623.
33. Nejati, K., Dadashpour, M., Gharibi, T., Mellatyar, H., & Akbarzadeh, A. (2022). *J. Cluster Sci., 33*, 1–16. https://doi.org/10.1007/s10876-022-02256-6.
34. Tiwari, P. M., Vig, K., Dennis, V. A., & Singh, S. R. (2011). *Nanomaterials, 1*, 31–63. https://doi.org/10.3390/nano1010031.
35. Nobuo, U. (2010). *Int. J. Japan Soc. Anal. Chem., 26*, 1219–1228. https://doi.org/10.2116/analsci.26.1219.
36. (a) Díez-Pascual, A. M. (2021). *Polymer, 13*, 2978. https://doi.org/10.3390/polym13182978. (b) Díez-Pascual, A. M. (2021). *Macromol, 1*, 64–83. https://doi.org/10.3390/macromol1010007. (c) Díez-Pascual, A. M. (2021). *Int. J. Mol. Sci., 22*, 7726. https://doi.org/10.3390/ijms22147726.
37. Liu, S., Höldrich, M., Sievers-Engler, A., Horak, M., & Lämmerhofer, M. (2017). *Anal. Chim. Acta, 963*, 33–43. https://doi.org/10.1016/j.aca.2017.01.036.

38. (a) Simon, J., Flahaut, E., & Golzio, M. (2019). *Materials, 12*, 624. https://doi.org/10.3390/ma12040624. (b) Díez-Pascual, A. M. (2021). *Int. J. Mol. Sci., 22*, 10511. https://doi.org/10.3390/ijms222010511. (c) Naffakh, M., Díez-Pascual, A. M., & Gómez-Fatou, M. A. (2011). *J. Mater. Chem., 21*, 7425–7430. https://doi.org/10.1039/c1jm10483a.
39. (a) Díez-Pascual, A. M., Martínez, G., González-Domínguez, J. M., Ansón, A., Martínez, M. T., & Gómez, M. A. (2010). *J. Mater. Chem., 20*, 8285–8292. https://doi.org/10.1039/c0jm01267j. (b) Díez-Pascual, A. M. (2019). *Int. J. Mol. Sci., 20*, 2321. https://doi.org/10.3390/ijms20102321.
40. (a) Díez-Pascual, A. M. (2012). Grafting of an aminated poly (phenylene sulphide) derivative to functionalized single-walled carbon nanotubes. *Carbon, 50*, 857–868. https://doi.org/10.1016/j.carbon.2011.09.006. (b) González-Domínguez, J. M., Castell, P., Bespin-Gascon, S., Anson-Casaos, A., Díez-Pascual, A. M., Gómez-Fatou, M. A., Benito, A., Maser, W. K., & Martínez, M. T. (2012). *J. Mater. Chem., 22*, 21285–21297. https://doi.org/10.1039/c2jm34153b.
41. (a) Zhang, X., Xu, Y., & Ye, B. (2018). *J. Alloys Compd., 767*, 651–656. https://doi.org/10.1016/j.jallcom.2018.07.237. (b) Mansouri Majd, S., & Salimi, A. (2018). *Anal. Chim. Acta, 1000*, 273–282. https://doi.org/10.1016/j.aca.2018.01.007.
42. (a) Kuźnik, N., & Tomczyk, M. M. (2016). *Beilstein J. Nanotechnol., 7*, 1086–1103. https://doi.org/10.3762/bjnano.7.104. (b) Delogu, L. G., Vidili, A., Ventureli, E., & Bianco, A. (2012). *PNAS, 109*, 16612–16617. https://doi.org/10.1073/pnas.1207728109.
43. (a) Son, K. H., Hong, J. H., & Lee, J. W. (2016). *Int. J. Nanomed., 11*, 5163–5185. https://doi.org/10.2147/IJN.S108448. (b) Wang, C., Xu, L., Liang, C., Xiang, J., Peng, R., & Liu, Z. (2014). *Adv. Mater., 26*, 8154–8162. https://doi.org/10.1002/adma.201402368. (c) Wang, S., Lin, Q., Chen, J., Gao, H., Fu, D., & Shen, S. (2017). *Carbon, 112*, 53–62. https://doi.org/10.1016/j.carbon.2016.10.010. (d) Zhu, Y., Sun, Q., Liu, Y., Ma, T., Su, L., Liu, S., Shi, X., Han, D., & Liang, F. (2018). *R. Soc. Open Sci., 5*, 180159. https://doi.org/10.1098/rsos.180159.
44. (a) Ahadian, S., Yamada, S., Ramón-Azcón, J., Estili, M., Liang, X., Nakajima, K., Shiku, H., Khademhosseini, A., & Matsue, T. (2016). *Acta Biomater., 31*, 134–143. https://doi.org/10.1016/j.actbio.2015.11.013. (b) Yu, H., Zhao, H., Huang, C., & Du, Y. (2017). *ACS Biomater. Sci. Eng., 3*, 3017–3021. https://doi.org/10.1021/acsbiomaterials.7b00309.
45. (a) Srivastava, V., Gusain, D., & Sharma, Y. C. (2015). *Ind. Eng. Chem. Res., 54*, 6209–6233. https://doi.org/10.1021/acs.iecr.5b01588. (b) Madani, S. Y., Mandel, A., & Seifalian, A. M. (2013). *Nano Rev., 4*, 21521. https://doi.org/10.3402/nano.v4i0.21521. (c) Katsumiti, A., Berhanu, D., Howard, K. T., Arostegui, I., Oron, M., Reip, P., Valsami-Jones, E., & Cajaraville, M. (2015). *Nanotoxicology, 9*, 543–553. https://doi.org/10.3109/17435390.2014.971695. (d) Sukhanova, A., Bozrova, S., Sokolov, P., Berestovoy, M., Karaulov, A., & Nabiev, I. (2018). *Nanoscale Res. Lett., 13*, 1–21. https://doi.org/10.1186/s11671-018-2495-0.
46. Singh, A., & Amiji, M. M. (2022). *Curr. Opin. Biotechnol., 74*, 241–246. https://doi.org/10.1016/j.copbio.2021.11.011.
47. (a) Imamura, Y., Yamada, S., Tsuboi, S., Nakane, Y., Tsukasaki, Y., Komatsuzaki, A., & Jin, T. (2016). *Molecules, 21*, 1080. https://doi.org/10.3390/molecules21081080. (b) Tian, X., Zhang, L., Yang, M., Bai, L., Dai, Y., Yu, Z., & Pan, Y. (2018). *Interdiscip. Rev. Nanomed. Nanobiotechnol., 1*, e1476. https://doi.org/10.1002/inn2.1476. (c) Ding, Y.,

Zeng, L., Xiao, X., Chen, T., & Pan, Y. (2021). *ACS Appl. Bio Mater., 15*, 1066–1076. https://doi.org/10.1021/acsabm.0c01312.

48. (a) Nassireslami, E., & Ajdarzade, M. (2018). *Adv. Pharm. Bull., 8*, 201–209. https://doi.org/10.15171/apb.2018.023. (b) Wang, D., Fei, B., Halig, L. V., Qin, X., Hu, Z., Xu, H., Wang, Y. A., Chen, Z., Kim, S., Shin, D. M., & Chen, Z. (2014). *ACS Nano, 8*, 6620–6632. https://doi.org/10.1021/nn5014795. (c) Silva, A. H., Lima, E., Mansilla, M. V., Zysler, R. D., Troiani, H., Pisciotti, M. L. M., Locatelli, C., Benech, J. C., Oddone, N., Zoldan, V. C., Winter, E., Pasa, A. A., & Creczynski-Pasa, T. B. (2016). *Nanomed. Nanotechnol. Biol. Med., 12*, 909–919. https://doi.org/10.1016/j.nano.2016.01.016.
49. (a) Zare, H., Ahmadi, S., Ghasemi, A., Ghanbari, M., Rabiee, N., Bagherzadeh, M., Karimi, M., Webster, T. J., Hamblin, M. R., & Mostafavi, E. (2021). *Int. J. Nanomed., 16*, 1681–1706. https://doi.org/10.2147/IJN.S296226. (b) Xie, L., Wang, G., Zhou, H., Zhang, F., Guo, Z., Liu, C., Zhang, X., & Zhu, L. (2016). *Biomaterials, 103*, 219–228. https://doi.org/10.1016/j.biomaterials.2016.06.012. (c) Eldridge, B. N., Xing, F., Fahrenholtz, C. D., & Singh, R. N. (2017). *Toxicol. in Vitro, 41*, 223–231. https://doi.org/10.1016/j.tiv.2016.12.009. (d) Sargazi, S., Mukhtar, M., Rahdar, A., Barani, M., Pandey, S., & Díez-Pascual, A. M. (2021). *Int. J. Mol. Sci., 22*, 10319. https://doi.org/10.3390/ijms221910319.
50. Shao, W., Paul, A., Rodes, L., & Prakash, S. (2015). *Cell Biochem. Biophys., 71*, 1405–1414. https://doi.org/10.1007/s12013-014-0272-5.
51. McCarroll, J., Baigude, H., Yang, C. S., & Rana, T. M. (2010). *Bioconjugate Chemistry, 21*(1), 56–63. https://doi.org/10.1021/bc900247x.
52. Li, H., Hao, Y., Wang, N., Wang, L., Jia, S., Wang, Y., Yang, L., & Zhang, Y. (2016). *Drug Delivery, 23*(6), 830–838. https://doi.org/10.3109/10717544.2014.1001577.
53. Li, Z., de Barros, A. L. B., Soares, D. C. F., Moss, S. N., & Alisaraie, L. (2017). *International Journal of Pharmaceutics, 524*(1–2), 41–54. https://doi.org/10.1016/j.ijpharm.2017.02.026.
54. (a) Kapat, K., Shubhra, Q. T., Zhou, M., & Leeuwenburgh, S. (2020). *Advanced Functional Materials, 30*(19), 1909045. https://doi.org/10.1002/adfm.201909045. (b) Gong, T., Xie, J., Liao, J., Zhang, T., Lin, S., & Lin, Y. (2015). *Bone Research, 3*, 15029. https://doi.org/10.1038/boneres.2015.29. (c) McMahon, R. E., Wang, L., Skoracki, R., & Mathur, A. B. (2013). *Journal of Biomedical Materials Research Part B: Applied Biomaterials, 101*(3), 387–397. https://doi.org/10.1002/jbm.b.32871.
55. (a) Zhang, Y., Venugopa, J. R., El-Turki, A., Ramakrishna, S., Su, B., & Lim, C. T. (2008). *Biomaterials, 29*(29), 4314–4322. https://doi.org/10.1016/j.biomaterials.2008.05.012.
56. (a) Liang, X. Y., Duan, P. G., Gao, J. M., Guo, R. S., Qu, Z. H., Li, X. F., He, Y., Yao, H. Q., & Ding, J. D. (2018). *ACS Biomaterials Science & Engineering, 4*(10), 3506–3521. https://doi.org/10.1021/acsbiomaterials.8b00719. (b) Naffakh, M., & Díez-Pascual, A. M. (2015). *RSC Advances, 5*(96), 65514. https://doi.org/10.1039/c5ra11722h. (c) Cui, Y., Li, H., Li, Y., & Mao, L. (2022). *Nanoscale Advances, 4*(1), 334–352. https://doi.org/10.1039/d1na00877j. (d) Shakir, M., Jolly, R., Khan, M. S., Iran, N., Sharma, T. K., & Al-Resayes, S. I. (2015). *Polymer Advances Technologies, 26*(1), 41–48. https://doi.org/10.1002/pat.3393. (e) Fu, S. Z., Wang, X. H., Guo, G., Shi, S., Fan, M., Liang, H., Luo, F., & Qian, Z. Y. (2011). *Journal of Biomedical Materials Research Part B: Applied Biomaterials, 97*(1), 74–83. https://doi.org/10.1002/jbm.b.31773.
57. Park, D., Cho, Y., Goh, S. H., & Choi, Y. (2014). *Chemical Communications, 50*(112), 15014–15017. https://doi.org/10.1039/c4cc06594d.

58. Zhao, G., Long, G. L., Zhang, L., Peng, M., Cui, T., Wen, X., Zhou, X., Sun, L., & Che, L. (2017). *Scientific Reports, 7*(1), 3383. https://doi.org/10.1038/s41598-017-03672-5.
59. Yang, G., Phua, S. Z. F., Bindra, A. K., & Zhao, Y. (2019). *Advanced Materials, 31*(22), 1805730. https://doi.org/10.1002/adma.201805730.
60. Díez-Pascual, A. M., & Rahdar, A. (2022). *ChemMedChem, 17*(2), e202200142. https://doi.org/10.1002/cmdc.202200142.

CHAPTER 4

Bioactivity and Biocompatibility of Chitosan-Based Biocomposites

NANCY JASWAL,[1] PURNIMA JUSTA,[1] HEMANT KUMAR,[2] SUJEET KUMAR CHAURASIA,[3] ADESH KUMAR,[4] BALARAM PANI,[5] and PRAMOD KUMAR[1]

[1]*Department of Chemistry and Chemical Science, School of Physical and Material Sciences, Central University of Himachal Pradesh, Dharamshala, Himachal Pradesh, India*

[2]*Department of Chemistry, Ramjas College, University of Delhi, Delhi, India*

[3]*Center for Nanoscience and Technology, Prof. Rajendra Singh Institute of Physical Sciences for Study and Research, V.B.S. Purvanchal University, Jaunpur, Uttar Pradesh, India*

[4]*Department of Chemistry, University of Delhi, Delhi, India*

[5]*Bhaskaracharya College of Applied Sciences, Department of Chemistry, University of Delhi, Delhi, India*

ABSTRACT

Finding a reliable alternative for conventional polymers has been a top priority for the plastics industry, as industrially generated plastic trash, mostly traditional food packaging, has escalated into a global environmental problem. Researchers are interested in biodegradable polymers as a potential replacement for plastics made from fossil fuels. A current emphasis for the biodegradable food packaging industry is chitosan-based packaging materials because of their biodegradability, non-toxicity, and antibacterial

Bioabsorbable Polymers for Drug Carriers and Fixation Devices. Arbind Prasad and Sougata Jana (Eds.)

qualities. After cellulose, chitosan, which is made from chitin, is one of the most ubiquitous biopolymers existing in nature at present. Chitosan is the perfect biomaterial for active packaging since it can be made alone or in combination with other polymers and metallic antibacterial particles in the form of layers or coacervates for testing as functional parts of active packaging systems. The utilization of chitosan-based systems for food packaging, including barrier films, sensor films, as well as antimicrobial films, has seen significant advancements. This article thoroughly examines current progress in the creation and use of tailored chitosan-based systems in the realm of food packaging.

4.1 INTRODUCTION

In recent years, bio-based packaging methods have significantly improved in response to the substantial environmental issues brought on by petroleum-based, non-biodegradable packaging materials. It has become feasible to substitute the conventional non-biodegradable plastic packaging materials with cutting-edge, highly effective, lightweight green nanocomposite materials. After cellulose, chitosan is one of the biopolymers that is most often used. Chitosan-based materials are commonly employed across a range of industries because of their biological and physical characteristics, including biocompatibility, biodegradability, antibacterial properties, and ease of film production [1–3]. Although polysaccharides like chitosan and carboxymethyl cellulose have poor mechanical properties, low water resistance, and limited antibacterial effects, they do not pose any environmental problems. Therefore, while maintaining biodegradable and non-toxic properties, nanomaterials can be used to enhance the antibacterial activity, thermal, mechanical, and gas barrier capabilities of materials [4]. In a market report titled "Global Market Study on Nano-Enabled Packaging for Food and Beverages," according to Persistence Market Study's report, "Intelligent Packaging to Witness Highest Growth by 2020," the market for nano-sized food and beverage packaging is expected to grow at a compound annual growth rate (CAGR) of 12.7% from 2014 to 2020, with an expected value of USD 15.0 billion in 2020 [5]. Figure 4.1 shows function of food packaging.

Bio-composites made from chitin and chitosan have several remarkable benefits, such as being biocompatible with living organisms, having superior barrier and mechanical qualities, and being less expensive than

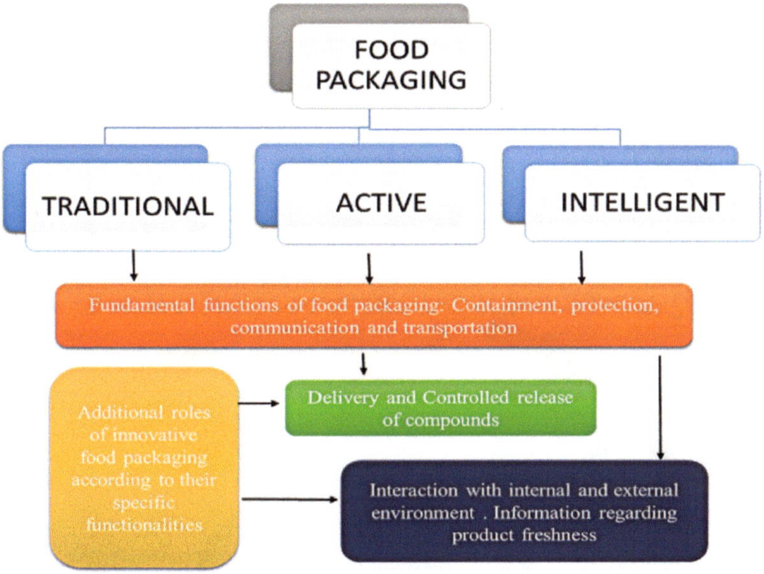

FIGURE 4.1 The main function of food packaging.

their synthetic counterparts. Additionally, their use in food packaging applications serves as a vehicle for antioxidant and antibacterial additives, which enhances food preservation by extending shelf life [6]. Following cellulose in terms of abundance, chitin has been shown to have a variety of uses in the biomaterials, water treatment, and other domains [7]. Chitin is a biopolymer that resembles cellulose and is found in the outer walls of fungi and yeast, as well as in the exoskeletons of crustaceans and insects. Similar to how cellulose serves as a structural component in plant cells, chitin also serves this purpose. It is a polymer that is mostly made of (1–4) linked, 2-acetamido-2-deoxy-D-glucose monomers, which is produced at a staggering rate of 10^{11} metric tons per year. The provenance of the chitin affects characteristics including the level of acetylation (DA), nitrogen content, N/C ratio, molecular size, and polydispersity. The nitrogen concentration of chitin is typically 7%, its N/C ratio is 0.146, and its DA is above 90%. Chitosan contains a nitrogen concentration of more than 7% and a DA lower than 40%. Chitosan has functional qualities because of the amino group; the electronegative amino group accepts protons, resulting in the generation of a positive charge, which leads to variation in the range of chemical, physical, and biological properties of chitosan. Due to its solubility, ability to form films, viscosity, ion binding, and other properties, chitosan is a versatile polymer that finds use in a variety of scientific domains, including food packaging [8]. The current chapter comprehensively reviews the future trends in the application of chitosan-based systems in the food packaging area (Figure 4.2).

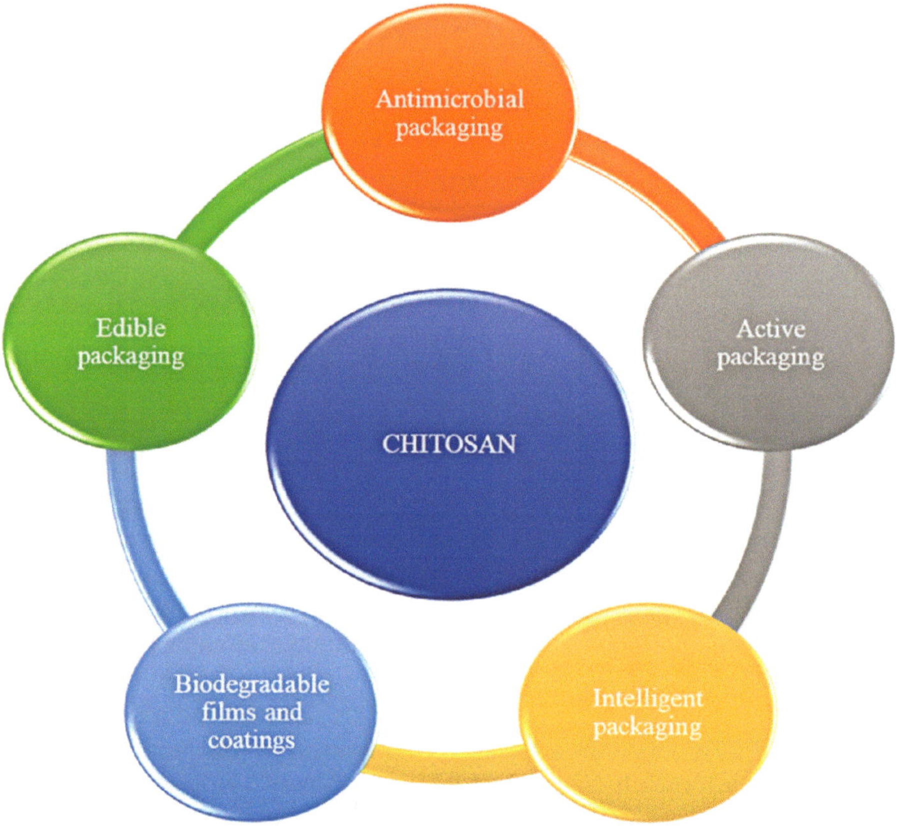
Antimicrobial packaging
Active packaging
Intelligent packaging
Biodegradable films and coatings
Edible packaging
CHITOSAN

FIGURE 4.2 Various food application of chitosan.

4.2 PROVENANCE OF CHITOSAN

The most frequent and efficient approach for isolating chitosan is by the deacetylation of chitin. However, certain fungi may also be used in the direct extraction of chitosan. Many different animal and fungal species use chitin as part of their structural framework. Table 4.1 Summarizes the sources from which chitin is extracted.

TABLE 4.1 Sources from Which Chitin is Extracted, Together the Proportion of Dry Mass in Each Source [8]

Organism	Chitin Content
Crustaceans	
Nephro	69.8
Euphasia superb	24.0
Homarus	60.0–75.0
Crangon crangon	17.8
Lepas	58.3
Chinoecetes opilio	26.6
Insects	
Blatella (cockroach)	18.4
Coleoptera (ladybird)	27.0–35.0
Diptera	54.8
Pieris (butterfly)	64.0
Bombyx (silkworm)	44.2
Galleria (wax worm)	33.7
Fungi	
Penicillium notatum	18.5
Penicillium chrysogenum	19.5–42.0
Saccharomyces gutulata	2.3
Mucrorrouxii	9.4
Siboglinidae	33.0
Cnidaria	3.0–30.0
Mollusks *Squid, cuttlefish, octopus*	6.0–40.0

4.3 EXTRACTION OF CHITIN

There are two techniques to remove chitin from animal waste: chemically and biologically. Due to its faster processing time, the chemical approach is the most commonly used commercial technique, despite its numerous drawbacks, such as being uneconomical and unfriendly to the environment. However, it has been shown that the yield of chitin produced from the shells of prawns as well as shrimp through the biological approach is greater than that of the chemical approach. The primary extraction procedure for chitin involves washing, drying, and crushing the raw material obtained from various sources into a fine powder. The powder is then put through a three-step process that includes demineralization, followed by deproteinization and decolorization (Figure 4.3). These three phases are used in both chemical and biological processes [9].

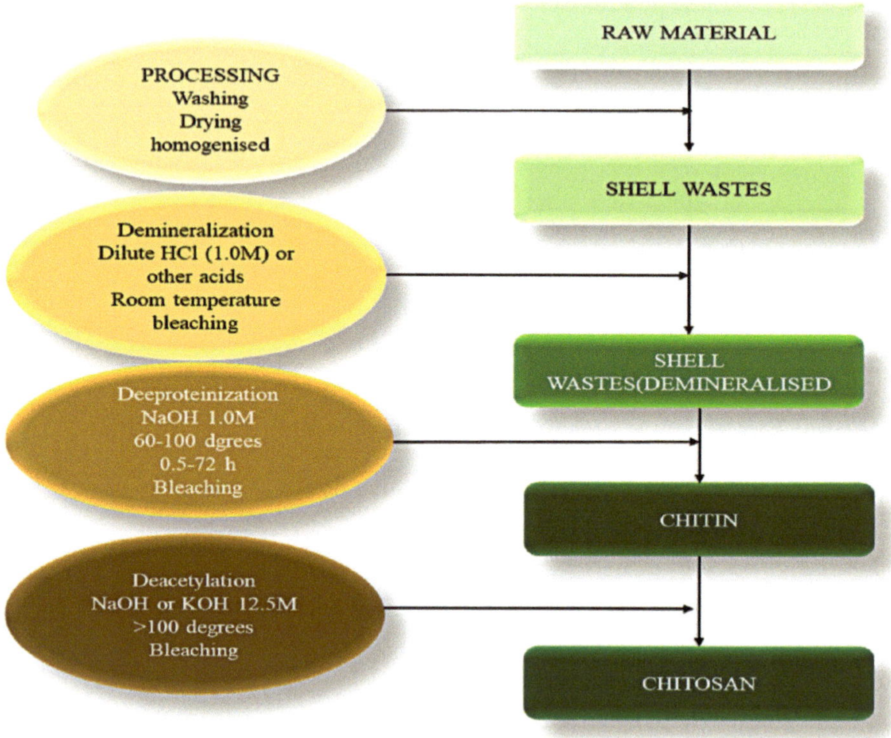

FIGURE 4.3 The process of extraction of chitosan from chitin.

4.4 CONVERSION OF CHITIN INTO CHITOSAN

By removing the acetyl groups by deacetylation process from chitin is then converted into chitosan (Figure 4.4.). Since the process of N-deacetylation is partially complete, multiple levels of deacetylated chitosan are produced. Chitin can be deacetylated using either the alkaline approach or the enzymatic method [10].

4.4.1 ALKALINE METHOD

A 40–50% NaOH solution is applied to the chitin powder. Through this process, acetyl groups are hydrolyzed, and N-acetyl-D-glucosamine units have been converted to D-glucosamine units containing free amine groups. The reaction duration, temperature, and alkali solution concentration all affect how much the chitosan is deacetylated (DD) as a result of this

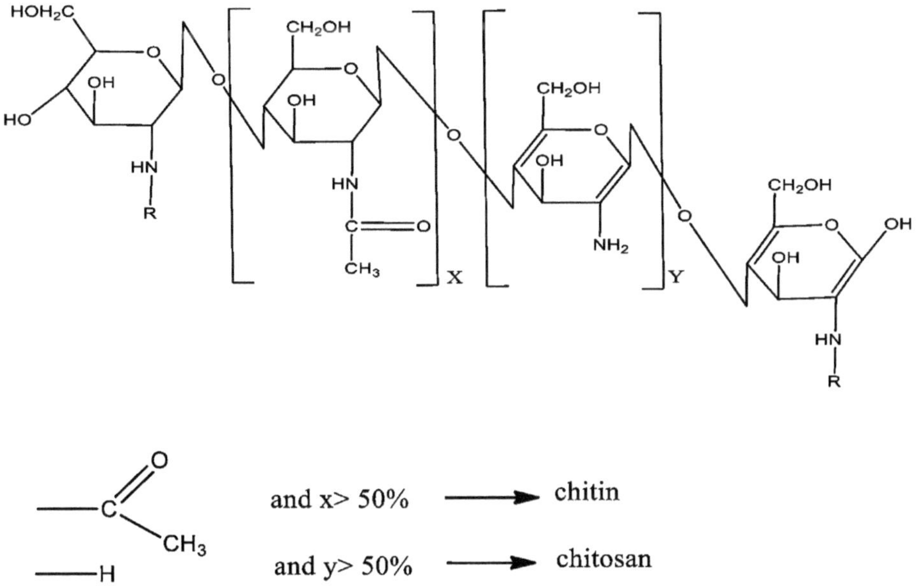

FIGURE 4.4 The effect on the production of chitin and chitosan on the basis of varying degrees of deacetylation.

process. The tendency is moving away from this technology in favor of a more environmentally friendly enzymatic approach since it utilizes a lot of energy and pollutes the environment [11].

4.4.2 ENZYMATIC METHOD

Chitin is transformed into chitosan by the chitin deacetylase enzyme. The enzyme was initially identified in 1974 in the fungus *Mucor rouxii*. Some fungi were discovered to have chitosan in their cell walls naturally. It has been discovered that the chitin deacetylase enzyme is the precursor that causes the conversion of chitin in their cell walls into chitosan. The chitin deacetylase-producing fungi, however, output very little enzyme and have difficult fermentation requirements. Additionally, compared to enzymes isolated from bacterial strains, those from fungal sources have lesser activity. Furthermore, large-scale fermentation systems promote quicker and simpler bacterial growth. Consequently, chitin deacetylase isolation from microbial isolates is becoming more and more common [12].

4.5 CHITOSAN-BASED FILMS

Due to their great performance, especially in the food business, in terms of the effects on the environment, research on chitosan films has been underway for years. Pure chitosan films, chitosan/biopolymer films, synthetic polymer films, and films designed and produced from chitosan derivatives all seem to be examples that may be utilized as food packaging materials to extend the shelf life of the product [13].

4.5.1 PURE CHITOSAN FILMS

Chitosan could be formed into various products, such as edible films, by dissolving it in a diluted acid solution (such as acetic acid and hydrochloric acid). Chitosan films have been used to preserve a variety of foods. The affected items, which have better storage stability following treatment, include banana, pomegranate, carrot, mango, tomato, salmon, papaya, and wolfberries. Additionally, it has been demonstrated that these pure chitosan films may maintain antioxidant activity, postpone changes in qualitative and nutraceutical features, stop the development of microorganisms, and extend shelf life. Films made from normal as well as submicron chitosan dispersions with diameters ranging from 600 nm to 1,000 nm showed superior food preservation, respectively [14].

Additionally, an acute amount of plasticizers, such as sorbitol and glycerol, might be added to increase chain mobility, extendibility, and strength. In order to create films with improved characteristics, emulsifiers or surfactants like Tween-80, Tween 20, Brij 56, and Span 20 can also be added to the chitosan solution [15]. Even though these films showed amazing qualities generally, some of them had high benefits in certain areas but low drawbacks in others, such as weight loss, and need unique circumstances like ultrasonography, which could not be helpful for practical mass application to food [16].

4.5.2 CHITOSAN-BIOPOLYMER-BASED FILMS

Chitosan/biopolymer films may indeed be produced by combining chitosan with naturally occurring biopolymers, as they are biodegradable, non-toxic, and biocompatible, among other qualities. These produced chitosan/biopolymer films have been extensively studied for use in food because of their combinational features. Polysaccharides, proteins, extracts, organic acids, and other substances make up these biopolymers [17].

4.5.3 CHITOSAN-POLYSACCHARIDES-BASED FILMS

Many researchers have looked into cellulose to create chitosan/cellulose films with better mechanical properties. The forces that propel the formation of films are created by hydrogen bonds between nanocellulose and chitosan. These films demonstrated outstanding optical, gas barrier, antibacterial, sustainability, and bioactivity properties [18]. These biodegradable chitosan/polysaccharide films, which have improved characteristics, might be used in food packaging in order to increase the shelf life of a variety of foods.

4.5.4 CHITOSAN-EXTRACTS-BASED FILMS

Natural and harmless plant extracts have been employed for decades in numerous industries, including food preservation. Regarding the chitosan film, it was discovered that the addition of plant extracts can significantly change the film's properties, such as its antimicrobial activity [19], antioxidant activity, barrier performances [20], mechanical property, thermal stability, and color property, resulting in the synergistic interaction between chitosan and plant extracts.

4.5.5 CHITOSAN-PROTEIN-BASED FILMS

Because of qualities including film-forming ability, biocompatibility, as well as high nutritional content, proteins derived from animals have attracted the attention of numerous researchers. Through ionic contact, caseinate, which has good thermoplastic and film-forming capabilities, will attach to the chitosan to create chitosan/caseinate film, improving the final film's features, including water vapor permeability [21].

4.6 CHITOSAN-BASED HYDROGELS

Hydrogels and composite films, two composite biomaterials with excellent biodegradability, are being considered as viable options for novel food packaging. Since they offer effective moisture barriers and antibacterial qualities, hydrogels have been employed in food packaging systems. The following benefits of hydrogel-based packaging materials include: (i) lowering food's water activity to inhibit harmful and spoilage bacteria; (ii) preventing dry food from consuming moisture; (iii) having good mechanical capacity in order to maintain its shape; (iv) being inexpensive and simple to prepare; and (v) having favorable biodegradability to reduce environmental issues [22].

4.7 MECHANICAL PROPERTIES

Predicting the behavior and integrity during handling, storage, as well as transportation has been made easier by studying the mechanical characteristics of biopolymers used as films (Table 4.2) for food packaging, for instance, tensile strength and percentage of elongation. Additionally, the packaged product with protuberances must be considered. Analysis of the axial mechanical parameters, such as puncture force and puncture deformation, is crucial even if it is uncommon. Evaluating the appropriateness and potential uses of the novel biopolymer is made easier by comparing these values to the mechanical characteristics of available synthetic polymers [23].

TABLE 4.2 Mechanical Characteristics of Pure Chitosan Films Under Distinct Conditions

Composition	Conditions	Acid Used	Tensile Strength (Mpa)	Chitosan Properties Mw	Percent of Elongation (%)	References
Chitosan 2%	25° 50%RH	Acetic	68.8–50.2	DD 95%	7.6–5.5	[24]
Chitosan 2%	25° 50%RH	Citric	6.7–17.4	37–920 kDa	41.9–117.8	[24]
Chitosan 2%	25° 50%RH	Lactic	17.1–62.6	37–920 kDa	19.6–31.1	[24]
Chitosan 2%	25° 50%RH	Malic	27.4–62.4	37–920 kDa	17.8–29.9	[24]
Chitosan 1%	25° 20%RH	Acetic	87.68	150 kDa	–	[25]
Chitosan 1%	25° 50%RH	Acetic	61.8	High	4.59	[26]
Chitosan 1%	25° 50%RH	Acetic	55.8	Low	4.58	[26]
Chitosan 2.5%	25° 60% RH	Acetic	~10.0	DD 85% Low Mw	~58.0	[27]
Chitosan 2.5%	25° 60% RH	Acetic	~18.0	DD 85% Medium Mw	~85.0	[27]
Chitosan 2.5%	25° 60% RH	Acetic	~60.0	DD 85% High Mw	~5.0	[27]

*The values enable analysis of the relationship between the film's characteristics and its deacetylation level, molecular weight, solvent method of production, chitosan content, and measuring parameters. DD: degree of deacetylation; RH: relative humidity; and Mw: molecular weight.

4.8 ANTIMICROBIAL PROPERTIES OF CHITOSAN

Chitosan may be used to prevent the growth of several fungi and bacteria. The bio-based polymer interacts with negatively charged residues during one of the stages and allows macromolecular adsorption onto the surface of bacteria, conceivable thanks to its polycationic properties [28]. By forcing a substance containing metal ions through the cell membrane of bacteria, chitosan also alters the permeability of the cell. In addition, chitosan and fungal DNA bond to prevent RNA production [29].

4.9 CHITOSAN AS PACKAGING MATERIAL

Table 4.3 summarizes the applications of chitosan-based nanocomposites.

4.10 RECENT DEVELOPMENT OF BIO-NANOCOMPOSITE FILMS IN THE FOOD PACKAGING APPLICATIONS

Table 4.4 shows the recent trends of nanocomposite films in the food packaging application.

4.11 CONCLUSION

Because petroleum-based packaging materials pose a serious risk to the environment and public health, bio-based polymeric materials have considerable promise in the realm of packaging. Technological advancements have made it possible to create chitosan-based films with several functions that show promise for use as packaging materials. The most complicated uses for chitosan-based films are in packaging, where antibacterial films, barrier films, and sensing films are used because chitosan has minimal cytotoxicity, biocompatibility, and antibacterial activity. However, much work is required to create chitosan-based packaging films that can compete with petroleum-based packaging films and fulfill practical requirements. To satisfy diverse packaging applications, for instance, specific measures must be taken to improve the mechanical strength of chitosan-based films.

The following characteristics of potential chitosan-based film innovations should be taken into account: (i) To suit specific requirements, more functional materials and chitosan derivatives must be researched and developed;

TABLE 4.3 Recent Applications of Chitosan-based Nanocomposites in Food Packaging Applications

Composites	Characteristics of Resultant Composites	Suppression of Microorganisms Well as Extension of Shelf Life	References
Chitosan–apple peel polyphenols (APP)	The films exhibit superior mechanical and antibacterial properties having: i. 0.5% apple peel polyphenols concentration in Chitosan–apple peel polyphenols film tensile strain as well as elongation ii. 1% APP at Chitosan–apple peel polyphenols, the film exhibits good mechanical and antibacterial capabilities. Reduction in the thermal stability	*Salmonella typhimurium, Bacillus cereus, Staphylococcus aureus*, and *Escherichia coli.* The resultant film may offer a viable substitute for synthetic materials, perhaps extending the shelf life of foods.	[30]
Chitosan–propolis extract (PE)	Propolis polyphenols and chitosan interacted in a few ways, resulting in mechanical qualities with antioxidant and antibacterial capabilities.	*Pseudomonas aeruginosa Staphylococcus aureus, Salmonella enteritidis & Escherichia coli.* The manufactured chitosan film has potential so that it can be used as active food packaging by the addition of PE.	[31]
Chitosan–Poly (caprolactone), i.e., grapefruit seed extract	Surface morphology, mechanical, along with the antibacterial characteristics of the films were all impacted by the varying GFSE/ chitosan ratios (0.5, 1.0, 1.5, 2.0, and 2.5 mL/g). As the concentration of GFSE rose above 1.0 ml/g in the *in-vitro* study, the resultant chitosan/PCL/GFSE films produced excellent bacteriostatic and bactericidal effects to defend food against pathogens.	*E. coli* and *Pseudomonas aeruginosa. Salmon* and bread were used in a packaging application test that demonstrated the major benefits of PCL//GFSE/ chitosan films for extending food shelf life and enhancing food safety.	[32]
Chitosan-gelatin–Quercetin (CH-ge, Q)	After the addition of Quercetin-starch to chitosan-gelatin, there is improvement in the surface morphology and water vapor barrier of bio-based polymer films. The Ch-ge film's antioxidant activity was greatly increased by the addition of Q. The tensile strength has also been improved.	*B. substilis–E. coli* Hence shelf life of the packaged food goods may be extended by using these chitosan-based films.	[4]

TABLE 4.3 *(Continued)*

Composites	Characteristics of Resultant Composites	Suppression of Microorganisms Well as Extension of Shelf Life	References
Chitosan–Proanthocyanidins (PA)	Barrier and mechanical characteristics were seen as a result of intermolecular bonding between the PA molecules & CS chains. The inclusion of PA considerably increased the ability of CS-based films' UV-vis light barrier, tensile strength, oxygen barrier as well as thermal stability.	*E. coli, Staphylococcus aureus, Listeria monocytogenes*, and *Salmonella.* Higher antibacterial & antioxidant properties can be found in CS-PA films. Therefore, CS-PA films can be utilised in food packaging as active packaging materials.	[33, 34]
Chitosan–Herba Lophatheri extract (HLE)	Chitosan/HLE films saw reductions in the following properties such as moisture content, water solubility, swelling degree, water vapor permeability, and oil absorption rate by the percentage of 14.81%, 38.97%, 48.03%, 69.23%, and 80%, respectively. HLE and chitosan's interactions also caused HLE/chitosan films to appear intense reddish & yellowish, have deeper tone shave a higher degree of opacity.	*Staphylococcus aureus & E. coli.* The resultant chitosan/HLE sheets showed excellent promise for usage in food packaging. There is still a need for more research, such that which examines the food's shelf life.	[34]
Chitosan–apricot kernel essential oil (AKEO)	When CH & Apricot Kernel Essential Oil (AKEO) are present in ratio of 1:1 then the increased water vapor barrier is increased by 41% while also improving water resistance. The elongation percentage value was dramatically raised by film having oil to chitosan ratio of 0.125. The tensile strength value was shown to rise with increasing AKEO content. When AKEO ratio and CH ratio were identical, a significant improvement (94%) was seen.	*E. coli–B. subtilis* The manufactured films extended bread's shelf life by limiting the growth of fungi.	[35]
Chitosan–kombucha tea (KT)	Water vapor permeability has been improved, along with the antioxidant and scavenging activity. Through addition of KT to chitosan film, the film's UV protection properties were improved.	*E. coli* and *Staphylococcus aureus.* The minced beef's shelf life is increased by 3 days with the help of chitosan/kombucha tea (KT) film, which also considerably reduces microbial development while maintaining quality of minced beef. This film might therefore be used for active food packing.	[36]

TABLE 4.3 *(Continued)*

Composites	Characteristics of Resultant Composites	Suppression of Microorganisms Well as Extension of Shelf Life	References
Chitosan–propolis extract (PE)–*Zataria multiflora* essential oil (ZEO)	The produced film's beneficial antibacterial and antioxidant effects against certain microorganisms improved the chicken breast meat's chemical properties and organoleptic qualities, including odor, color, taste, texture, and overall acceptability.	Lactic acid bacteria (LAB), *Pseudomonas* spp. & *Pseudomonas* spp. It could be a good way to slow down the degradation of freshly packaged chicken.	[37]
Chitosan–Cornstarch–different acids	The produced film's beneficial antibacterial and antioxidant effects against certain microorganisms improved the chicken breast meat's chemical as well as organoleptic qualities, including odor, texture, color, taste and overall acceptability.	*Staphylococcus aureus*. The obtained combinations might be used in packaging.	[38]
Chitosan–*Zataria multiflora* essential oil (hydroalcoholic extract of sumac)	The resultant displayed meat's preferable sensory qualities, including its color, flavor, texture, odor, and general appeal.	*Pseudomonas spp., Enterobacteriaceae,* lactic acid bacteria, and yeasts. These findings demonstrated ability of CH with the sumac hydro-alcoholic extract, & *Z. multiflora* essential oil to preserve biological qualities of beef when packaged normally with refrigeration.	[39]
Chitosan–grape seed extract (GSE)	WVP and opacity values for CH-GSE were greater, whereas transparency and brightness values were lower. The use of grape seed extract increased the film samples' flexibility while lowering their tensile strength. Chitosan-infused films from GS shown strong antibacterial and antioxidant effects.	*E. coli, Staphylococcus aureus Listeria monocytogenes,* and *Pseudomonas aeruginosa.* The shelf life of packed food was increased by using the ready-made Chitosan/grape seed extract films.	[40]
Chitosan–Capsaicin	Significant enhancement in biological, mechanical, and physicochemical qualities. The antibacterial activity, anti-quorum sensing, antioxidant capabilities, elasticity, transparency, as well as hydrophobicity all steadily improved when capsaicin concentration was raised.	*E. coli & Staphylococcus aureus* (*S. aureus*) ATCC 25923. The chitosan-capsaicin mix films that have been created can be utilised to pack food as well as to make patches for skin care and wound healing.	[41]

TABLE 4.3 *(Continued)*

Composites	Characteristics of Resultant Composites	Suppression of Microorganisms Well as Extension of Shelf Life	References
Chitosan–*Litsea cubeba* oil (LCO) (hard leaf oat chestnut starch (HOS)	When the amounts of CH, LCO, & HOS were in the right proportions, a special compatibility was seen. The ratio of the HOS content rose from 1:0 to 1:1, which leads to an increase in the TS, DPPH radical scavenging capacity & a decrease in WVP ability. LEO inclusion increased antibacterial characteristics and static water contact angle while decreasing mechanical properties, water vapor permeability, moisture content, & total soluble matter of such films.	*E. coli–S. aureus* Future food packaging has a lot of possibilities for the manufactured films.	[42]

TABLE 4.4 The Recent Trends of Nanocomposite Films in the Food Packaging Application

Nanoparticles	Materials	Preparation Methods	Properties	References
ZnO—NPs	Chitosan or acetate or cellulose or phthalate	Casting technique	Nano ZnO concentrations between 2 and 7.5% (w/w) associated with an improvement in barrier characteristics and thermal stability.	[43]
ZnO—NPs	Polyvinyl alcohol (PVA) or starch	Casting technique	Improved mechanical, antibacterial, and water barrier qualities	[44]
ZnO—NPs	Chitosan or carboxymethyl-cellulose (CMC)	Casting technique	Casting technique the bio-nanocomposite films' morphological, mechanical, and antimicrobial characteristics were assessed.	[45]
ZnO–NPs	Chitosan or polyethylene	Casting technique	Casting technique enhancing polyethylene's antibacterial capabilities by blocking 99.9% of live pathogenic microorganisms.	[46]
ZnO–NPs	Polyhydroxyalkanoates	Casting technique	Casting technique the tensile, Young's modulus, thermal stability, crystallinity, impact strength, and vapor barrier characteristics of the bio-based polymers were all improved.	[47]
ZnO–NPs	Polylactic acid	Coating technique	Coating technique because of the surface modification, the nanoparticle dispersion was uniform throughout the film surface, however some of them did agglomerate there.	[48]
ZnO–NPs Aluminum doped	Polylactic acid	Casting approach	High visual transparency and UV blocking qualities were demonstrated by the casting approach, and samples that had been sputter-coated had significant antibacterial action against bacteria.	[49]
Silver NPs	Polyvinyl alcohol (PVA)–Montmorillonite clay ginger extract	Casting technique	*S. aureus and Typhimurium,* two frequent foodborne pathogens, have clear antibacterial action. Additionally, it was water resistant and had excellent mechanical and light barrier qualities.	[50]
Silver NPs	Poly-3-hydroxybutyrate-co3-hydroxyvalerate (PHBV3)–Poly-3-hydroxybutyrate-co-3 mol-3-hydroxyvalerate (PHBV3)	Coating technique	Better oxygen barrier shown a potent and long-lasting bactericidal action.	[51]

TABLE 4.4 *(Continued)*

Nanoparticles	Materials	Preparation Methods	Properties	References
Silver NPs	Polyvinyl chloride	Casting technique	*Bacillus subtilis and Fusarium solani* with halos PVCAg1% and PVCAg2%, respectively, demonstrated superior antimicrobial activity.	[52]
Silver NPs	Carboxymethyl-cellulose or Sodium alginate	Coating technique	Excellent antibacterial activity was shown against both Gram +ve as well as Gram –ve microorganisms.	[53]
Ag-Cu	Fish skin gelatin	Casting technique	Mechanical as well as thermal properties have been improved. And demonstrated significant antibacterial-action against bacteria of both the Gram-+ve and Gram –ve types.	[54]
Titanium oxide NPs	Polyethylene or chitosan	Casting technique	Better tensile strength as well as barrier qualities than ethylene.	[55]
Titanium oxide NPs	Polyvinyl alcohol–chitosan	Coating technique	Boosted water vapor and gas barrier. Also advanced antibacterial and mechanical qualities.	[56]
Magnesium oxide (MgO)	Polylactic acid	Coating technique	Reinforced PLA–bio-based polymer, 2 weight percent	[57]
Polylactic acid nanofibers	Cinnamon essential oil β cyclodextrin inclusion complex	Coating technique	CEO has dramatically improved heat stability and antimicrobial action.	[58]
Magnesium-oxide (MgO)	Chitosan	Coating technique	Chitosan composites produced their best mechanical properties when the concentration of MgO is 5 (w/w%), where the tensile strength as elastic modulus has been increased significantly by 86% and 38%, respectively. These composites also show exceptional shielding against UV, thermal stability, and flame retardant, moisture barrier properties.	[59]

TABLE 4.4 *(Continued)*

Nanoparticles	Materials	Preparation Methods	Properties	References
Nano-cellulose	Chitosan or gelatine or Starch	Casting technique	By adding 10% more nanocellulose, the tensile strength increases to 8,121 MN/m^2 while the elongation decreases. Additionally, chitosan content can be increased up to 30% to improve preservation of food up to 15 days. Modulus and transparency improvements	[60]
Nano-cellulose	Polylactic acid or Rosin	Coating technique	Ideal mechanical characteristics were attained at an 8% R-CNF loading percolation threshold. Excellent antibacterial activity of RCNF/PLA/CHT.	[61]
Organo-clay	Polycaprolactone	–	PCL C0.4 G10 K25 An antibacterial effect was seen in the composite film. The addition of chitosan to composite films reduces the mechanical characteristics of PCL.	[62]
Chitosan Gelatin (nano)	Chitosan or gelatin–Moringa oil	–	Crosslinking with ions. Cheese has a strong antimicrobial effect in the temperature range of 4°C to 25°C, addition of gelatin will not affect the surface sensors, quality or color.	[63]
Lignin nanoparticles	Cellulose–Poly-lactic acid	–	By combining the two lignocellulosic nanofillers at two selected weight contents has been proved effective in the enhancement of nucleation as well as in the growth of crystal with respect to binary reference systems. This was confirmed by optically characterizing the films, which demonstrated a synergistic effect of LNP & CNC nanoparticles regarding transparency and UV light uptake capacity.	[64]
Layered double hydroxides	Pectin–Sodium salicylate	Coating technique	Coating. The proportion of glycerol in the mixture influence both the mechanical characteristics as well as behavior of thermal degradation. The most significant increase in water vapors barrier properties (sorption, diffusion, and permeability) was shown in the nanocomposite injection molded with 4 vol% glycerol (barrier properties).	[65]
Graphene mass	Chitosan cinnamaldehyde	–	Cinnamaldehyde as well as graphite mass were applied to CH substrates to increase their mechanical and antifungal properties.	[66]

(ii) to move closer to industrial production, these current technologies might be enhanced or merged with other useful technologies. In order to easily mass-produce the chitosan-based films with the requisite qualities to fulfill various packaging applications, new technologies are still needed; (iii) in order to be used more widely in the market, chitosan-based films need to undergo exhaustive toxicology tests when they come into contact with food; and (iv) more research must be done to determine how the films affect the environment and how they deteriorate over time. Despite the difficulties in realizing actual utilization, chitosan-based films should have a promising future in a variety of packaging applications.

KEYWORDS

- **antibacterial activity**
- **biocompatibility**
- **chitin**
- **chitosan**
- **cytotoxicity**
- **food packaging**
- **toxicology**

REFERENCES

1. Carvalho, R. A., Santos, T. A., de Azevedo, V. M., Felix, P. H. C., Dias, M. V., & Borges, S. V. (2018). Bio-nanocomposites for food packaging applications: Effect of cellulose nanofibers on morphological, mechanical, optical, and barrier properties. *Polymer International, 67*(4), 386–392. https://doi.org/10.1002/pi.5584.
2. Wang, H., Qian, J., & Ding, F. (2018). Emerging chitosan-based films for food packaging applications. *Journal of Agricultural and Food Chemistry, 66*(2), 395–413. https://doi.org/10.1021/acs.jafc.7b04338.
3. Cazón, P., & Vázquez, M. (2019). Applications of chitosan as food packaging materials. In *Advances in Food and Nutrition Research* (pp. 81–123). Elsevier. https://doi.org/10.1016/bs.afnr.2018.12.003.
4. Al-Tayyar, N. A., Youssef, A. M., & Al-hindi, R. (2020). Antimicrobial food packaging based on sustainable bio-based materials for reducing foodborne pathogens: A review. *Food Chemistry, 310*, 125850. https://doi.org/10.1016/j.foodchem.2019.125850.

5. Fortunati, E., Luzi, F., Yang, W., Kenny, J. M., Torre, L., & Puglia, D. (2018). Bio-based nanocomposites in food packaging. In *Nanomaterials for Food Packaging: Materials, Processing Technologies, and Safety Issues* (pp. 71–110). Elsevier. https://doi.org/10.1016/B978-0-12-812323-1.00006-4.
6. Zubair, M., Arshad, M., Pradhan, R. A., & Ullah, A. (2020). Chitosan/chitin-based composites for food packaging applications. In *Handbook of Chitin and Chitosan* (pp. 641–670). https://doi.org/10.1016/B978-0-12-819284-0.00024-4.
7. Zhu, K., Shi, S., Cao, Y., Lu, A., Hu, J., & Zhang, L. (2019). Robust chitin films with good biocompatibility and breathable properties. *Carbohydrate Polymers, 212*, 361–367. https://doi.org/10.1016/j.carbpol.2019.03.027.
8. Priyadarshi, R., & Rhim, J. W. (2020). Chitosan-based biodegradable functional films for food packaging applications. *Innovative Food Science & Emerging Technologies, 62*, 102346. https://doi.org/10.1016/j.ifset.2020.102346.
9. Kim, Y., & Park, R. D. (2015). Progress in bio extraction processes of chitin from crustacean biowastes. In *Journal of the Korean Society for Applied Biological Chemistry, 58*(4), 545–554. https://doi.org/10.1007/s13765-015-2032-x.
10. FallahDelavar, M., & Sedaghat, N. (2020). An overview of the functional and antimicrobial properties of chitosan in food preservation. *Journal of Food Science and Technology, 11*(41), 16–25. https://doi.org/10.1007/s11483-020-09750-w.
11. Jung, J., & Zhao, Y. (2011). Characteristics of deacetylation and depolymerization of β-chitin from jumbo squid (*Dosidicus gigas*) pens. *Carbohydrate Research, 346*(13), 1876–1884. https://doi.org/10.1016/j.carres.2011.05.008.
12. Kaur, S., & Dhillon, G. S. (2015). Recent trends in biological extraction of chitin from marine shell wastes: A review. In *Critical Reviews in Biotechnology, 35*(1), 44–61. https://doi.org/10.3109/07388551.2014.893746.
13. Sun, L., Sun, J., Chen, L., Niu, P., Yang, X., & Guo, Y. (2017). Preparation and characterization of chitosan film incorporated with thinned young apple polyphenols as an active packaging material. *Carbohydrate Polymers, 163*, 81–91. https://doi.org/10.1016/j.carbpol.2017.01.021.
14. Ali, A., Zahid, N., Manickam, S., Siddiqui, Y., & Alderson, P. G. (2014). Double layer coatings: A new technique for maintaining physico-chemical characteristics and antioxidant properties of dragon fruit during storage. *Food and Bioprocess Technology, 7*(8), 2366–2374. https://doi.org/10.1007/s11947-014-1337-6.
15. Vimaladevi, S., Panda, S. K., Xavier, K. A. M., & Bindu, J. (2015). Packaging performance of organic acid incorporated chitosan films on dried anchovy (*Stolephorus indicus*). *Carbohydrate Polymers, 127*, 189–194. https://doi.org/10.1016/j.carbpol.2015.03.015.
16. Mustafa, M. A., Ali, A., Manickam, S., & Siddiqui, Y. (2014). Ultrasound-assisted chitosan-surfactant nanostructure assemblies: Towards maintaining postharvest quality of tomatoes. *Food and Bioprocess Technology, 7*(7), 2102–2111. https://doi.org/10.1007/s11947-014-1309-x.
17. Talón, E., Trifkovic, K. T., Nedovic, V. A., Bugarski, B. M., Vargas, M., Chiralt, A., & González-Martínez, C. (2017). Antioxidant edible films based on chitosan and starch containing polyphenols from thyme extracts. *Carbohydrate Polymers, 157*, 1153–1161. https://doi.org/10.1016/j.carbpol.2016.10.020.
18. Bansal, M., Chauhan, G. S., Kaushik, A., & Sharma, A. (2016). Extraction and functionalization of bagasse cellulose nanofibers to Schiff-base based antimicrobial

membranes. *International Journal of Biological Macromolecules, 91*, 887–894. https://doi.org/10.1016/j.ijbiomac.2016.06.009.
19. Wang, L., Wang, Q., Tong, J., & Zhou, J. (2017). Physicochemical properties of chitosan films incorporated with honeysuckle flower extract for active food packaging. *Journal of Food Process Engineering, 40*(1). https://doi.org/10.1111/jfpe.12304.
20. Genskowsky, E., Puente, L. A., Pérez-Álvarez, J. A., Fernandez-Lopez, J., Muñoz, L. A., & Viuda-Martos, M. (2015). Assessment of antibacterial and antioxidant properties of chitosan edible films incorporated with maqui berry (Aristotelia chilensis). *LWT–Food Science and Technology, 64*(2), 1057–1062. https://doi.org/10.1016/j.lwt.2015.06.039.
21. Khwaldia, K., Basta, A. H., Aloui, H., & El-Saied, H. (2014). Chitosan-caseinate bilayer coatings for paper packaging materials. *Carbohydrate Polymers, 99*, 508–516. https://doi.org/10.1016/j.carbpol.2013.08.020.
22. Batista, R. A., Espitia, P. J. P., Quintans, J. de S. S., Freitas, M. M., Cerqueira, M. Â., Teixeira, J. A., & Cardoso, J. C. (2019). Hydrogel as an alternative structure for food packaging systems. *Carbohydrate Polymers, 205*, 106–116. https://doi.org/10.1016/j.carbpol.2018.10.055.
23. Rouhi, M., Razavi, S. H., & Mousavi, S. M. (2017). Optimization of crosslinked poly (vinyl alcohol) nanocomposite films for mechanical properties. *Materials Science and Engineering C, 71*, 1052–1063. https://doi.org/10.1016/j.msec.2016.10.016.
24. Park, S. Y., Marsh, K. S., & Rhim, J. W. (2002). Characteristics of different molecular weight chitosan films affected by the type of organic solvents. *Journal of Food Science, 67*(6). https://doi.org/10.1111/j.1365-2621.2002.tb08583.x.
25. Li, J., Zivanovic, S., Davidson, P. M., & Kit, K. (2010). Characterization and comparison of chitosan/PVP and chitosan/PEO blend films. *Carbohydrate Polymers, 79*(3), 786–791. https://doi.org/10.1016/j.carbpol.2009.09.003.
26. Leceta, I., Guerrero, P., & de La Caba, K. (2013). Functional properties of chitosan-based films. *Carbohydrate Polymers, 93*(1), 339–346. https://doi.org/10.1016/j.carbpol.2012.07.043.
27. Bof, M. J., Bordagaray, V. C., Locaso, D. E., & García, M. A. (2015). Chitosan molecular weight effect on starch-composite film properties. *Food Hydrocolloids, 51*, 281–294. https://doi.org/10.1016/j.foodhyd.2015.06.021.
28. Youssef, A. M., Assem, F. M., Abdel-Aziz, M. E., Elaaser, M., Ibrahim, O. A., Mahmoud, M., & Abd El-Salam, M. H. (2019). Development of bio nanocomposite materials and its use in coating of Ras cheese. *Food Chemistry, 270*, 467–475. https://doi.org/10.1016/j.foodchem.2018.07.013.
29. de Farias, B. S., Junior, T. R. S. A. C., & de Almeida Pinto, L. A. (2019). Chitosan-functionalized nanofibers: A comprehensive review on challenges and prospects for food applications. *International Journal of Biological Macromolecules, 123*, 210–220. https://doi.org/10.1016/j.ijbiomac.2018.11.161.
30. Riaz, A., Lei, S., Akhtar, H. M. S., Wan, P., Chen, D., Jabbar, S., Abid, M., Hashim, M. M., & Zeng, X. (2018). Preparation and characterization of chitosan-based antimicrobial active food packaging film incorporated with apple peel polyphenols. *International Journal of Biological Macromolecules, 114*, 547–555. https://doi.org/10.1016/j.ijbiomac.2018.03.099.
31. Siripatrawan, U., & Vitchayakitti, W. (2016). Improving functional properties of chitosan films as active food packaging by incorporating with propolis. *Food Hydrocolloids, 61*, 695–702. https://doi.org/10.1016/j.foodhyd.2016.05.021.

32. Wang, K., Lim, P. N., Tong, S. Y., & Thian, E. S. (2019). Development of grapefruit seed extract-loaded poly(ε-caprolactone)/chitosan films for antimicrobial food packaging. *Food Packaging and Shelf Life, 22*. https://doi.org/10.1016/j.fpsl.2019.01.002.
33. Bi, F., Zhang, X., Bai, R., Liu, Y., Liu, J., & Liu, J. (2019). Preparation and characterization of antioxidant and antimicrobial packaging films based on chitosan and proanthocyanidins. *International Journal of Biological Macromolecules, 134*, 11–19. https://doi.org/10.1016/j.ijbiomac.2019.05.072.
34. Wang, L., Guo, H., Wang, J., Jiang, G., Du, F., & Liu, X. (2019). Effects of *Herba Lophatheri* extract on the physicochemical properties and biological activities of chitosan film. *International Journal of Biological Macromolecules, 133*, 51–57. https://doi.org/10.1016/j.ijbiomac.2019.04.126.
35. Priyadarshi, R., Sauraj, Kumar, B., Deeba, F., Kulshreshtha, A., & Negi, Y. S. (2018). Chitosan films incorporated with apricot (Prunus armeniaca) kernel essential oil as active food packaging material. *Food Hydrocolloids, 85*, 158–166. https://doi.org/10.1016/j.foodhyd.2018.07.029.
36. Ashrafi, A., Jokar, M., & Mohammadi Nafchi, A. (2018). Preparation and characterization of bio composite film based on chitosan and kombucha tea as active food packaging. *International Journal of Biological Macromolecules, 108*, 444–454. https://doi.org/10.1016/j.ijbiomac.2017.11.082.
37. Mehdizadeh, T., & Mojaddar Langroodi, A. (2019). Chitosan coatings incorporated with propolis extract and Zataria multiflora Boiss oil for active packaging of chicken breast meat. *International Journal of Biological Macromolecules, 141*, 401–409. https://doi.org/10.1016/j.ijbiomac.2019.07.053.
38. Pavoni, J. M. F., Luchese, C. L., & Tessaro, I. C. (2019). Impact of acid type for chitosan dissolution on the characteristics and biodegradability of cornstarch/chitosan-based films. *International Journal of Biological Macromolecules, 138*, 693–703. https://doi.org/10.1016/j.ijbiomac.2019.07.044.
39. Mojaddar Langroodi, A., Tajik, H., Mehdizadeh, T., Moradi, M., Moghaddas Kia, E., & Mahmoudian, A. (2018). Effects of sumac extract dipping and chitosan coating enriched with Zataria multiflora Boiss oil on the shelf-life of meat in modified atmosphere packaging. *LWT–Food Science and Technology, 98*, 372–380. https://doi.org/10.1016/j.lwt.2018.08.026.
40. Sogut, E., & Seydim, A. C. (2018). The effects of chitosan and grape seed extract-based edible films on the quality of vacuum packaged chicken breast fillets. *Food Packaging and Shelf Life, 18*, 13–20. https://doi.org/10.1016/j.fpsl.2018.05.007.
41. Akyuz, L., Kaya, M., Mujtaba, M., Ilk, S., Sargin, I., Salaberria, A. M., & Islek, C. (2018). Supplementing capsaicin with chitosan-based films enhanced the anti-quorum sensing, antimicrobial, antioxidant, transparency, elasticity, and hydrophobicity. *International Journal of Biological Macromolecules, 115*, 438–446. https://doi.org/10.1016/j.ijbiomac.2018.03.053.
42. Zheng, K., Li, W., Fu, B., Fu, M., Ren, Q., Yang, F., & Qin, C. (2018). Physical, antibacterial and antioxidant properties of chitosan films containing *Hardleafoatchestnut* starch and *Litsea cubeba* oil. *International Journal of Biological Macromolecules, 118*, 707–715. https://doi.org/10.1016/j.ijbiomac.2018.06.037.
43. Indumathi, M. P., Saral Sarojini, K., & Rajarajeswari, G. R. (2019). Antimicrobial and biodegradable chitosan/cellulose acetate phthalate/ZnO nanocomposite films with optimal oxygen permeability and hydrophobicity for extending the shelf life of black

grape fruits. *International Journal of Biological Macromolecules, 132*, 1112–1120. https://doi.org/10.1016/j.ijbiomac.2019.03.062.
44. Jayakumar, A., K. V., H., T. S., S., Joseph, M., Mathew, S. G., P., Nair, I. C., & E. K., R. (2019). Starch-PVA composite films with zinc-oxide nanoparticles and phytochemicals as intelligent pH sensing wraps for food packaging application. *International Journal of Biological Macromolecules, 136*, 395–403. https://doi.org/10.1016/j.ijbiomac.2019.05.136.
45. Youssef, A. M., El-Sayed, S. M., El-Sayed, H. S., Salama, H. H., & Dufresne, A. (2016). Enhancement of Egyptian soft white cheese shelf life using a novel chitosan/carboxymethyl cellulose/zinc oxide bio nanocomposite film. *Carbohydrate Polymers, 151*, 9–19. https://doi.org/10.1016/j.carbpol.2016.04.014.
46. Al-Naamani, L., Dobretsov, S., & Dutta, J. (2016). Chitosan-zinc oxide nanoparticle composite coating for active food packaging applications. *Innovative Food Science & Emerging Technologies, 38*, 231–237. https://doi.org/10.1016/j.ifset.2016.10.007.
47. Díez-Pascual, A. M. (2017). Biodegradable food packaging nanocomposites based on ZnO-reinforced polyhydroxyalkanoates. In *Food Packaging* (pp. 185–221). Elsevier. https://doi.org/10.1016/B978-0-12-803822-0.00011-5.
48. Zhang, R., Lan, W., Ji, T., Sameen, D. E., Ahmed, S., Qin, W., & Liu, Y. (2021). Development of polylactic acid/ZnO composite membranes prepared by ultrasonication and electrospinning for food packaging. *LWT, 135*. https://doi.org/10.1016/j.lwt.2020.110188.
49. Valerini, D., Tammaro, L., di Benedetto, F., Vigliotta, G., Capodieci, L., Terzi, R., & Rizzo, A. (2018). Aluminum-doped zinc oxide coatings on polylactic acid films for antimicrobial food packaging. *Thin Solid Films, 645*, 187–192. https://doi.org/10.1016/j.tsf.2017.12.046.
50. Mathew, S., S., S., Mathew, J., & Radhakrishnan, E. K. (2019). Biodegradable and active nanocomposite pouches reinforced with silver nanoparticles for improved packaging of chicken sausages. *Food Packaging and Shelf Life, 19*, 155–166. https://doi.org/10.1016/j.fpsl.2018.11.006.
51. Castro-Mayorga, J. L., Fabra, M. J., & Lagaron, J. M. (2016). Stabilized nano silver based antimicrobial poly(3-hydroxybutyrate-co-3-hydroxyvalerate) nanocomposites of interest in active food packaging. *Innovative Food Science & Emerging Technologies, 33*, 524–533. https://doi.org/10.1016/j.ifset.2015.10.013.
52. Braga, L. R., Rangel, E. T., Suarez, P. A. Z., & Machado, F. (2018). Simple synthesis of active films based on PVC incorporated with silver nanoparticles: Evaluation of the thermal, structural and antimicrobial properties. *Food Packaging and Shelf Life, 15*, 122–129. https://doi.org/10.1016/j.fpsl.2017.10.004.
53. Su, C. H., Velusamy, P., Kumar, G. V., Adhikary, S., Pandian, K., & Anbu, P. (2017). Studies of antibacterial efficacy of different biopolymer protected silver nanoparticles synthesized under reflux condition. *Journal of Molecular Structure, 1128*, 718–723. https://doi.org/10.1016/j.molstruc.2016.12.095.
54. Arfat, Y. A., Ahmed, J., Hiremath, N., Auras, R., & Joseph, A. (2017). Thermo-mechanical, rheological, structural and antimicrobial properties of bio nanocomposite films based on fish skin gelatin and silver-copper nanoparticles. *Food Hydrocolloids, 62*, 191–202. https://doi.org/10.1016/j.foodhyd.2016.07.007.
55. Kaewklin, P., Siripatrawan, U., Suwanagul, A., & Lee, Y. S. (2018). Active packaging from chitosan-titanium dioxide nanocomposite film for prolonging storage life of tomato

fruit. *International Journal of Biological Macromolecules, 112*, 523–529. https://doi.org/10.1016/j.ijbiomac.2018.01.149.
56. Lian, Z., Zhang, Y., & Zhao, Y. (2016). Nano-TiO_2 particles and high hydrostatic pressure treatment for improving functionality of polyvinyl alcohol and chitosan composite films and nano-TiO_2 migration from film matrix in food simulants. *Innovative Food Science & Emerging Technologies, 33*, 145–153. https://doi.org/10.1016/j.ifset.2015.10.007.
57. Swaroop, C., & Shukla, M. (2018). Nano-magnesium oxide reinforced polylactic acid biofilms for food packaging applications. *International Journal of Biological Macromolecules, 113*, 729–736. https://doi.org/10.1016/j.ijbiomac.2018.01.010.
58. Wen, P., Zhu, D. H., Feng, K., Liu, F. J., Lou, W. Y., Li, N., & Wu, H. (2016). Fabrication of electrospun polylactic acid nanofilm incorporating cinnamon essential oil/β-cyclodextrin inclusion complex for antimicrobial packaging. *Food Chemistry, 196*, 996–1004. https://doi.org/10.1016/j.foodchem.2015.09.036.
59. de Silva, R. T., Mantilaka, M. M. M. G. P. G., Goh, K. L., Ratnayake, S. P., Amaratunga, G. A. J., & de Silva, K. M. N. (2017). Magnesium oxide nanoparticles reinforced electro spun alginate-based nanofibrous scaffolds with improved physical properties. *International Journal of Biomaterials, 2017*. https://doi.org/10.1155/2017/1696845.
60. Noorbakhsh-Soltani, S. M., Zerafat, M. M., & Sabbaghi, S. (2018). A comparative study of gelatin and starch-based nano-composite films modified by nano-cellulose and chitosan for food packaging applications. *Carbohydrate Polymers, 189*, 48–55. https://doi.org/10.1016/j.carbpol.2018.02.063.
61. Niu, X., Liu, Y., Song, Y., Han, J., & Pan, H. (2018). Rosin modified cellulose nanofiber as a reinforcing and co-antimicrobial agent in polylactic acid/chitosan composite film for food packaging. *Carbohydrate Polymers, 183*, 102–109. https://doi.org/10.1016/j.carbpol.2018.01.068.
62. Cesur, S., Köroğlu, C., & Yalçın, H. T. (2018). Antimicrobial and biodegradable food packaging applications of polycaprolactone/organonanoclay/chitosan polymeric composite films. *Journal of Vinyl & Additive Technology, 24*(4), 376–387. https://doi.org/10.1002/vnl.21560.
63. Lin, D., Zheng, Y., Huang, Y., Ni, L., Zhao, J., Huang, C., & Xing, B. (2020). Investigation of the structural, physical properties, antioxidant, and antimicrobial activity of chitosan-nano-silicon aerogel composite edible films incorporated with okara powder. *Carbohydrate Polymers, 250*, 116842. https://doi.org/10.1016/j.carbpol.2020.116842.
64. Yang, W., Owczarek, J. S., Fortunati, E., Kozanecki, M., Mazzaglia, A., Balestra, G. M., Kenny, J. M., Torre, L., & Puglia, D. (2016). Antioxidant and antibacterial lignin nanoparticles in polyvinyl alcohol/chitosan films for active packaging. *Industrial Crops and Products, 94*, 800–811. https://doi.org/10.1016/j.indcrop.2016.09.030.
65. Gorrasi, G., & Bugatti, V. (2016). Edible bio-nano-hybrid coatings for food protection based on pectin's and LDH-salicylate: Preparation and analysis of physical properties. *LWT–Food Science and Technology, 69*, 139–145. https://doi.org/10.1016/j.lwt.2016.01.013.
66. Demitri, C., de Benedictis, V. M., Madaghiele, M., Corcione, C. E., & Maffezzoli, A. (2016). Nanostructured active chitosan-based films for food packaging applications: Effect of graphene stacks on mechanical properties. *Measurement: Journal of the International Measurement Confederation, 90*, 418–423. https://doi.org/10.1016/j.measurement.2016.05.016.

CHAPTER 5

Degradation Studies of Bioabsorbable Polymeric Composites

ATANU KUMAR PAUL,[1] GOURHARI CHAKRABORTY,[1]
SHASANKA SEKHAR BORKOTOKY,[2] and ARBIND PRASAD[3]

[1]*Department of Chemical Engineering, National Institute of Technology, Tadepalligudem, West Godavari District, Andhra Pradesh, India*

[2]*Department of Chemical Engineering, Assam Engineering College, Jalukbari, Guwahati, Assam, India*

[3]*Mechanical Engineering Department, Katihar Engineering College (Under Department of Science, Technology and Technical Education, Government of Bihar), Katihar, Bihar, India*

ABSTRACT

Bioabsorbable polymers have become essential in the biomedical industry due to their ability to degrade in the body over time, eliminating the need for surgical removal after healing. The use of polymers in biomedical implants has expanded to include various applications, including sutures, pins, screws, and drug delivery systems. Biomaterials, including polymers, are commonly used to improve the functionality of medical implants. There are four types of biomaterials: polymer-based biomaterials, ceramic-based biomaterials, metal-ceramic-based biomaterials, and polymer-ceramic-based biomaterials. Researchers worldwide focus on diverse composite materials for various biomedical applications, including orthopedics, skin regeneration, cardio-vascular applications, and wound healing. The degradation of bioabsorbable materials can result in new chemical bonds and chemical decomposition, which allows for reabsorption by surrounding tissues. Bone tissue typically

Bioabsorbable Polymers for Drug Carriers and Fixation Devices. Arbind Prasad and Sougata Jana (Eds.)

grows into bioabsorbable scaffolds as implant materials degrade. Laminated composite materials have been found to have combined advantages, such as higher tensile strength, elongation at break, and elastic modulus. These composites also have adequate thermal stability, lower water absorption capacity, and antimicrobial activity, making them suitable for use as bone implants. The prospects of bioabsorbable polymeric composites and their degradation studies and thermal stability will continue to be researched and discussed in the biomedical industry.

5.1 INTRODUCTION

Bioabsorbable polymeric composites have gained significant consideration in recent times because of their potential use in various biomedical applications. These composites typically comprise a polymeric matrix augmented with bioabsorbable fillers or reinforcements such as fibers or particles to improve mechanical properties. Using bioabsorbable materials in composites has various advantages, including the potential of the materials to break down and be absorbed by the body over time, eliminating the need for surgical removal and lowering the risk of long-term consequences. The complexity of the degradation behavior of bioabsorbable polymeric composites is a subject of numerous studies. The degradation behavior of these materials depends on several features, such as the category of the polymer matrix, the nature and composition of the reinforcements, the processing conditions, and the environmental conditions where the composites are used. Understanding the behavior of these materials over time and their performance in different environments is crucial to optimizing their attributes for specific applications. Thus, degradation studies play a significant role in developing bioabsorbable polymeric composites for various biomedical applications.

The capacity of bioabsorbable polymeric composites to disintegrate *in vivo* eliminates the need for surgical removal or long-term presence in the body. This makes them ideal for transitory applications such as scaffolds for tissue engineering, where they can offer temporary mechanical support to damaged tissue while progressively dissolving and being replaced by newly created tissue. The controlled deterioration of these composites can be customized by selecting appropriate biodegradable polymers with varied degradation rates, allowing for precise control over the material's lifespan in the body.

Mechanical strength is an essential factor for orthopedic implants and sutures. Reinforcements are typically incorporated into bioabsorbable polymeric composites to increase their tensile strength, modulus, and toughness.

Reinforcements can be made from various materials in nanofibers, nanoparticles, or fibers, including ceramics, metals, and polymeric substances. Incorporating reinforcements can significantly enhance the mechanical performance of bioabsorbable composites, allowing them to be used in load-bearing applications. Using bioabsorbable composites in such applications eliminates the need for surgical removal, reducing the risk of long-term complications [57–61]. The bioabsorbable-based composite specifically used for bioimplants must be compatible with the body and also bioactive in nature so that the neo-generation of the bone takes place during the bone remodeling process [62–67]. The degrading behavior of bioabsorbable polymeric composites is an essential component that must be studied for them to be successfully applied in biomedical domains. Deterioration studies are carried out to evaluate the kinetics of deterioration, mass loss, changes in mechanical properties, and changes in chemical and physical properties of composites over time. Environmental variables (e.g., temperature, humidity), pH, and the presence of enzymes or other biological components can all influence how bioabsorbable composites degrade. Understanding how these composites degrade is critical for optimizing their performance and safety in biomedical applications.

The degradation behavior of bioabsorbable polymeric composites is a complex phenomenon that requires standardized protocols for reproducible and trustworthy results. A lack of such standardization poses issues in comparing results across different research groups, which impedes our understanding of the degrading behavior of bioabsorbable composites. Standardization can help to address this issue and enable comparison of results from various investigations, providing a better understanding of these materials. This chapter offers an overview of the degradation studies of bioabsorbable polymeric composites, including the approaches used, the factors influencing degradation, and the characterization techniques used to evaluate these materials' degradation behavior.

5.2 CHARACTERISTICS OF POLYMER-BASED BIOABSORBABLE MATERIALS

5.2.1 POLYGLYCOLIC ACID (PGA)

PGA is a bioabsorbable polymer initially developed for bone surgery, specifically for pins, screws, and plates. Its most notable characteristics are its strength, durability, and highly crystalline structure. PGA has a typical molecular weight range from 2.0×10^4 to [1.45×10^5] and a melting temperature of approximately 224°C. However, despite its 6–12 month clearance period, PGA loses its mechanical strength early in the *in vivo* environment, usually within 4–7 weeks after implantation, due to its rapid degradation [1]. This has led to complications in orthopedic surgery, such as fluid accumulation and sinus formation [2]. As a result, the use of PGA has been primarily limited to some instances in craniofacial surgery [3].

5.2.2 POLY-LACTIC ACID (PLA): PLLA AND PDLA

PLA is a biodegradable polymer that has a high molecular weight [(1.8×10^5 to 5.3×10^5)]. It contains optically active carbon in lactate, which gives rise to two stereoisomeric forms: Poly-L-Lactic Acid (PLLA) and Poly-D-Lactic Acid (PDLA) [4]. PLLA is a light-colored polymer melting from 174°C to 184°C. PLLA was utilized as a bioabsorbable osteosynthetic material in maxillofacial surgery later in the early 1990s, representing the first generation of this type of material. Due to its hydrophobic nature, PLLA exhibits greater resistance to hydrolysis than PGA.

PLLA has a long degradation period *in vitro*—about two years [1, 5] and over 3.5 years in a clinical context. When used for zygomatic fracture fixation, it was observed to cause adverse body reactions and unfavorable tissue reactions due to delayed disintegration [6]. In comparison to PLLA, PDLA has lesser crystallinity and hydrolysis resistance. PDLA, conversely, has a comparatively extended disintegration phase, and its crystalline elements may produce some inciting reactions [7]. There has been no research into using pure PDLA for maxillofacial osteo fixation.

5.2.3 COPOLYMERS OF PGA, PLLA, AND PDLA

The second generation of bioabsorbable osteosynthetic material comprises PGA, PLLA, and PDLA copolymers that degrade faster than their first-generation counterparts. Copolymerization of different acid derivatives allows for varying mechanical characteristics and degradation rates. Generally, higher levels of glycolide result in faster deterioration rates. Carbon dioxide and water, byproducts of the polymerization process through the citric acid cycle, are expelled from the body *via* the lungs [8, 9] (Figure 5.1). Unlike pure polymers, copolymers do not produce crystalline elements, and their degradation rate is sluggish enough to ensure outstanding biocompatibility [10, 11]. Poly-L-CO-DL-Lactide (PLDLA) copolymers and PLLA and glycolic acid (PLGA) copolymers are commonly used to create the bulk of copolymer-based devices. PLDLA copolymers have a high biodegradation rate but possess mechanical properties similar to PLA. Absorption for SR-PLDLA takes two to three years. PLGA was created in order to provide early, controlled absorption and stability. It has a decent resorption length of 9–15 months and provides strength for 6–8 weeks [12–14].

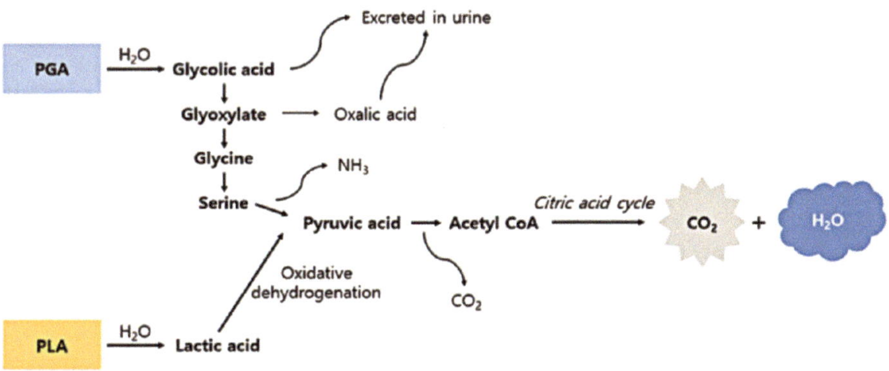

FIGURE 5.1 A schematic diagram is presented to depict the breakdown process of PGA and PLA polymers and copolymers.

5.3 DEGRADATION MECHANISMS

There are two types of degradation mechanisms for bioabsorbable polymeric composites: chemical degradation and physical degradation. Chemical degradation of bioabsorbable polymers is a complicated process in which various chemical reactions can occur, leading to deviations in the composite's molecular weight, polymer structure, and mechanical properties [15, 16]. Factors, for example, the polymer matrix type, reinforcing fillers, and environmental conditions, can all affect the rate and mechanism of chemical degradation. Enzymes or other biological agents can also play a role in breaking down the polymer matrix. The pH and temperature of the surrounding environment are critical parameters that can influence the degradation rate.

Physical deterioration of composites refers to the physical changes that can occur, such as swelling, hydrolysis, erosion, or crystallization. These changes can be due to moisture or fluid absorption, temperature fluctuations, or mechanical forces. Physical degradation can also affect various aspects of the composite, such as its mechanical properties, porosity, and mass loss.

5.4 FACTORS AFFECTING DEGRADATION

Several factors can influence the degradation behavior of bioabsorbable polymeric composites. Some of the key elements include:

1. **Polymer Composition:** The polymer type used as the composite's matrix can significantly impact the degradation behavior. Different bioabsorbable polymers, such as poly(lactic acid) (PLA), poly(glycolic acid) (PGA), poly(caprolactone) (PCL), and their copolymers, have different degradation rates and mechanisms due to differences in their chemical structures and properties [17, 18].
2. **Reinforcement Type and Content:** The nature and composition of the reinforcements used in the composites can affect their degradation behavior. For example, the use of bioabsorbable fibers, such as poly(lactic acid) (PLA) or poly(glycolic acid) (PGA) fibers, as reinforcements can alter the degradation rate and mechanism of the composites compared to composites without reinforcements.
3. **Processing Conditions:** The processing conditions used during the fabrication of the composites, such as temperature, pressure, and curing time, can affect their degradation behavior. For instance, higher processing temperatures or longer curing times can result in increased crystallinity, which may affect the degradation rate of the composites.
4. **Environmental Conditions:** The environmental conditions in which the composites are used, such as temperature, pH, and the presence of enzymes or other biological agents, can significantly influence the degradation behavior of bioabsorbable polymeric composites [19]. For example, composites used in the body may experience different degradation rates and mechanisms depending on the location of the implant, such as in bone, soft tissue, or the bloodstream, and the physiological conditions at that site.
5. **Composite Architecture:** The architecture of the composites, such as the arrangement and orientation of the reinforcements, can also impact their degradation behavior [20]. For example, composites with aligned fibers may degrade differently than composites with randomly dispersed fibers, as the fiber orientation can affect the diffusion of degradation agents into the composite.

5.5 CONVENTIONAL BIOABSORBABLE PLATES AND SCREWS

Bioabsorbable materials from polymers have made significant progress since the first trial in 1971, which used such materials to stabilize a fractured facial bone in the maxillofacial area [21]. The plates, which are absorbable, and the screws' low strength initially necessitated a large and robust design to provide adequate mechanical stability. Nevertheless, with the development of self-reinforcing technology, it has become possible to produce bioabsorbable devices that are stronger, longer-lasting, and more biocompatible [22]. The self-reinforcement technique entails aligning polymeric fibers and mixing polymers to achieve an oriented structure. Self-reinforcement is a phenomenon that causes polymers' toughness, mechanical strength, and modulus to increase significantly. According to research, self-reinforced (SR) biodegradable plates and screws provide enough strength and stability to treat fractures in high-stress locations like the mandible [23]. Bioabsorbable polymer plates and screws are currently utilized in maxillofacial trauma surgery, orthognathic surgery, and pediatric surgery as a direct outcome of advancements in medical technology and research, as indicated in Table 5.1.

TABLE 5.1 System of Polymer-based Bioabsorbable Plates and Screws Applied for Osteofixation in Maxillofacial Bone Surgery

Product Name	Manufacturer	Polymer Composition	Degradation Time
Biofixfi SR-PGA	Bionx implants, Tampere, Finland	SR-PGA	6 weeks
Biofixfi SR-PLLA	Bionx implants, Tampere, Finland	SR-PLLA	5–7 years
Resomerfi LR708	Evonik Industries, Darmstadt, Germany	PLLA (70%) + PDLLA (30%)	2–3 years
MacroPore	MacroPore Biosurgery Inc., San Diego, CA, USA	PLLA (70%) + PDLLA (30%)	2–3 years
Macrosorb	MacroPore Biosurgery Inc., San Diego, CA, USA	PLLA (70%) + PDLLA (30%)	2–3 years
Biosorb FX	Linvatec Biomaterials Ltd., Tampere, Finland	PLLA (70%) + PDLLA (30%)	2–3 years
Resorb X	KLS Martin Group, Tuttlingen, Germany	PLLA (50%) + PDLLA (50%)	12–30 months
PolyMax	Synthes, Oberdorf, Switzerland	PLLA (70%) + PDLLA (30%)	2 years

TABLE 5.1 *(Continued)*

Product Name	Manufacturer	Polymer Composition	Degradation Time
PolyMax	RAPID Synthes, Oberdorf, Switzerland	PLLA (85%) + PGA (15%)	12 months
Rapidsorb	DePuy Synthes, West Chester, PA, USA	PLLA (85%) + PGA (15%)	12 months
Lactosorb	Lorenz, Jacksonville, FL, USA	PLLA (82%) + PGA (18%)	12 months
Delta	Stryker Leibinger Corp., Kalamazoo, MI, USA	PLLA (85%), PGA (10%), PDLA (5%)	8–13 months
Inion CPS	Inion Inc., Tampere, Finland	PLLA, PGA, TMC–proportion varies	2–4 years
Inion CPS	Baby Inion Inc., Tampere, Finland	PLLA, PGA, TMC–proportion varies	2–3 years
Osteotrans-MX	TEIJIN Medical corp., Osaka, Japan	PLLA (60–70 wt%), u-HA (30–40 wt%)	4.5–5.5 years

5.6 THERMAL PROPERTIES

Various reports indicate that information about the breakdown due to the thermal degradation of poly(lactic acid) or PLA is ambiguous and subject to debate. Vogel et al. [24] reported the production of water, carbon dioxide, carbon monoxide, methane, and acetaldehyde during the thermal breakdown of PLA. However, Aoyagi et al. [25] perceived that the breakdown study of PLA leads to the release of acetaldehyde, lactide monomer, and oligomers. As the temperature rises, lactide emerges as the principal byproduct of degradation. Additionally, Kopinke et al. [26] suggested that the degradation of this polymer takes place above 200°C through intramolecular transesterification, yielding lactide and cyclic oligomers, as well as cis-elimination that generates acrylic acid and acyclic oligomers. On the contrary, as indicated by Aoyagi et al. [25]; and Vogel et al. [24], crotonic acid and its oligomers are primarily produced through an arbitrary chain scission reaction of the ester groups during the thermal degradation of polyhydroxybutyrate (PHB). However, Li et al. [27] discovered that the thermal breakdown of PHB results in the formation of not only esters such as propenyl-2-butenoate and butyric-2-butenoate, but also carboxylic acids such as 2-butenoic acid (crotonic acid) and even propene.

Thermal analysis is a widely used method to investigate the effect of temperature on a substance's chemical, physical, and structural properties.

Temperature is a fundamental parameter crucial in determining the behavior of chemical reactions, physical attributes, and structural alterations. Thermodynamic analysis can therefore be considered any method of evaluating a substance that manipulates temperature [28]. However, this term has traditionally been restricted to methods that exploit thermogravimetric and calorimetric phenomena [29]. Thermal analysis typically employs three primary techniques, namely differential thermal analysis (DTA), thermogravimetry analysis (TGA), and differential scanning calorimetry (DSC). The DTA technique determines the temperature variance between a studied sample and a reference material, while TGA determines weight loss as measured by thermogravimetry. DSC measures the heat flow during temperature changes [29, 30]. Thermogravimetry is a commonly employed technique to evaluate the heat endurance of composites, including natural fibers and polymers. The stability of such composites, which are made up of natural fibers and polymers, has been exhaustively analyzed using TG/DTG research. The characteristics of lignocellulosic fibers can be considerably affected by temperature [29].

In their study, Yao et al. [31] investigated the kinetics of thermal degradation of 10 distinct types of natural fibers. These organic materials comprised wood, bamboo, agricultural waste, and bast fibers. The authors depicted the entire thermogravimetric degradation process of these natural fibers in Figures 5.2(a) and (b), utilizing a heating rate of 2°C/min. Cellulose thermal degradation often results in a distinct DTG peak with a visible shoulder (indicated by an arrow), frequently caused by hemicellulose thermal decomposition under inert conditions. Nonetheless, in some cases, the shoulder peaks of low-temperature hemicelluloses coincide with the prominent peaks of cellulose, as illustrated in Figure 5.2(b), rendering them indistinguishable. Lignin breakdown usually occurs at higher temperatures, as evidenced in Figures 5.2(a) and (b). As natural fibers are composed of lignocellulosic materials, their TG and DTG profiles are similar, implying that they have comparable thermal degradation characteristics.

Herrera-Kao et al. [32] used TGA to examine the heat degradation of three popular biodegradable polyesters: polycaprolactone (PCL), polylactic acid (PLA), and polyhydroxybutyrate (PHB). PCL and PLA degradation curves indicated a single decomposition level. However, PHB's TGA showed two different degradations. Figures 5.2(c) and (d) depict each biopolymer's TGA mass loss curve and the related derivative curve (DTGA). The maximum rate of breakdown temperature varied with polymer type.

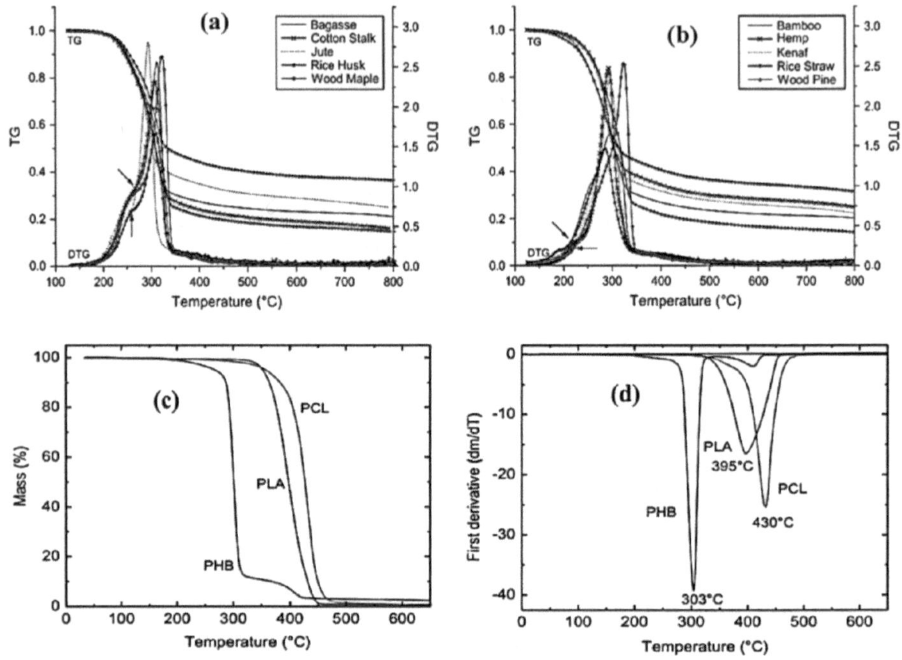

FIGURE 5.2 Thermogravimetric decomposition of natural fibers and biodegradable polymers. (a) Natural fibers with prominent hemicellulose shoulders; and (b) not prominent hemicellulose shoulders; (c) TGA for PCL, PLA; and PHB (d) DTGA for PCL, PLA, and PHB.

5.7 THERMAL DEGRADATION OF BIO-NANOCOMPOSITES

Biopolymers are renewable natural source polymers that provide a viable foundation for adding various additives such as antioxidants, antimicrobials, antifungal agents, and other nutrients [33, 34]. Natural biopolymers, synthetic biodegradable polymers, and biopolymers created through microbial fermentation can be classified depending on the raw materials utilized and the developed method [35]. Carbon nanotubes, nanoclays, cellulose nanowhiskers, and ultrafine layered titanate are examples of inorganic nanoparticles that have been used to improve the characteristics of several biopolymers [36–38].

Biopolymers represent a class of biologically sourced polymers with the potential for diverse functionalities by incorporating various additives, encompassing antioxidants, antimicrobials, antifungal agents, and other nutrients [33, 34]. Raw materials and production processes provide a basis for classifying polymers into three categories: natural biopolymers, synthetic biodegradable polymers, and biopolymers produced through microbial fermentation [35]. Additionally, inorganic nanoparticles, including carbon nanotubes, nanoclays, cellulose nanowhiskers, and ultrafine layered titanate, have been employed to enhance the characteristics of multiple biopolymers [36–38].

To overcome these shortcomings, mixing, copolymerization, and filling procedures have been used to improve the thermomechanical characteristics of biopolymers [39]. Bio-nanocomposites, a new hybrid material class incorporating diverse nanofillers into the biopolymer matrix, provide exceptional material characteristics [20, 40]. Good thermal stability is essential for many industrial applications, which can be obtained with a minimal proportion of filler, such as clay. Clay nanofillers are excellent insulators and mass transport barriers for volatile compounds produced during decomposition [38]. Because clay minerals like montmorillonite (MMT) are thermally stable up to 900°C, thermal gravimetric analysis (TGA) is used to quantify the clay content of bio-nanocomposites. Combining polylactic acid (PLA) with organically adapted fluorohectorite (FH) or MMT clay was the first study to indicate an improvement in the thermal stability of bio-nanocomposites.

Carrasco et al. [41] found that the thermal stability of polylactic acid (PLA) can be enhanced by increasing the crystallinity of the polymer through annealing or by blending it with other polymers such as poly(butylene succinate) (PBS). They also found that PLA processed by injection molding had higher thermal stability than PLA processed by extrusion or blow molding. Additionally, residual moisture in the PLA decreased its thermal stability, indicating the importance of controlling the moisture content during processing.

The researchers discovered that untreated PLA was more stable than PLA that had been processed and thermally treated. According to de Paula et al. [42], adding cellulose nanowhiskers to poly(D,L-lactide) increased thermal stability by raising the onset decomposition temperature by 12 and 26°C for 1% and 5% loadings, respectively. On the other hand, the effect of cellulose nanowhiskers on PLA thermal stability was minor [43].

5.7 SOME CASE STUDIES

5.7.1 CASE STUDY 1: DEGRADATION OF POLYLACTIC ACID (PLA) REINFORCED WITH NATURAL FIBERS

PLA is a type of polymer that can naturally break down and has been widely utilized in medical fields due to its ability to work well with biological systems and be absorbed by them. Lately, there has been an increasing focus on producing PLA composites strengthened with natural fibers such as cellulose. The appeal of these composites stems from the sustainable and renewable nature of their reinforcing fibers. In an investigation, it was reported by Daud et al. [44] that the degradation of PLA composites reinforced with cellulose fibers occurs under various environmental conditions [44].

According to the study led by Daud et al. [44], incorporating cellulose fibers in PLA composites increased their hydrophilicity and resulted in faster degradation due to increased water uptake. The degradation caused a decline in the tensile strength and modulus of the composites, which was due to the breakdown of ester bonds in PLA and the plasticization caused by the diffusion of water into the composite. SEM analysis of the degraded composites revealed increased porosity and surface roughness, indicating the degradation of the polymer matrix and the release of cellulose fibers from the composite.

The study also looked into the results of environmental variables on the degrading behavior of PLA composites reinforced with cellulose fibers. The composites degraded faster in acidic environments due to the acid's hydrolysis of ester linkages in PLA. In alkaline circumstances, however, the cellulose fibers themselves stained, resulting in a loss of the mechanical capabilities of the composites. According to the findings, the degrading behavior of PLA composites reinforced with cellulose fibers is influenced not only by the hydrophilicity of the fibers and the interaction between the fibers and the polymer matrix but also by environmental factors.

5.7.2 CASE STUDY 2: DEGRADATION OF POLY(LACTIC-CO-GLYCOLIC ACID) (PLGA) REINFORCED WITH BIOCERAMIC PARTICLES

Poly(lactic-co-glycolic acid) (PLGA) is a popular bioabsorbable polymer for bone tissue engineering, and PLGA composites reinforced with hydroxyapatite (HA) bioceramic particles have been studied as potential bone substitute materials [45]. The observed composites demonstrated a reduced rate of degradation in comparison to pure PLGA, as evidenced by a more gradual decline in molecular weight. Additionally, these composites exhibited greater uniformity in their surface morphology, with a diminished presence of cracks and pores. The sustained release of calcium ions from the hydroxyapatite (HA) particles during degradation suggests that they remained stable and have the potential to promote bone tissue regeneration by stimulating osteoblast cell proliferation and differentiation. The reading highlights the possibility of PLGA/HA composites as a promising material for bone tissue engineering.

5.7.3 CASE STUDY 3: DEGRADATION OF POLY(E-CAPROLACTONE) (PCL) REINFORCED WITH NANOFILLERS

Poly(ε-caprolactone) (PCL) is another commonly used bioabsorbable polymer that has been investigated for various biomedical applications [46–49]. PCL composites reinforced with nanofillers, such as nanoparticles or nanofibers, have gained attention due to their potential to improve PCL's mechanical properties and biodegradation behavior.

The investigation found that adding CNFs to PCL meaningfully improved the tensile strength and modulus of the composites. The existence of CNFs, nevertheless, expedited the deterioration of PCL, evident from a swifter decline in molecular weight and mechanical characteristics when juxtaposed with untainted PCL. The CNFs were found to create additional pathways for water penetration into the composites, leading to increased hydrolysis of the ester bonds in PCL and faster degradation [47].

The study also investigated the morphological changes of the composites during degradation using SEM analysis [48]. It was observed that the PCL/CNF composites showed a rougher surface with more cracks and voids compared to pure PCL, indicating the degradation of the polymer matrix and the discharge of CNFs from the composite. The CNFs were more resistant to degradation than PCL, suggesting that the composites exhibited a selective degradation behavior, with the CNFs remaining in the degraded matrix.

Furthermore, the study investigated the cytocompatibility of the PCL/CNF composites employing *in vitro* cell culture experiments. The composites presented good cytocompatibility and supported the proliferation of human mesenchymal stem cells, representing their potential for tissue engineering applications.

5.7.4 CASE STUDY 4: DEGRADATION OF POLYDIOXANONE (PDO) REINFORCED WITH FIBERGLASS

Polydioxanone (PDO) is a bioabsorbable polymer used for various biomedical applications, such as sutures and tissue scaffolds [50]. PDO composites reinforced with fiberglass have been inspected for potential use in orthopedic applications. An investigation by Bisht et al. [62] suggested the degradation behavior of PDO composites reinforced with fiberglass in different environmental conditions.

The study found that adding fiberglass to PDO expressively upgraded the mechanical properties of the composites, including tensile strength, modulus, and toughness [51]. However, fiberglass's presence also accelerated PDO's degradation, as indicated by a faster decrease in molecular weight and mechanical properties than pure PDO. The study attributed the accelerated degradation to the amplified hydrophilicity of the composites due to fiberglass, which facilitated water penetration and hydrolysis of the ester bonds in PDO.

The study also investigated the morphological changes of the composites during degradation using SEM analysis. It was observed that the PDO/fiberglass composites showed a more porous surface and a higher degree of fiber exposure compared to pure PDO, indicating the degradation of the polymer matrix and the discharge of fiberglass from the composite.

Furthermore, the study evaluated the *in vivo* degradation behavior of the PDO/fiberglass composites in a rat model [51]. The composites gradually lost mechanical properties over time and were absorbed within 12 weeks without causing any adverse inflammatory responses. The study concluded that adding fiberglass to PDO can improve the mechanical properties of the composites but also accelerates their degradation, which can be advantageous for specific biomedical applications where a faster absorption rate is desired.

5.7.5 CASE STUDY 5: BIODEGRADATION OF BIOCOMPOSITES WITH DIFFERENT AMOUNTS OF WOOD FLOUR

Wood flour is a plentiful and renewable natural substance with desired qualities such as low density, high stiffness, and biodegradability, making it a cost-effective candidate for use in composites [52]. Using a micro-extruder MiniLab II, composites were created by integrating wood flour (WF) as a natural filler into a P(3HB-co-4HB) polymer matrix. The present study delved into an inquiry into the impact of filler type and filler content on the mechanical properties of composites. The inclusion of wood flour caused the polymer matrix to be disrupted during tensile stress. The observed development in thermal stability was attributable to the acidic byproducts of hydrolytic breakdown and the chemicals derived from the filler.

Tensile and flexural testing were performed to evaluate the influence of filler type and content on the mechanical properties of the composites. The following parameters were measured: tensile strength (σ_m), Young's modulus

(E_t), and elongation at break (ε_b). The results showed that using wood flour as a filler decreased tensile strength values compared to the neat matrix, with the decrease directly proportional to the filler quantity. This was attributed to the filler's poor adherence to the polymer matrix. The absence of a coupling agent during processing lowered tensile strength even further as filler content rose. Furthermore, the wood flour filler created a tensile load rupture in the polymer matrix.

This work aimed to investigate the degrading behavior of composites formed from P(3HB-co-4HB) and wood flour in laboratory and industrial composting conditions and the antibacterial characteristics of some materials when treated with nisin. The results revealed that the accumulation of wood flour hastened the abiotic deterioration of the composites. Furthermore, including wood flour influenced the thermal properties of the studied materials throughout degradation. The addition of filler also affected the composites' mechanical properties, resulting in higher stiffness when compared to the pure matrix. Based on these findings, it is proposed that P(3HB-co-4HB) composites containing wood flour could be used in food packaging applications. Furthermore, by applying a nisin coating on the external surface of the chosen material, it may be feasible to improve the protective characteristics of such packaging.

- **Case study 6:** Degradation of Polymer-based Composites in Corrosive Media: Amini [53] noted that over the last 20 years, research efforts have concentrated on utilizing unsaturated polyester resin to develop engineering composites. In order to assess the performance of these composites in the presence of hydrogen chloride solutions, this study evaluated their bending, tensile, and hardness properties. Maintaining the mechanical properties and minimizing the degradation of these materials under these circumstances is critical; hence, understanding their behavior in contact with acidic media is crucial. The study identified a correlation between the composite samples' exposure time, temperature, and mechanical properties.

  The study's findings highlight the importance of considering the effects of chemical exposure on the mechanical properties of composites, primarily when they are intended for use in harsh environments such as the oil and chemical industries. The results indicate that using glass fiber/PE composites may not be suitable for prolonged exposure to acidic media, as the mechanical properties degrade significantly over time. This information can aid in selecting materials for specific applications and designing appropriate maintenance and replacement schedules. Overall, the study underscores the need for a comprehensive understanding of the behavior of composite materials in harsh environments to ensure their long-term performance and reliability.

- **Case Study 7: Morphology, Thermal Properties, Mechanical Properties and Degradation of PLGA/PTMC Composites:** The morphology, thermal properties, mechanical properties, and degrading behavior of composites produced from poly(lactic-co-glycolic acid) (PLGA) and poly(trimethylene carbonate) (PTMC) were studied by Qi et al. [54]. When placed in the human body, metallic implants used for bone regeneration have potential dangers. To solve this problem, solution co-precipitation was used to create PLGA/PTMC composites. It was discovered that adding PTMC to the composites decreased their tensile strength and tensile modulus. The study aimed to explore the effects of altering PTMC concentration on the miscibility, fracture morphology, thermodynamic characteristics, mechanical properties, and degrading behavior of the PLGA/PTMC composites to create a variety of new biodegradable materials.

  Risks associated with using metal implants as bone repair materials include bone corrosion, a stress shielding effect, and non-degradation, which could necessitate additional surgery. To address these problems, PLGA/PTMC composites were created using a solution co-precipitation technique. The shape, thermodynamic properties, mechanical characteristics, crystallization characteristics, surface water wettability, and degradation characteristics of PLGA/PTMC/PLT composites were all examined in this work regarding variable PTMC concentration. The phase separation study revealed that PLGA and PTMC were physically mixing and were thermodynamically immiscible. The composites' tensile strength and tensile modulus were reduced due to the inclusion of PTMC.

- **Case study 8: Thermal, Mechanical, and Degradation Behavior of Banana Fibers Reinforced Polypropylene Composites:** The phase separation study revealed that PLGA and PTMC were physically mixing and were thermodynamically immiscible [55]. The composites' tensile strength and tensile modulus were reduced due to the inclusion of PTMC. The degradation investigation showed a decrease in intrinsic viscosity concerning the soaking period, and after 8 weeks and 12 weeks, respectively, the tensile strength and mass loss dramatically reduced. These results indicate the potential of PLGA/PTMC composites as biodegradable bone healing materials. The low density, low cost, renewable resources, biodegradability, and minimal health risks of natural fibers are only a few of their benefits. However, they also have certain drawbacks, including lower thermal stability and incompatibility with hydrophobic polymers. Securing the structural and functional stability of natural fiber-reinforced composites during their service life and their degradability after service life is one of the hurdles in creating them.

An investigation on the effects of chemical treatment on the thermal, mechanical, and degrading properties of polymer composites reinforced with banana fibers was undertaken by Komal [55]. Natural fibers, like those found in bananas, have several benefits, including low cost, low density, being a renewable resource, and posing few health risks. They do not mix well with hydrophobic polymers and have decreased thermal stability, among other drawbacks. Developing natural fiber-reinforced composites is difficult because they must be structurally and functionally stable throughout their service life and degradable at the end. According to the study, alkaline treatment successfully removed non-cellulosic components from banana fibers, which caused the peak seen at 245°C for untreated fibers to vanish. Compared to PUBF composites, the PTBF composites' tensile and flexural strengths were enhanced by 3.8% and 5.17%, respectively, by adding treated fibers to the polypropylene matrix [56]. There was no difference in the tensile modulus between PTBF composites and PUBF composites. However, the flexural modulus of the former was increased by 5.3%. For the investigation, extrusion-injection molding was used to create PP composites reinforced with banana fibers.

Komal [55] investigated the impact of chemical behavior on the thermal, mechanical, and degrading behavior of composites reinforced with banana fibers. Natural fibers, such as banana fibers, are low-cost, low-density, renewable resources, and pose few health risks; however, when combined with hydrophobic polymers, they exhibit lower thermal stability and incompatibility. Making natural fiber reinforced composites structurally and operationally robust throughout their service life while ensuring they are disposal-friendly at the end of their service life is a challenge. The research demonstrated that the alkaline treatment of banana fibers efficiently eliminated non-cellulosic materials, causing the peak at 245°C for untreated banana fibers to vanish. The tensile and flexural strength of PTBF composites increased by 3.8% and 5.17%, respectively, when treated fibers were added to the polypropylene matrix [56]. In contrast to PUBF composites, the flexural modulus of PTBF composites was also increased by 5.3%, with no change in the tensile modulus. In the investigation, PP composites reinforced with banana fibers were created utilizing the extrusion-injection molding technique.

5.8 CONCLUSION

Bioabsorbable polymeric composites are promising biomedical materials with advantages such as biodegradability, customized degradation rates, and mechanical reinforcement. However, degradation studies of these composites are complicated, necessitating extensive research to comprehend their degradation behavior, mechanical property changes, and long-term consequences on host tissue. Addressing the challenges associated with bioabsorbable composite degradation studies would contribute to developing safe and reliable materials for biomedical applications, potentially revolutionizing various fields of medicine such as tissue engineering, drug delivery, and medical implants. Degradation studies of bioabsorbable polymeric composites are critical for understanding how these materials behave over time and optimizing their characteristics for biomedical applications. Researchers can gain valuable insights into how these materials behave in different environmental conditions by conducting comprehensive investigations of the degradation mechanisms, rate, and extent of bioabsorbable composites, which can inform the design and development of bioabsorbable composites with tailored properties.

The degrading behavior of bioabsorbable polymeric composites is a complicated and diverse phenomenon impacted by various factors. More study is needed in this area to improve our understanding of the degradation behavior of bioabsorbable composites and optimize their characteristics for biomedical applications. Standardization of testing methodologies, long-term degradation research, *in vivo* evaluations, multiscale modeling, and the study of novel reinforcement materials are just a few of the topics that need to be looked at further. Continued study in these areas will help to develop advanced bioabsorbable composites with improved characteristics, performance, and biocompatibility, opening the path for their widespread use in biomedical sectors.

KEYWORDS

- **biocompatibility**
- **biomedical applications**
- **biomedical sectors**
- **polymeric composites**
- **polymers**
- **polypropylene matrix**

REFERENCES

1. Schumann, P., Lindhorst, D., Wagner, M. E. H., Schramm, A., Gellrich, N. C., & Rücker, M. (2013). Perspectives on resorbable osteosynthesis materials in craniomaxillofacial surgery. *Pathobiology, 80*(4), 211–217. https://doi.org/10.1159/000348328.
2. Vasenius, J., Vainionpää, S., Vihtonen, K., Mäkelä, A., Rokkanen, P., Mero, M., & Törmälä, P. (1990). Comparison of in vitro hydrolysis, subcutaneous, and intramedullary implantation to evaluate the strength retention of absorbable osteosynthesis implants. *Biomaterials, 11*(7), 501–504. https://doi.org/10.1016/0142-9612(90)90065-X.
3. Bostman, O., Hirvensalo, E., Makinen, J., & Rokkanen, P. (1990). Foreign-body reactions to fracture fixation implants of biodegradable synthetic polymers. *Journal of Bone and Joint Surgery–Series B, 72*(4), 592–596. https://doi.org/10.1302/0301-620X.72B4.2199452.
4. Chakraborty, G., Katiyar, V., & Pugazhenthi, G. (2021). Improvisation of polylactic acid (PLA)/exfoliated graphene (GR) nanocomposite for detection of metal ions (Cu^{2+}). *Composites Science and Technology, 213*, 108877. https://doi.org/10.1016/j.compscitech.2021.108877.
5. Pihlajamaki, H., Bostman, O., Hirvensalo, E., Tormala, P., & Rokkanen, P. (1992). Absorbable pins of self-reinforced poly-L-lactic acid for fixation of fractures and osteotomies. *Journal of Bone and Joint Surgery–British Volume, 74-B* (6), 853–857. https://doi.org/10.1302/0301-620X.74B6.1447246.
6. Bergsma, E. J., Rozema, F. R., Bos, R. R. M., & Bruijn, W. C. (1993). Foreign body reactions to resorbable poly(L-lactide) bone plates and screws used for the fixation of unstable zygomatic fractures. *Journal of Oral and Maxillofacial Surgery, 51*(6), 666–670. https://doi.org/10.1016/S0278-2391(10)80267-8.

7. Bergsma, J. E., de Bruijn, W. C., Rozema, F. R., Bos, R. R. M., & Boering, G. (1995). Late degradation tissue response to poly(L-lactide) bone plates and screws. *Biomaterials, 16*(1), 25–31. https://doi.org/10.1016/0142-9612(95)91092-D.
8. Edwards, R. C., Kiely, K. D., & Eppley, B. L. (2001). The fate of resorbable poly-L-lactic/poly-glycolic acid (LactoSorb) bone fixation devices in orthognathic surgery. *Journal of Oral and Maxillofacial Surgery, 59*(1), 19–25. https://doi.org/10.1053/joms.2001.19267.
9. Peltoniemi, H., Ashammakhi, N., Kontio, R., Waris, T., Salo, A., Lindqvist, C., Grätz, K., & Suuronen, R. (2002). The use of bioabsorbable osteofixation devices in craniomaxillofacial surgery. *Oral Surgery, Oral Medicine, Oral Pathology, Oral Radiology, and Endodontics, 94*(1), 5–14. https://doi.org/10.1067/moe.2002.122160.
10. Park, Y. W. (2015). Bioabsorbable osteofixation for orthognathic surgery. *Maxillofacial Plastic and Reconstructive Surgery, 37*(1), 6. https://doi.org/10.1186/s40902-015-0003-7.
11. Schumann, P., Lindhorst, D., Wagner, M. E. H., Schramm, A., Gellrich, N. C., & Rücker, M. (2013). Perspectives on resorbable osteosynthesis materials in craniomaxillofacial surgery. *Pathobiology, 80*(4), 211–217. https://doi.org/10.1159/000348328.
12. Eppley, B. L., & Reilly, M. (1997). Degradation characteristics of PLLA-PGA bone fixation devices. *Journal of Craniofacial Surgery, 8*(2), 116–120. https://doi.org/10.1097/00001665-199703000-00010.
13. Pietrzak, W. S., Sarver, D. R., & Verstynen, M. L. (1997). Bioabsorbable polymer science for the practicing surgeon. *Journal of Craniofacial Surgery, 8*(2), 87–91. https://doi.org/10.1097/00001665-199703000-00004.
14. Pietrzak, W. S., Verstynen, M. L., & Sarver, D. R. (1997). Bioabsorbable fixation devices: Status for the craniomaxillofacial surgeon. *Journal of Craniofacial Surgery, 8*(2), 92–96. https://doi.org/10.1097/00001665-199703000-00005.
15. Borkotoky, S. S., Chakraborty, G., & Katiyar, V. (2018). Thermal degradation behavior and crystallization kinetics of poly (lactic acid) and cellulose nanocrystals (CNC) based microcellular composite foams. *International Journal of Biological Macromolecules, 118*, 1518–1531. https://doi.org/10.1016/j.ijbiomac.2018.06.202.
16. Chakraborty, G., Valapa, R. B., Pugazhenthi, G., & Katiyar, V. (2018). Investigating the properties of poly (lactic acid)/exfoliated graphene-based nanocomposites fabricated by versatile coating approach. *International Journal of Biological Macromolecules, 113*, 1080–1091. https://doi.org/10.1016/j.ijbiomac.2018.03.037.
17. Marras, S. I., Zuburtikudis, I., & Panayiotou, C. (2007). Nanostructure vs. microstructure: Morphological and thermomechanical characterization of poly (L-lactic acid)/layered silicate hybrids. *European Polymer Journal, 43*(6), 2191–2206. https://doi.org/10.1016/j.eurpolymj.2007.03.013.
18. Eslami, H., Azimi Lisar, H., Jafarzadeh Kashi, T. S., Tahriri, M., Ansari, M., Rafiei, T., Bastami, F., Shahin-Shamsabadi, A., Mashhadi Abbas, F., & Tayebi, L. (2018). Poly (Lactic-Co-Glycolic Acid) (PLGA)/TiO_2 nanotube bioactive composite as a novel scaffold for bone tissue engineering: In vitro and in vivo studies. *Biologicals, 53*, 51–62. https://doi.org/10.1016/j.biologicals.2018.02.004.
19. Chen, C. X., & Yoon, J. S. (2005). Morphology and thermal properties of poly(L-lactide)/poly (butylene succinate-co-butylene adipate) compounded with twice functionalized clay. *Journal of Polymer Science Part B: Polymer Physics, 43*(4), 478–487. https://doi.org/10.1002/polb.20345.

20. Yang, K. K., Wang, X. L., & Wang, Y. Z. (2007). Progress in nanocomposite of biodegradable polymer. *Journal of Industrial Engineering Chemistry, 13*(4), 485–500. https://doi.org/10.1016/j.jiec.2007.03.002.
21. Cutright, D. E., Hunsuck, E. E., & Beasley, J. D. (1971). Fracture reduction using a biodegradable material, polylactic acid. *Journal of Oral Surgery, 29*(6), 393–397.
22. Toermaelae, P. (1992). Biodegradable self-reinforced composite materials: Manufacturing structure and mechanical properties. *Clinical Materials, 10*(1), 29–34.
23. Kallela, I., Iizuka, T., Salo, A., & Lindqvist, C. (1999). Lag-screw fixation of anterior mandibular fractures using biodegradable polylactide screws: A preliminary report. *Journal of Oral and Maxillofacial Surgery, 57*(2), 113–118. https://doi.org/10.1016/S0278-2391(99)90220-3.
24. Vogel, C., & Siesler, H. W. (2008). Thermal degradation of poly(ε-caprolactone), poly (L-lactic acid) and their blends with poly(3-hydroxy-butyrate) studied by TGA/FT-IR spectroscopy. *Macromolecular Symposia, 265*(1), 183–194. https://doi.org/10.1002/masy.200850520.
25. Aoyagi, Y., Yamashita, K., & Doi, Y. (2002). Thermal degradation of poly[(R)-3-hydroxybutyrate], poly[ε-caprolactone], and poly[(S)-lactide]. *Polymer Degradation and Stability, 76*(1), 53–59. https://doi.org/10.1016/S0141-3910(01)00265-8.
26. Kopinke, F. D., & Mackenzie, K. (1997). Mechanistic aspects of the thermal degradation of poly (lactic acid) and poly (β-hydroxybutyric acid). *Journal of Analytical and Applied Pyrolysis, 40–41*, 43–53. https://doi.org/10.1016/S0165-2370(97)00022-3.
27. Li, S. D., He, J. D., Yu, P. H., & Cheung, M. K. (2003). Thermal degradation of poly(3-hydroxybutyrate) and poly(3-hydroxybutyrate-co-3-hydroxyvalerate) as studied by TG, TG-FTIR, and Py-GC/MS. *Journal of Applied Polymer Science, 89*(8), 1530–1536. https://doi.org/10.1002/app.12249.
28. Sagar, S., Iqbal, N., Maqsood, A., Shahid, M., Shah, N. A., Jamil, T., & Bassyouni, M. I. (2015). Fabrication and thermal characteristics of functionalized carbon nanotubes impregnated polydimethylsiloxane nanocomposites. *Journal of Composite Materials, 49*(8), 995–1006. https://doi.org/10.1177/0021998314528733.
29. Monteiro, S. N., Calado, V., Rodriguez, R. J. S., & Margem, F. M. (2012). Thermogravimetric behavior of natural fibers reinforced polymer composites—An overview. *Materials Science and Engineering: A, 557*, 17–28. https://doi.org/10.1016/j.msea.2012.05.109.
30. Gholampour, A., & Ozbakkaloglu, T. (2020). A review of natural fiber composites: Properties, modification and processing techniques, characterization, applications. *Journal of Materials Science, 55*(2), 829–892. https://doi.org/10.1007/s10853-019-03990-y.
31. Yao, F., Wu, Q., Lei, Y., Guo, W., & Xu, Y. (2008). Thermal decomposition kinetics of natural fibers: Activation energy with dynamic thermogravimetric analysis. *Polymer Degradation and Stability, 93*(1), 90–98. https://doi.org/10.1016/j.polymdegradstab.2007.10.012.
32. Herrera-Kao, W. A., Loría-Bastarrachea, M. I., Pérez-Padilla, Y., Cauich-Rodríguez, J. V., Vázquez-Torres, H., & Cervantes-Uc, J. M. (2018). Thermal degradation of poly(caprolactone), poly (lactic acid), and poly(hydroxybutyrate) studied by TGA/FTIR and other analytical techniques. *Polymer Bulletin, 75*(11), 4191–4205. https://doi.org/10.1007/s00289-017-2260-3.

33. Halleux, J., & Clarinval, A. M. (2005). Classification of biodegradable polymers. In *Biodegradable Polymers: Industrial Applications* (pp. 1–24). https://doi.org/10.1201/9781439823699.pt1.
34. Kümmerer, K. (2007). Sustainable from the very beginning: Rational design of molecules by life cycle engineering as an important approach for green pharmacy and green chemistry. *Green Chemistry, 9*(9), 899–907. https://doi.org/10.1039/B703825E.
35. Rhim, J. W., Park, H. M., & Ha, C. S. (2013). Bio-nanocomposites for food packaging applications. *Progress in Polymer Science, 38*(10), 1629–1652. https://doi.org/10.1016/j.progpolymsci.2013.05.008.
36. Kumar, A. P., Depan, D., Singh Tomer, N., & Singh, R. P. (2009). Nanoscale particles for polymer degradation and stabilization—Trends and future perspectives. *Progress in Polymer Science, 34*(4), 479–515. https://doi.org/10.1016/j.progpolymsci.2009.01.002.
37. Raquez, J. M., Habibi, Y., Murariu, M., & Dubois, P. (2013). Polylactide (PLA)-based nanocomposites. *Progress in Polymer Science, 38*(11), 1504–1542. https://doi.org/10.1016/j.progpolymsci.2013.05.014.
38. Ray, S. S., & Bousmina, M. (2005). Biodegradable polymers and their layered silicate nanocomposites: In greening the 21st century materials world. *Progress in Materials Science, 50*(9), 962–1079. https://doi.org/10.1016/j.pmatsci.2005.05.002.
39. Bikiaris, D. (2011). Can nanoparticles really enhance thermal stability of polymers? Part II: An overview on thermal decomposition of polycondensation polymers. *Thermochimica Acta, 523*(1–2), 25–45. https://doi.org/10.1016/j.tca.2011.06.012.
40. Mohanty, A. K., Wibowo, A., Misra, M., & Drzal, L. T. (2003). Development of renewable resource-based cellulose acetate bioplastic: Effect of process engineering on the performance of cellulosic plastics. *Polymer Engineering and Science, 43*(3), 1151–1161. https://doi.org/10.1002/pen.10097.
41. Carrasco, F., Pagès, P., Gámez-Pérez, J., Santana, O. O., & Maspoch, M. L. (2010). Processing of poly (lactic acid): Characterization of chemical structure, thermal stability and mechanical properties. *Polymer Degradation and Stability, 95*(1), 116–125. https://doi.org/10.1016/j.polymdegradstab.2009.11.045.
42. Luiz De Paula, E., Mano, V., & Pereira, F. V. (2011). Influence of cellulose nano whiskers on the hydrolytic degradation behavior of poly(d,l-lactide). *Polymer Degradation and Stability, 96*(12), 1631–1638. https://doi.org/10.1016/j.polymdegradstab.2011.06.006.
43. Hossain, K. M. Z., Ahmed, I., Parsons, A. J., Scotchford, C. A., Walker, G. S., Thielemans, W., & Rudd, C. D. (2012). Physico-chemical and mechanical properties of nanocomposites prepared using cellulose nanowhiskers and poly (lactic acid). *Journal of Materials Science, 47*(6), 2675–2686. https://doi.org/10.1007/s10853-011-6093-4.
44. Daud, Y. M., Yee, T. G., Adnan, S. A., & Zaidi, N. H. A. (2018). Tensile and thermal degradation properties of poly (lactic acid)/Typha latifolia bio-composites. *AIP Conference Proceedings, 2030*. https://doi.org/10.1063/1.5066689.
45. Lanao, R. P. F., Jonker, A. M., Wolke, J. G. C., Jansen, J. A., van Hest, J. C. M., & Leeuwenburgh, S. C. G. (2013). Physicochemical properties and applications of poly (lactic-co-glycolic acid) for use in bone regeneration. *Tissue Engineering Part B: Reviews, 19*(5), 380–390. https://doi.org/10.1089/ten.teb.2012.0443.
46. Terzopoulou, Z., Baciu, D., Gounari, E., Steriotis, T., Charalambopoulou, G., & Bikiaris, D. (2018). Biocompatible nanobioglass reinforced poly(ε-caprolactone) composites synthesized via in situ ring opening polymerization. *Polymers, 10*(4), 381. https://doi.org/10.3390/polym10040381.

47. Amirian, M., Nabipour Chakoli, A., Cai, W., & Sui, J. H. (2012). In vitro degradation of poly(l-lactide)/poly(ε-caprolactone) blend reinforced with MWCNTs. *Iranian Polymer Journal, 21*(2), 165–174. https://doi.org/10.1007/s13726-012-0014-5.
48. Bouakaz, B. S., Habi, A., Grohens, Y., & Pillin, I. (2018). Effect of combinations of nanofillers on rheology-structure relations in biodegradable poly(ε-caprolactone) nanocomposites. *Applied Clay Science, 161*, 35–47. https://doi.org/10.1016/j.clay.2018.04.006.
49. Vandamme, T. F., & Legras, R. (1995). Physio-mechanical properties of poly(ε-caprolactone) for the construction of rumino-reticulum devices for grazing animals. *Biomaterials, 16*(18), 1395–1400. https://doi.org/10.1016/0142-9612(95)96875-Z.
50. Suárez, D., de Maldonado, G. J. V., Ortiz, R., Garcia-Guevara, V., & Miller-Kobisher, B. (2019). In vitro degradation of polydioxanone (PDO) lifting threads in hyaluronic acid (HA). *Journal of Surgical Clinical Research, 10*, 1–13. https://doi.org/10.20398/jscr.v10i1.15790.
51. Suarez-Vega, D., Velazco De Maldonado, G., Ortiz, R., García-Guevara, V., & Miller-Kobisher, B. (2019). In vitro degradation of polydioxanone lifting threads in hyaluronic acid. *Journal of Cutaneous and Aesthetic Surgery, 12*(3), 145–148. https://doi.org/10.4103/JCAS.JCAS_150_18.
52. Musiol, M., Jurczyk, S., Sobota, M., Klim, M., Sikorska, W., Zieba, M., Janeczek, H., Rydz, J., Kurcok, P., Johnston, B., et al. (2020). (Bio)degradable polymeric materials for a sustainable future—Part 3: Degradation studies of the PHA/wood floor-based composites and preliminary tests of antimicrobial activity. *Materials, 13*(9), 2200. https://doi.org/10.3390/ma13092200.
53. Amini, M., & Khavandi, A. (2019). Degradation of polymer-based composites in corrosive media: Experimental attempts towards underlying mechanisms. *Mechanics of Time-Dependent Materials, 23*(1), 153–172. https://doi.org/10.1007/s11043-018-09408-7.
54. Qi, J., Feng, S., Liu, X., Xing, L., Chen, D., & Xiong, C. (2020). Morphology, thermal properties, mechanical property and degradation of PLGA/PTMC composites. *Journal of Polymer Research, 27*(1), 1–14. https://doi.org/10.1007/s10965-020-2018-8.
55. Komal, U. K., Verma, V., Ashwani, T., Verma, N., & Singh, I. (2020). Effect of chemical treatment on thermal, mechanical and degradation behavior of banana fiber reinforced polymer composites. *Journal of Natural Fibers, 17*(6), 1026–1038. https://doi.org/10.1080/15440478.2018.1550461.
56. Ye, C., Ma, G., Fu, W., & Wu, H. (2015). Effect of fiber treatment on thermal properties and crystallization of sisal fiber reinforced polylactide composites. *Journal of Reinforced Plastics and Composites, 34*(8), 718–730. https://doi.org/10.1177/0731684415579090.
57. Gupta, A., Singh, A., Sharma, S., Sinha, S., & Joshi, S. (2017). Multifunctional nanohydroxyapatite-promoted toughened high-molecular-weight stereo complex poly (lactic acid)-based bio nanocomposite for both 3D-printed orthopedic implants and high-temperature engineering applications. *ACS Omega, 2*(7), 4039–4052. https://doi.org/10.1021/acsomega.7b00224.
58. Prasad, A. (2021a). Bioabsorbable polymeric materials for biofilms and other biomedical applications: Recent and future trends. *Materials Today: Proceedings, 44*, 2447–2453. https://doi.org/10.1016/j.matpr.2020.12.489.
59. Prasad, A. (2021b). State of art review on bioabsorbable polymeric scaffolds for bone tissue engineering. *Materials Today: Proceedings, 44*, 1391–1400. https://doi.org/10.1016/j.matpr.2020.11.622.

60. Prasad, A., Bhasney, S., Katiyar, V., & Sankar, M. R. (2017). Biowastes processed hydroxyapatite filled poly (lactic acid) bio-composite for open reduction internal fixation of small bones. *Materials Today: Proceedings, 4*(9), 10153–10157. https://doi.org/10.1016/j.matpr.2017.08.025.
61. Prasad, A., Devendar, B., Sankar, M. R., & Robi, P. S. (2015). Micro-scratch based tribological characterization of hydroxyapatite (HAp) fabricated through fish scales. *Materials Today: Proceedings, 2*(4–5), 1216–1224. http://linkinghub.elsevier.com/retrieve/pii/S2214785315002795 (accessed on 8 August 2024).
62. Prasad, A., Sankar, M. R., & Katiyar, V. (2017). State of art on solvent casting particulate leaching method for orthopedic scaffolds fabrication. *Materials Today: Proceedings, 4*(2), 898–907. http://dx.doi.org/10.1016/j.matpr.2017.01.101.
63. Prasad, A., Chakraborty, G., & Kumar, A. (2022). Bio-based environmentally benign polymeric resorbable materials for orthopedic fixation applications. In *Advanced Materials for Biomedical Applications* (pp. 251–266). CRC Press.
64. Prasad, A. (2022). Biomaterial-based nanofibers scaffolds in tissue engineering application. In *Functional Biomaterials* (pp. 245–264). Springer, Singapore.
65. Prasad, A., Bhasney, S. M., Prasannavenkadesan, V., et al. (2023). Polylactic acid reinforced with nano-hydroxyapatite bioabsorbable cortical screws for bone fracture treatment. *Journal of Polymer Research, 30*, 177. https://doi.org/10.1007/s10965-023-03542-8.
66. Sarkar, K., Dutta, K., Chatterjee, A., Sarkar, J., Das, D., Prasad, A., Chattopadhyay, D., Acharya, K., Das, M., Verma, S. K., & De, S. (2023). Nanotherapeutic potential of antibacterial folic acid-functionalized nanoceria for wound-healing applications. *Nanomedicine, 18*(2). https://doi.org/10.2217/nnm-2022-0233.
67. Katiyar, V., Prasad, A., Sankar, M. R., & Bhasney, S. M. (2022). Process for the preparation of polymer composite-based cancellous screw and pins (Indian Patent No. 401811).

CHAPTER 6

Biopolymer and Bio-Ceramics Composite for Orthopedic Applications

YUSUF OLATUNJI WAIDI,[1] SAMIR DAS,[2] and SUDIPTO DATTA[1]

[1]*Indian Institute of Science, C.V. Raman Avenue, Bangalore, Karnataka, India*

[2]*Indian Institute of Technology, Kharagpur, West Bengal, India*

ABSTRACT

Compared to the first and second generations, biomaterials for orthopedic applications, third-generation biomaterials are now being used because they closely match the mechanical properties of natural human bones. These two biomaterials are combined to develop a composite material with good mechanical properties due to their intrinsic higher strength and stiffness. Among all the biomaterials for orthopedic applications, calcium phosphate ceramics are commonly used for bone replacement because they mimic the mineral composition of bone. Additionally, they have further advantages such as nontoxicity, bioactivity, and biocompatibility. This book chapter will briefly cover a few biopolymer-ceramic composites and their biological and physical properties. These composite materials are ideal for bone substitution because they have a good reputation in controlled delivery devices and bone augmentation, which transforms the hard tissue engineering field.

6.1 INTRODUCTION

Annually, many people suffer from bone defects due to tumor rejections, bone disease, trauma, and congenital irregularities. Adverse effects of motorization also increase the number of patients due to changes in lifestyle

Bioabsorbable Polymers for Drug Carriers and Fixation Devices. Arbind Prasad and Sougata Jana (Eds.)

and unhygienic habits. Research reports indicate that the value of the US \$58.1 billion biomaterials market is emerging, which represents a 15% increase from the year 2009 to the year 2014. The entire orthopedic implant, device, and drug market is assessed to be 25 billion per year. Orthopedic surgery, bone healing, and stabilization are the most important parameters for repairing bone defects after a surgical process. Different metallic fixations, such as screws and plates, have been used as conventional treatment strategies in past decades. The most commonly used fixation plates are 316 stainless steel, cobalt and chromium-based alloys, and titanium alloys. However, using metal plates decreases bone density due to the lack of mechanical stimulation at the fracture site. As metal plates are stiffer, the stress received after implantation in this system leads to osteoporosis in the localized bones during fracture healing or stress shielding. Stress shielding weakens the bones after implant removal, which may lead to bone fractures at the implant site and osteoporosis in the later stages of fracture healing. Metallic implants are prone to metallic oxidization and the formation of infections due to the colonization of the epidermis by bacteria. The removal of metallic plates and screws by surgery after they have fulfilled their stabilization role can lead to significant trauma and suffering. Non-metallic bond fixation has less stress shielding and allows for flexible fixation after implantation, which increases its appeal at the implant site. Polymeric biomaterials play a crucial role because they can easily restore the function of native tissue after implantation and improve quality of life. This review addresses the numerous polymer-ceramic composite materials that can be used in orthopedic applications.

6.2 HYDROXYAPATITE

Heterogeneous structures of the native bone tissue can be established through a natural growth, resorption process, and mechanical stimuli to the surrounding tissue. Different organic and inorganic ceramic composites with varying weight ratios can easily mimic the natural bone tissue made up of 45–60% minerals, 20–30% matrix, and 10–20% water. The natural bones consist of collagen fibers with a thickness of 80 nm that are arranged in a nanocrystalline rod-like structure measuring 25 to 50 nanometers longitudinally. The matrix of the bone is an organic constituent that mainly contains anisotropic, triple helix type 1 collagen [1–3]. Organic materials show good flexibility after implantation, while inorganic minerals provide good mechanical properties in bones. Bone can be considered as having two types of mechanical properties: one is compact, and the other is spongy. Inorganic mineral constituents are replaced by calcium phosphate, which is analogous in conformation and structure to hydroxyapatite (HA). HA is a unique class of calcium phosphate with excellent cytocompatibility, and it promotes greater tissue growth by developing an organically active carbonate hydroxylapatite layer on its surface under conditions similar to *in vivo* [4–6]. However, among the different calcium orthophosphates, only certain calcium-to-phosphate ratios can be used for biomedical applications, as Ca/P ratios less than 1 are very acidic and soluble, hence cannot be suitable for implantation. Calcium-to-phosphate ratios can vary from 1.5 to 1.67 in some cases. The stable phase of calcium phosphate is dependent on the presence of water and the temperature at the time of handling or in the location where it is used [7–9]. Hydroxyapatite (HA) is also compatible with our body temperature, pH < 42, as well as other biologically active parameters. Hydroxyapatite ($Ca_{10}(PO_4)6(OH)_2$) is the most stable calcium phosphate phase at body temperature, at pH 7.4 and 37°C, that can be used for ceramic bone substitutes. Tricalcium phosphate is one of the common bone substitutes that exhibit dissimilar features under *in vivo* conditions. Though they both have the same calcium-to-phosphate ratio within the range of 1.5 to 1.67, they can promote bone tissue after implanting the HA bond with the native bone tissue directly within the pH range of 4.6 to 12.4. Metal, ceramic, natural and synthetic polymers, and a variety of calcium phosphate-based materials are used for bone tissue engineering. Metallic biomaterials have excellent mechanical properties, but stress shielding limits their application. Whereas natural and synthetic polymers have greater cellular viability and cytocompatibility, they are mechanically inferior for load-bearing applications [9]. Different biomaterials have various drawbacks, such as lesser mechanical reliability, lack of flexibility, and high density, which ultimately lead to failure in the development of orthopedic prostheses. Polymer and ceramic bioglass composites are now considered 3rd-generation orthopedic materials for greater bioactivity and the ability to closely match natural bone properties when compared with the 1st-generation and 2nd-generation bone tissue substitutes during the development of bone tissue analogs. Our body tissue is much more heterogeneous and complex, and variations in mechanical properties can be seen based on body location and daily activities. Therefore, the ceramic composite and polymer blends can be used with better mechanical properties because of their greater strength and stiffness, making them suitable for applications such as bone augmentation and repair [10, 11].

For example, nano and micro-HA can be mixed with artificial polymers to generate materials with greater mechanical properties, characteristics comparable to bone tissue. These composite scaffolds comprising polyethylene, poly-methylmethacrylate, alginate, chitosan, etc., can promote identical cell seeding, cell ingrowth, and tissue formation. Further variation in porosity is one of the major concerns for the development of successful tissue analogs. Macro and micro porous ceramic and polymer composite scaffolds can promote tissue growth with excellent mechanical properties and osteoconductivity, which ultimately lead to the osteointegration of the implant with the native tissue.

6.3 COMPOSITES OF BIOSTABLE POLYMERS

6.3.1 COMPOSITES BASED ON POLYETHYLENE

Polyethylene (PE) is widely explored as a reference polymer in various polymer research to examine innovation in other polymers because of its simple molecular structure, especially low-density polyethylene (LDPE). Thin LDPE films were sulfonated to enhance hydrophilicity, blood compatibility, and protein adsorption. The findings demonstrate that surface treatment can decrease albumin and fibrinogen-mediated platelet adhesion. Since the early 1980s, high-density polyethylene (HDPE) reinforced with hydroxyapatite (HA) composite has been established as a bone substitute equivalent and joint load-bearing end prostheses [16]. Recently, Bonfield et al. suggested the use of HDPE composites as a bone mimic approach [17, 18].

The inclusion of HA in the composites facilitates mechanical strength, improved creep, and better bioactivity and biocompatibility. Furthermore, ultra-high molecular weight polyethylene (UHMWPE) possesses enormous merits, such as excellent sliding characteristics, high fatigue resistance, outstanding impact strength, and biocompatibility. A 40% composite by volume of HA has been observed to give an optimal balance of biological and mechanical characteristics [17, 18]. This combination possesses a modulus close to cortical bone and has improved bioactivity and toughness. The modulus figures suggest a promising solution to mechanically induced bone resorption in traditional implants with greater modulus values than bone. Figure 6.1 shows the hierarchical structure of natural bone.

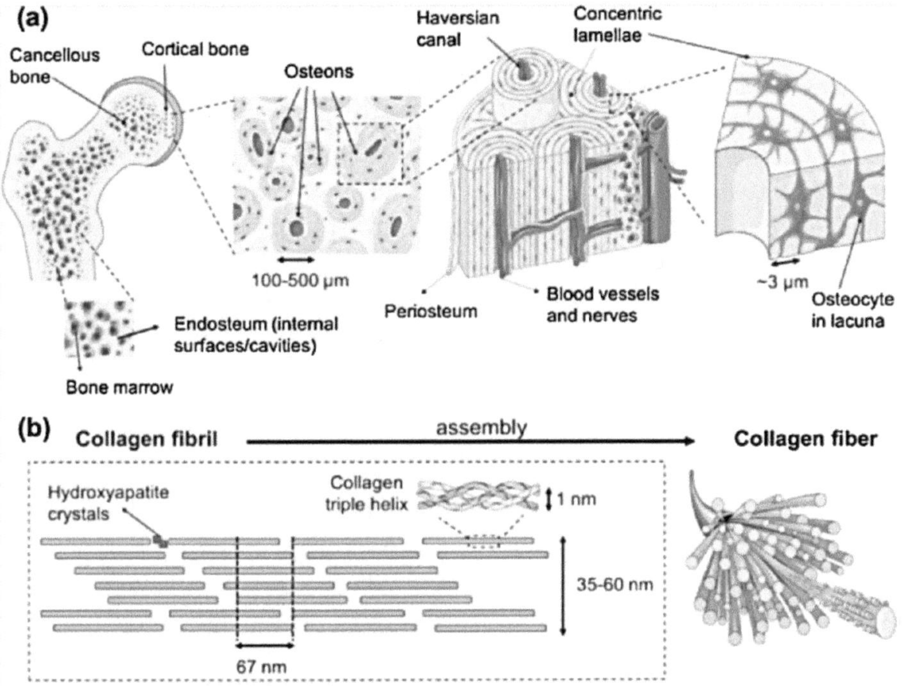

FIGURE 6.1 Natural bone hierarchical structure: (a) cancellous and cortical bone, a multiple-layer structure with complicated components at macro to micro levels; and (b) constitution of bone tissue, having fibers of collagen and nucleated with crystals of HAP.

Source: Reproduced with permission from Ref. [53], Copyright © 2020 Elsevier B.V.

Furthermore, instead of the fibrous encapsulation seen with other implant materials, this means that these composites favored bone apposition [19]. Fabrication processes are crucial in determining the mechanical characteristics of composites. The only feasible fabrication method for UHMWPE is powder compression molding. In contrast, HDPE composites may be produced by hydrostatic extrusion and compounding [20, 21]. High-density polyethylene composite reinforced with hydroxyapatite (HAPEX™) displays a remarkable modulus of elasticity, manufactured by the combination of compression molding and hydrostatic extrusion [20]. Furthermore, controlled shear orientation molding injection can induce anisotropic features [22]. In another study, high shear forces were observed in HDPE-reinforced HA using twin-screw compounding extrusion [23]. However, when HA levels exceeded 40%, tensile strength decreased, resulting in brittle fracture. According to Bonfield and colleagues [24, 25], the observed poor efficacy of reinforcing agents (HA particles) is mainly attributable to their intrinsic small aspect ratio and limited level of polymer matrix reaction. Several efforts have been made to improve mechanical performance by creating an appropriate coupling group for chemical interactions using silane agents and acrylic acid grafting. The researchers next explored the role of varying the size and shape of HA particles and homogeneous mixtures on the tensile strength of the composite. To investigate the variations in tensile strength, two classes of dried HA spray with average particle diameters of 4 and 8 microns, with a few surface area changes, were explored [21]. The smaller-sized HA particles had increased tensile and torsional stiffness, yielding stronger composites. Even though HA particles improve creep properties and promote material stiffness, an increase in HA concentration leads to more polymer-ceramic interfaces. Therefore, the amount of interface must be considered because failure predominantly develops at the interface once mechanical force is applied to the implant [22]. Joseph et al. [26], on the other hand, looked at the effects of HA-sintered powder and spray-dried materials having equal particle dimensions but different specific surface areas. The dried HA spray composite has a much greater viscosity than the HA composite that is sintered. The disparity was attributed to the influence of the specific surface area that coincides with the quantity of available PE that functions as the coated surfaces matrix. Recently, the Selective Laser Sintering (SLS) fabrication method was employed to fabricate HA/PE porous composite constructs [27, 28]. By adjusting laser intensity and particle size, 20% HA/PE and 30% HA/PE composites were effectively sintered. The preliminary HAPEX biological evaluation *in vivo* revealed great biocompatibility. In addition, the *in vitro* investigations demonstrated that cells grew quicker on particles containing 40% HA/PE than on particles containing 20% HA/PE [24]. Downes et al. [30] implanted HAPEX in patients and employed it in orbital floor procedures, and the results showed enhanced bone bonding. Meijer et al. [31] stated in another clinical application research that the reactions to implantation were deemed satisfactory two and a half years post-implantation. Figure 6.2 represents bone scaffolds with different types of morphologies.

6.3.2 POLY(METHYL METHACRYLATE) (PMMA)-BASED COMPOSITES

For more than 40 years, PMMA has been widely explored for bone reconstruction applications. Because of its intrinsic flexibility and fast liquid-to-solid phase transition, it was first utilized in paste form to fill the defect site [32].

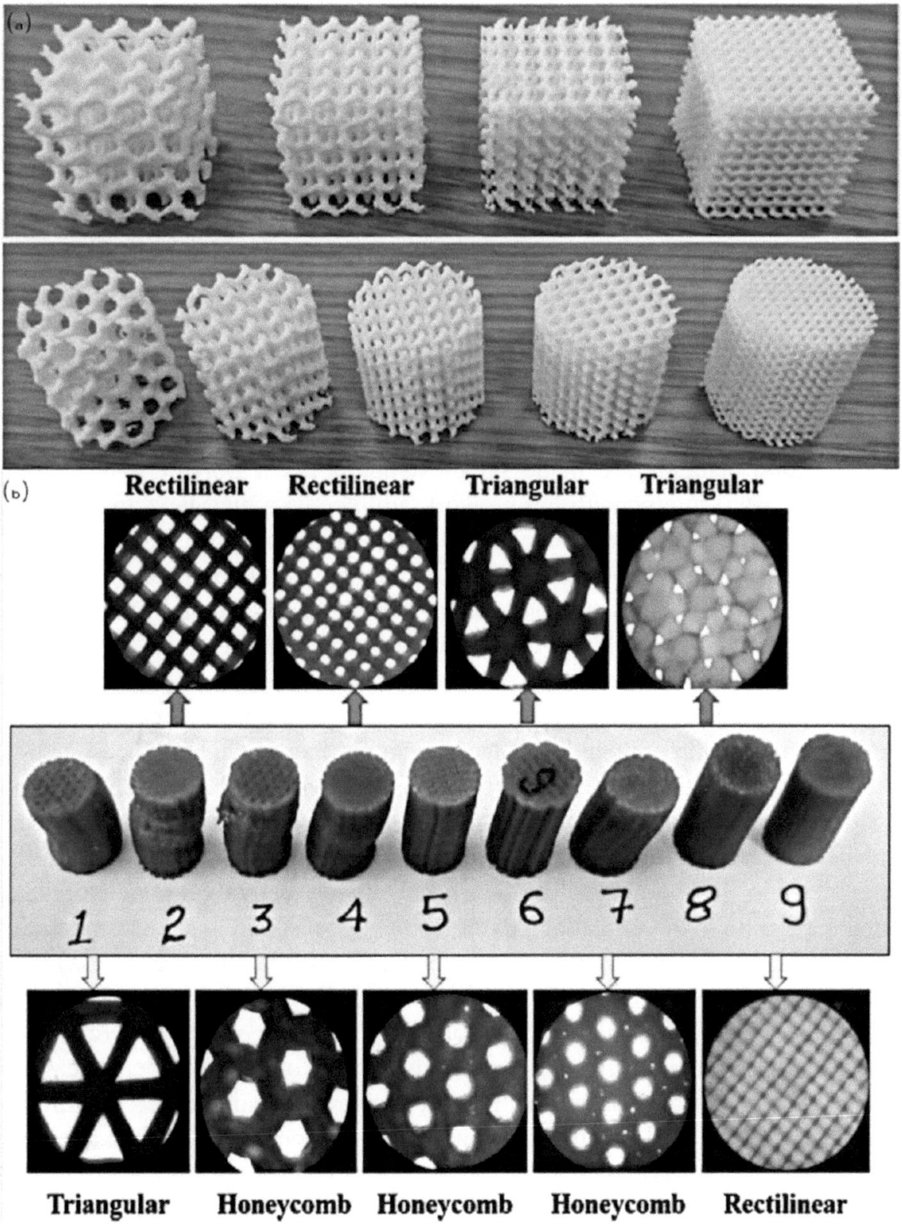

FIGURE 6.2 Various morphologies of the scaffold of bone (a) FDM fabricated bone scaffold having cylindrical and cubic configuration; and (b) various scaffold types having variable parentage of infill and thickness of layers.

Source: Reproduced with permission from Ref. [53]; Copyright © 2020 Elsevier B.V.

Percutaneous vertebroplasty is a new prevalent method for treating lesions and spinal fractures. PMMA has been widely employed for percutaneous vertebroplasty despite many limitations. Some PMMA-based cement products are already on the market, including Mendec Spine (M/S Tecres S.p.A) and Simplex Radiopaque (K032945) (M/S Stryker). The types of cement for bone reconstruction currently commercially available are composed of (a) PMMA polymer or related block copolymers in powder form; and (b) methyl methacrylate (MMA) in liquid form or monomer-associated liquids. Commercially available PMMA types of cement typically comprise benzoyl peroxide, barium sulfate, and PMMA oligomers [1]. Both powder and liquid constituents are mixed to create bone cement. The powder constituents are introduced into the monomer phase for proper dissolution and subsequently auto-polymerize to generate a thick, moldable dough that cures to obtain cement. PMMA-based bone cements are made up of standard linear polymers structurally. Although semi-interpenetrating network architectures may be achieved using cross-linkers such as ethylene glycol dimethacrylate, the PMMA cement extravasation resulting in nerve root radiculopathy and compression has been documented in several situations using PMMA-based cement in percutaneous vertebroplasty in the epidural or foraminal area. PMMA cement extravasation in perivertebral veins results in pulmonary embolism and mortality. The high exothermic temperature (86°C to 107°C inside the core of the cement) during the polymerization of methyl methacrylate monomer might harm nearby tissue, such as nerve roots and the spinal cord, causing an inflammatory response along with temporary worsening of discomfort. Due to its cardiotoxic and arrhythmogenic features, absorption of PMMA monomer after injection might result in hypotension. The monomer residue's toxic impacts, activation of macrophages, and the failure to directly attach to the bone have resulted in significant clinical consequences [34, 35]. M/S Kyphon Inc., Sunnyvale, California, has developed balloon kyphoplasty using bone cement made from PMMA-based materials [Kyphx HV-R] with a balloon kyphoplasty kit as an alternative to percutaneous vertebroplasty. Unfortunately, the disadvantages of high-temperature levels derived from inflammation and methyl methacrylate monomer polymerization, which is caused by unreacted hazardous monomer, may not be alleviated using the kyphoplasty balloon. Exothermic temperatures of 60°C to 70°C have been seen during the polymerization of methyl methacrylate monomer during the balloon kyphoplasty technique, resulting in tissue necrosis. Secondary osteoporotic individuals are more likely than primary osteoporotic patients to have a spinal compression fracture after undergoing balloon kyphoplasty. Nevertheless, in most situations, PMMA-based types of cement have been used in orthopedic surgery for years. As a result, there has been increased interest in producing better biocompatible PMMA-based types of cement. One suggestion was to create PMMA-based bone types of cement that were more bioactive and tissue-friendly. Consequently, bioactive cement was developed by including ceramics at the proper concentrations. Compared to pure PMMA cement, these bioactive PMMA types have considerably greater bone-bonding strength [36, 37]. However, including high concentrations of ceramics in PMMA might result in poor mechanical qualities, especially if the ceramic (filler) and PMMA (matrix) do not adhere well. Harper38 combined PMMA and HA (17 wt%) to induce bioactivity without compromising mechanical characteristics. The composite cellular reaction was examined, and thus, HA addition improved the resulting materials' cellular activities, such as actin filament organization. As a result, numerous bioactive fillers, including HA, titania, [40] bioactive glass [41], β-tricalcium phosphate (β-TCP) [39], and bioactive glass ceramics [42], have been used with matrix PMMA. When implanted *in vivo*, these bioactive composites exhibit appropriate bioactivity by generating an apatite layer [43]. Co-precipitation [44] has also introduced covalently bound HEMA into non-stoichiometric hydroxyapatite to improve mechanical characteristics. Jayabalan et al. [45] discovered that polypropylene fumarate/phloroglucinol triglycidyl methacrylate might be explored as a partly degradable polymeric cement for orthopedic purposes. Two oligomers containing a 50:50 blend might yield an optimal setup time. A 50:50 combination of composite cement and hydroxyapatite granules was discovered to have enough bioactivity. Ishhara et al. [44] then showed that MMA bone cement containing 4-methacryloyloxyethyl trimellitic anhydride could attach to HA and had improved tensile characteristics. Another study observed that surfaces treated with HA increased dental composites' diametral tensile strength [42, 43]. Recently, it was identified that glass-ceramic heat-treated at 950°C could be a commercial PMMA bone cement bioactive filler (PALACOS® LV) [44]. The findings revealed appropriate bioactive behavior. The Micro CT [45] investigation on the bone healing quantitative variables at the PMMA bone-implant boundary, including calcium phosphate, reveals complementary histology, morphological information, and precise creation of freshly produced bone.

6.4 COMPOSITES BIODEGRADABLE POLYMERS

6.4.1 COMPOSITE BASED ON POLYESTER

Polymeric biodegradable composites are novel advances in bone disease therapy and fracture healing. The benefits of biodegradable materials include

(i) they do not need to be removed by subsequent surgery after usage since the by-products produced can be eliminated via natural processes from the human body; (ii) the gradual degradation of implanted biodegradable material will result in bone rebuilding by osteoclasts and osteoblasts; and (iii) biodegradable cement has the potential to eliminate the requirement for revisiting surgery for the removal of stainless steel bone screws, plates, and other bone guiding devices. Interestingly, polymeric biodegradable composites might also be programmed to break down in a controlled fashion *in vivo* for a certain duration. The full recovery of function with new bone development must be achieved for the restoration of bone disease to be successful. Biodegradable polymeric composites are potential orthopedic implant materials, including spinal cord arthrodesis intersomatic cages and fracture repair plates for osteosynthesis treatments. As a result, modeling and creating polymeric biodegradable composites with suitable monomers to obtain optimal bioactivity, mechanical characteristics, and biodegradability for treating fracture disorders and healing bone is necessary. Polyester-based composites have been widely researched among the numerous materials tested for bone treatments and correcting skeletal problems. An unsaturated linear polyester, Poly(propylene fumarate) (PPF), is one of the interesting polymers that degrades by hydrolysis mechanism, yielding fumaric acid and propylene glycol as finished products. Furthermore, the biodegradable polymer contains numerous unsaturated bonds, especially double bonds that may get cross-linked. In addition, it has been demonstrated to be noncytotoxic, osteoconductive, and biocompatible. Jayabalan et al. [46] investigated a PPF co-polymer with ethylene glycol/hydroxyapatite as a bone tissue engineering injectable bone cement. The biodegradation investigations *in vitro* show a sluggish and progressive breakdown trend. Previous research has also demonstrated that neat PPF possesses compressive properties that mimic bone; therefore, it is an excellent option for orthopedic remedies. PPF/TCP polymeric materials exhibit mechanical characteristics comparable to trabecular bone. Furthermore, the heat produced during the cross-linking process in PPF is less than that of the marketed PMMA bone cement. The influence of TCP concentrations and polymer bond ratios on cross-linking and mechanical properties of injectable PPF-based composites was investigated by He et al. [47]. They observed that the introduction of TCP and an increase in the double-bond ratio led to an enhancement in mechanical characteristics. The *in vitro* investigations of the composites showed that increasing the PPF molecular weight improved mechanical characteristics and aided human trabecular bone regeneration in 7 weeks [48].

Gerhart et al. [49] evaluated and compared the mechanical qualities and antibiotic delivery of MMA and PPF to a commercially available methacrylate cement. The investigation revealed that the MMA and PPF bone cement possessed higher mechanical features and maintained antimicrobial concentrations for longer than the commercially available cement. Although the types of cement's initial mechanical characteristics were acceptable, they degraded by a proportion of 12 merely 4 weeks post-implantation. In another study, PPF/calcium sulfate/TCP composites were produced to study the *in vivo* breakdown and tissue reaction to implantation with the help of histological examination and radiography [50]. No inflammation was discovered, and the osteogenic constructs may produce pores *in situ*. The composite's pore formation rate may be modified by adjusting its content. The influences of HA on the biological features of polymeric composites composed of a hydroxy-terminated unsaturated polyester high molecular weight PPF were studied [51]. Various biodegradable polymeric composites containing HA particles were fabricated, i.e., (i) <100 nm sized calcined HA nanoparticles; (ii) HA nanoparticles (<100 nm) precipitated; and (iii) nanopowder of HA (<200 nm) available commercially with a reinforcement concentration of 30% wt. The findings showed that HA calcined nanoparticles with rod-like morphologies influenced the matrix resin's strong cross-linking, exhibiting great interfacial polymer bonding and high cross-linking density. The buffering action of hydroxyapatite controlled and reduced biodegradation. The tissue compatibility was then investigated for 3 months in a rabbit intramuscular implantation animal model based on ISO standard 10993/6. The rabbit animal model was also used for *in vivo* femoral bone regeneration per ISO standard 10993/6. In addition, the composite was demonstrated to be a potential option for dimensional stability, stress shielding prevention, and allowing new normal tissue to develop on the biodegraded implant composite for fixative bone device scaffolds. In another work, calcium phosphate cement (CPC) reinforced PPF was fabricated to offer enough mechanical strength for femoral head osteonecrosis [52]. The findings show that the fabricated cement has reduced cytotoxicity, and the CPC fraction increase boosts the modulus, lowers the cross-linking temperature, and decreases extreme cement swelling. The addition of ginsenoside Rg1 had an angiogenic impact, and the antigenicity of produced Rg1 was validated by tube growth in HUVEC cells. This freshly formed angiogenic bone cement composite has exceptional development prospects for repairing femoral head osteonecrosis [56]. Zhongyu et al. [50] examined PPF/$CaSO_4$/β-TCP composite biodegradability for bone regeneration. This work aimed to examine the impact of the $CaSO_4$/β-TCP molar ratio and the molecular weight of PPF on *in vivo* biodegradation and bone tissue reaction to the composite [32]. The prepared specimens were inserted at segmental imperfections, collected at various breaks, and examined to evaluate the composites' *in vivo* deterioration and consequent effects on the implants. All the samples maintained their initial form, as observed by the *in vivo* degradation data. They were proficient in in-situ pore creation, with the pore formation rate changing with the content of the composite. Tissue penetration was found near the surface of the composites in the holes produced by the breakdown of the $CaSO_4$/β-TCP spheres, but no inflammatory responses were observed. Poly(hydroxybutyrate) (PHB) esters and their co-polymer poly(hydroxyvalerate) (PHV) have already been investigated as biodegradable polymers with tensile qualities similar to bone. PHB has a greater modulus than many other degradable polymers, making it an excellent matrix material. Doyle et al. created a porous composite of hydroxyapatite/poly(hydroxybutyrate) (HA-PHB) by infusing PHB particles into stiff constructs of HA. The resultant HA-PHB composites' mechanical characteristics, HA/PHB volume fractions, surface adhesion, and porosity were related to the pure constructs of HA [25]. The addition of PHB to the fabricated composites (HA-PHB) resulted in a significant improvement in strength. The inclusion of PHB did not affect the stiffness of the filled composites. However, the coated composites increased stiffness from 35 MPa to 105 MPa above the initial HA scaffolds. Strong interactions between the HA and PHB component phases increased strength in the coated composites. The Young's modulus of PHB alone was 4 GPa, which was enhanced to 11 GPa with 40% HA. The 40 vol% HA/PHB formulation enhances bone ingrowth formation, and high-resolution TEM analyses revealed that bone bonding occurred throughout the interface. Furthermore, PHB has recently been employed in bioactive reinforced compounds with short fibers of 5% and 15% wt of HA by Coskun et al. [54] and Chen et al. [55], who reinforced PHB/PHV along with 14 vol% nano-HA. Additionally, adding some PHV co-polymer increases ductility while decreasing strength and stiffness.

6.4.2 COMPOSITES BASED ON CHITOSAN

Chitosan is an amino polysaccharide having a linear chain generated by the chitin deacetylation, comprising (1→4) D-glucosamine randomly dispersed and N-acetyl-D-glucosamine parts. Chitosan's cellular connections have been demonstrated in tissue healing, and its adaptability allows it to be molded into porous structures for tissue engineering applications. Furthermore, it is appropriate for various tissue engineering applications due to its greater tissue compatibility, functionality, non-antigenicity, and architectural resemblance to glycosaminoglycans in the extracellular matrix. Many manufacturing processes have been used to create 3D biodegradable chitosan composite constructs, including solvent casting, freeze-drying, melt molding, and particle leaching. The manner and direction of applied stress, water content, shape, porosity, and ceramic particle dimension determine the mechanical characteristics of these scaffolds. The amount of bone mineralization has been observed to improve the mechanical strength of chitosan composites. Although real bones have far greater mechanical characteristics than chitosan ceramic composite scaffolds, porosity promotes mechanical adherence to the neighboring tissue by offering a platform for bone development. Furthermore, the bone quality around implants of porous composites is superior to that of dense composites [56]. Many bioactive chitosan composites using ceramic materials like HA have been explored for hard tissue regeneration remedies for musculoskeletal ailments [57]. Several bone-filling solutions have been created in recent years using chitosan in conjunction with calcium phosphates, coupled with biological components, or as a binding agent. Various surface-adherent dependent cells, notably bone cells, are grown on chitosan-based 2D and 3D frameworks for tissue engineering [58, 59]. It has been observed during surgery that chitosan/HA composites are more moldable and manageable than neat HA granules or powder. However, compared to normal bone, the fundamental drawbacks of biodegradable materials are their significantly lower modulus. As a result, they can be used only for high-load-bearing skeleton-related applications. Nevertheless, various novel materials based on chitosan, including films, hydrogels, sponges, and microspheres, have been created to improve bone joining and repair. MCCh, a functionalized chitosan form developed based on the amino glucose macromolecule clustering process, is one of the most interesting chitosan derivatives. MCCh is distinguished by its inherent chitosan qualities and specific features, such as direct film formation and the formation of super-molecular and molecular structures during its manufacture. However, their uses are restricted because they hinder disintegration at pH 7 and the considerably large produced biocomposites' crystallinity. [60] Wan et al. [61] created a composite by evenly dispersing and effectively mixing HA with chitin bio-ink although the mechanical features were unsatisfactory, microscopic studies indicated that the particles of HA interfered with polymer chains, degrading their connections and diminishing their modulus. Yamaguchi et al. [62] produced the composites with chitosan mixed in various organic acids via a co-precipitation technique. They discovered that the formation of elliptic agglomerations and alignment with the chitosan molecule prevented the development of HA crystals. Histological examination revealed the formation of new bone surrounding the composite and no inflammation. Furthermore, they developed a 3D composite containing chitosan/HA composite scaffolds with geometry based on the chitosan hydrogel structure [62]. The amount of HA included in the composite scaffolds might regulate their swelling. TCP was also mixed into the chitosan matrix by separating the solvent sublimation and polymer bio-ink in the solid-liquid phase [33]. The fabricated composite exhibited bioactivity in SBF and had increased compressive modulus and strength. These composites were proposed as tissue engineering materials, with porosity in the constructs based on parameters such as TCP concentration and ratio of ceramic to chitosan. To ensure the effectiveness of biodegradable orthopedic implants, the mechanical features of the biomaterial must be matched to those of bone while also preventing dimensional degradation. Those parameters can prohibit stress protection while allowing for the slow formation of scaffolds, enabling natural tissue to develop over the progressively biodegraded composite, thus avoiding necrosis. Polymeric nanocomposites with molecular reinforcement are potential materials for bone fixation devices. This type of composite guarantees that nano-sized filler is dispersed throughout the three-dimensional cross-linked biodegradable polymer. Warping caused by differential deterioration rates on the material surfaces interacting with the tissue fluid and those close to the bone might be prevented by molecularly fortified biodegradable polymeric nanocomposites with excellent dimensional stability.

6.5 FUTURE SCOPE

Despite the volume of reported articles dedicated to polymer ceramic composites in the past, there is still much room for advancement in the subject. Composites containing a polymer matrix have the benefit of being extremely adaptable, permitting their ultimate customizing characteristics. Several composites may be created and manufactured to meet particular needs by utilizing a variety of reinforcements, manufacturing techniques, and polymeric matrices. The primary prerequisites involve improved mechanical qualities, increased bioactivity, the creation of biomimetic composites, growth factor and protein delivery methods, and a general grasp of biological system foundations. Gene-triggering composite scaffolds customized to specific illnesses could be achievable in the future. When paired with smart materials, manufacturing, and surgical advancements, all these ideas might result in the development of next-generation scaffolds for skeletal rebuilding employed in regenerative therapy.

6.6 CONCLUSION

Complex tissue repair and restoration techniques have received much interest in recent decades, significantly increasing quality of life. Many results have been achieved and published in articles and patents in recent years. This demonstrates the steps taken to establish materials and processes for developing artificial tissues such as cartilage, bones, nerves, skin, and blood vessels, which help regain the features of damaged hard tissues. Many solutions for both short- and long-term uses have been offered. Almost all of these devices are biocompatible and are expected to function normally after being implanted. However, creating an appropriate material for bone scaffolds with adequate mechanical strength and porosity to allow cell attachment, growth, migration, and proliferation, leading to effective surrounding tissue integration, remains challenging in complex tissue engineering. With fresh contributions from tissue engineering coupled with nanotechnology, these composites may change the field of complex tissue regeneration, from bone augmentation and repair to structured delivery systems.

KEYWORDS

- **bio-ceramics**
- **bio-polymer**
- **bone augmentation**
- **bone tissue engineering**
- **nanotechnology**
- **scaffolds**
- **tissue regeneration**

REFERENCES

1. Sikavitsas, V. I., Temenoff, J. S., & Mikos, A. G. (2001). Biomaterials and bone mechano transduction. *Biomaterials, 22*(24), 2581–2593.
2. Katz, E. P. (1973). Structure and function of bone collagen fibrils. *Journal of Molecular Biology, 80*(1), 1–21.
3. Rho, J. Y., Kuhn-Spearing, L., & Zioupos, P. (1998). Mechanical properties and the hierarchical structure of bone. *Medical Engineering & Physics, 20*(2), 92–102.
4. Hench, L. L. (1991). Bio ceramics, from concept to clinic. *Journal of the American Ceramic Society, 74*(7), 1482–1517.
5. Daculsi, G. (1998). Biphasic calcium phosphate concept applied to artificial bone, implant coating and injectable bone substitute. *Biomaterials, 19*(14), 1473–1486.
6. Sampath Kumar, T. S., Manjubala, I., & Gunasekharan, K. (2000). Synthesis of carbonated calcium phosphate ceramics using microwave irradiation. *Biomaterials, 21*(16), 1623–1630.
7. Wang, M., Deb, S., Tanner, K. E., & Bonfield, W. (1996). Hydroxyapatite polyethylene composites for bone substitution: Effects of silanation and polymer grafting. In *ECCM-7* (pp. 455–460). Woodhead Publishing Ltd., Cambridge.
8. Ladizesky, N. H., Pirhonen, E. M., Appleyard, D. B., Ward, I. M., & Bonfield, W. (1998). Fiber reinforcement of ceramic/polymer composites for a major load bearing bone substitute material. *Composites Science and Technology, 58*(3), 419–427.
9. Heller, M. O., Mehta, M., Taylor, W. R., Kim, D. Y., Speirs, A., Duda, G. N., & Perka, C. (2011). Influence of prosthesis design and implantation technique on implant stresses after cementless revision total hip replacement. *Journal of Orthopedic Surgery and Research, 13*, 6.
10. Liu, F., Jin, Y., Lin, X., & Jia, D. (2006). Properties and morphology of bio ceramics/ poly (D, L-lactide) composites modified by in situ computerizing extrusion. *Journal of Applied Polymer Science, 102*(5), 4085–4092.
11. Collins, A. M., Skaer, N. J. V., Gheysens, T., Knight, D., Bertram, C., & Mann, S. (2009). Bone-like resorbable silk-based scaffolds for load-bearing osteoregenerative applications. *Advanced Materials, 21*(1), 75–80.
12. Bonfield, W., Grynpas, M. D., Tully, A. E., Bowman, J., & Abram, J. (1981). Hydroxyapatite reinforced polyethylene—A mechanically compatible implant. *Biomaterials, 2*(3), 185–192.
13. Bonfield, W. (1988). Composites for bone replacement. *Journal of Biomechanical Engineering, 10*(6), 522–528.
14. Huang, J., Di Silvio, L., Wang, M., Tanner, K. E., & Bonfield, W. (1997). In vitro mechanical and biological assessment of hydroxyapatite reinforced polyethylene composites. *Journal of Materials Science: Materials in Medicine, 8*(9), 775–784.
15. Huang, J., Di Silvio, L., Wang, M., Rehman, I., Ohtsuki, I. C., & Bonfield, W. (1997). Evaluation of in-vitro bioactivity and biocompatibility of bio glass reinforced polyethylene composite. *Journal of Materials Science: Materials in Medicine, 8*(9), 809–814.
16. Wang, M., Ladizesky, N. H., Tanner, K. E., Ward, I. M., & Bonfield, W. (2000). Hydrostatically extruded HAPEX(TM). *Journal of Materials Science, 35*(5), 1023–1028.

17. Nazhat, S. N., Joseph, R., Wang, M., Smith, R., Tanner, K. E., & Bonfield, W. (2000). Dynamic mechanical characterization of hydroxyapatite reinforced polyethylene: Effect of particle size. *Journal of Materials Science: Materials in Medicine, 11*(10), 621–627.
18. Bonfield, W., Grynpas, M., Tully, A. E., Bowman, J., & Abram, J. (1981). Hydroxyapatite reinforced polyethylene: A mechanically compatible implant material for bone replacement. *Biomaterials, 2*(3), 185–192.
19. Wang, M., Porter, D., & Bonfield, W. (1994). Processing, characterization and evaluation of hydroxyapatite reinforced polyethylene composites. *British Ceramic Transactions, 93*(2), 91–96.
20. Wang, M., Joseph, R., & Bonfield, W. (1998). Hydroxyapatite/polyethylene composites for bone substitution: Effects of ceramic particle size and morphology. *Biomaterials, 19*(23), 2357–2365.
21. Suwanprateeb, J., Tanner, K. E., Turner, S., & Bonfield, W. (1997). Influence of sterilization by gamma irradiation and of thermal annealing on creep of hydroxyapatite-reinforced polyethylene composites. *Journal of Biomedical Materials Research, 39*(1), 16–23.
22. Joseph, R., Martyn, M. T., Tanner, K. E., Coates, P. D., & Bonfield, W. (2001). Rheological characterization of hydroxyapatite filled polyethylene composites. Part 1. Shear and extensional behavior. *Plastics, Rubbers and Composites, 30*(5), 197–204.
23. Zhang, Y., & Tanner, K. E. (2003). Impact behavior of hydroxyapatite reinforced polyethylene composites. *Journal of Materials Science: Materials in Medicine, 14*(1), 63–69.
24. Deb, S., Wang, M., Tanner, K. E., & Bonfield, W. (1996). Hydroxyapatite–polyethylene composites: Effect of grafting and surface treatment of hydroxyapatite. *Journal of Materials Science: Materials in Medicine, 7*(3), 191–195.
25. Doyle, C., Tanner, E. T., & Bonfield, W. (1991). *In vitro* and *in vivo* evaluation of polyhydroxybutyrate and polyhydroxybutyrate reinforced with hydroxyapatite. *Biomaterials, 12*(11), 841–848.
26. Downes, R. N., Vardy, S., Tanner, K. E., & Bonfield, W. (1991). Hydroxyapatite-polyethylene composite in ophthalmic surgery. In W. Bonfield, G. W. Hastings, & K. E. Tanner (Eds.), *Proceedings of the 4th International Symposium on Ceramics in Medicine* (pp. 239–246). Butterworth-Heinemann Ltd., London.
27. Meijer, A. G. W., Segenhout, H. M., Albers, F. W. J., & van de Want, H. J. L. (2002). Histopathology of biocompatible hydroxylapatite-polyethylene composite in ossiculoplasty. *ORL: Journal for Otorhinolaryngology and Related Specialties, 64*(3), 173–178.
28. Boyd, D., Towler, M. R., Wren, A., & Clarkin, O. M. (2008). Comparison of an experimental bone cement with surgical Simplex® P, Spineplex® and Cortoss®. *Journal of Materials Science: Materials in Medicine, 19*(4), 1745–1752.
29. Puska, M., Korventausta, L., Garoushi, S., Seppälä, J., Vallittu, P. K., & Aho, A. (2009). Preliminary in vitro biocompatibility of injectable calcium ceramic polymer composite bone cement. *Key Engineering Materials, 396–398*, 273–276.
30. Leeson, M. C., & Lippitt, S. B. (1993). Thermal aspects of the use of PMMA in large metaphyseal defects in bone: A clinical review and laboratory study. *Clinical Orthopedics and Related Research, 295*, 239–248.

31. Horowitz, S. M., Doty, S. B., Lane, J. M., & Burstein, A. H. (1993). Studies of the mechanism by which the mechanical failure of polymethylmethacrylate leads to bone resorption. *Journal of Bone and Joint Surgery, 75*(6), 802–810.
32. Deb, S., & Vazquez, B. (2001). The effect of cross-linking agents on acrylic bone cements containing radiopacifies. *Biomaterials, 22*(12), 2177–2184.
33. Zhang, Y., & Zhang, M. (2001). Synthesis and characterization of macroporous chitosan/ calcium phosphate composite scaffolds for tissue engineering. *Journal of Biomedical Materials Research, 55*(2), 304–310.
34. Dalby, M. J., Di Silvio, L., Harper, E. J., & Bonfield, W. (1999). In vitro evaluation of a new polymethylmethacrylate cement reinforced with hydroxyapatite. *Journal of Materials Science: Materials in Medicine, 10*(7), 793–798.
35. Canul-Chuil, A., Vargas-Coronado, R., Cauich-Rodríguez, J. V., Martinez-Richa, A., Fernandez, E., & Nazhat, S. N. (2003). Comparative study of bone cements prepared with either HA or β-TCP and functionalized methacrylates. *Journal of Biomedical Materials Research, 64*(1), 27–34.
36. Goto, K., Hashimoto, M., Takadama, H., Tamura, J., Fujibayashi, S., Kawanabe, K., Kokubo, T., & Nakamura, T. (2008). Mechanical setting and biological properties of bone cements containing micron-sized titania particles. *Journal of Materials Science: Materials in Medicine, 19*(3), 1009–1017.
37. Shinzato, S., Nakamura, T., Kokubo, T., & Kitamura, Y. (2001). Effect of glass bead filler content on mechanical and biological properties. *Journal of Biomedical Materials Research, 54*(3), 491–496.
38. Mousa, W. F., Kobayashi, M., Shinzato, S., Kamimura, M., Neo, M., Yoshihara, S., & Nakamura, T. (2000). Biological and mechanical properties of PMMA-based bioactive bone cement. *Biomaterials, 21*(21), 2137–2145.
39. Kokubo, T. (1991). Bioactive glass-ceramics: Properties and application. *Biomaterials, 12*(3), 155–163.
40. Ishihara, K., & Nakabayashi, N. (1989). Adhesive bone cement both to bone and metals: 4-META in MMA initiated with tri-n-butyl borane. *Journal of Biomedical Materials Research, 23*(12), 1475–1489.
41. Jayabalan, M., Thomas, V., & Rajesh, P. N. (2001). Polypropylene fumarate/ phloroglucinol triglycidyl methacrylate blend for use as partially biodegradable orthopedic cement. *Biomaterials, 22*(12), 2749–2760.
42. Misra, D. N. (1985). Adsorption of zirconyl salts and their acids on hydroxyapatite: Use of salts as coupling agents to dental polymer composites. *Journal of Dental Research, 12*(4), 1405–1410.
43. Delpech, V., & Lebugle, A. (1990). Calcium phosphate and interfaces in orthopedic cement. *Clinical Orthopedics and Related Research, 5*, 209–216.
44. Abd Samad, H., Jaafar, M., Othman, R., Kawashita, M., & Abdul Razak, N. H. (2011). New bioactive glass-ceramic: Synthesis and application in PMMA bone cement composites. *Biomedical Materials Engineering, 21*(3), 247–257.
45. Cuijpers, V. M., Jaroszewicz, J., Anil, S., Al Farraj Aldosari, A., Walboomers, X. F., & Jansen, J. A. (2013). Resolution, sensitivity, and in vivo application of high-resolution computed tomography for titanium-coated polymethyl methacrylate (PMMA) dental implants. *Clinical Oral Implants Research*. https://doi.org/10.1111/clr.12128.

46. Jayabalan, M., Thomas, V., & Sreelatha, P. K. (2000). Studies on poly (propylene fumarate-co-ethylene glycol) based bone cement. *Bio-Medical Materials and Engineering, 10*(1), 57–66. PMID: 11086840.
47. He, S., Yaszemski, M. J., Yasko, A. W., Engel, P. S., & Mikos, A. G. (2000). Injectable biodegradable polymer composites based on poly (propylene fumarate) crosslinked with poly (ethylene glycol) dimethacrylate. *Biomaterials, 21*(12), 2389–2396.
48. Yaszemski, M. J., Payne, R. G., Hayes, W. C., Langer, R., Aufdemorte, T. B., & Mikos, A. G. (1995). The ingrowth of new bone tissue and initial mechanical properties of a degradable polymeric composite scaffold. *Tissue Engineering, 1*(1), 41–52.
49. Gerhart, T. N., Roux, R. D., Horowitz, G., Miller, R. L., Hanff, P., & Hayes, W. C. (1988). Antibiotic releases from an experimental biodegradable bone cement. *Journal of Orthopedic Research, 6*(5), 585–591.
50. Cai, Z., Zhang, T., Di, L., Xu, D. M., Xu, D. H., & Yang-An, D. A. (2011). Morphological and histological analysis on the in vivo degradation of poly (propylene fumarate)/(calcium sulfate/tricalcium phosphate). *Biomedical Microdevices, 13*(4), 623–632.
51. Jayabalan, M., Shalumon, K. T., Mitha, M. K., Ganesan, K., & Epple, M. (2010). Effect of hydroxyapatite on the biodegradation and biomechanical stability of polyester nanocomposites for orthopedic applications. *Acta Biomaterialia, 6*(2), 763–772.
52. Chang, C. H., Liao, T. C., Hsu, Y. M., Fang, H. W., Chen, C. C., & Lin, F. H. (2010). A poly (propylene fumarate)-calcium phosphate based angiogenic injectable bone cement for femoral head osteonecrosis. *Biomaterials, 31*(15), 4048–4056.
53. Shuaia, C., Yua, L., Fenga, P., Gaoa, C., & Pengd, S. (2020). Interfacial reinforcement in bioceramic/biopolymer composite bone scaffold: The role of coupling agent. *Colloids and Surfaces B: Bio Interfaces, 193*, 111146.
54. Coskun, S., Korkusuz, F., & Hasirci, V. (2005). Hydroxyapatite reinforced poly(3-hydroxybutyrate) and poly(3-hydroxybutyrate-co-3-hydroxyvalerate) based degradable composite bone plate. *Journal of Biomedical Materials Research: Part A, 16*(11), 1485–1495.
55. Chen, D. Z., Tang, C. Y., Chan, K. C., Tsui, C. P., Yu, P. H. F., Leung, M. C. P., & Uskokovic, P. S. (2007). Dynamic mechanical properties and in vitro bioactivity of PHBHV/HA nanocomposite. *Composites Science and Technology, 67*(8–9), 1617–1623.
56. Kong, L., Yuan, G., Guangyuan, L., Yandao, G., Nanming, Z., & Xiufang, Z. (2006). A study on the bioactivity of chitosan/nanohydroxyapatite composite scaffolds for bone tissue engineering. *European Polymer Journal, 42*(12), 3171–3182.
57. Francis, S. J. K., & Matthew, W. T. H. (2000). Application of chitosan-based polysaccharide biomaterials in cartilage tissue engineering: A review. *Biomaterials, 21*(24), 2589–2596.
58. Pillai, C. K. S., Willi, P., & Chandra, P. S. (2012). Chitin and chitosan polymers: Chemistry, solubility and fiber formation. *Progress in Polymer Science, 34*(7), 641–678.
59. Dahlan, K., Dewi, S. U., Nurlaila, A., & Soejako, D. (2012). Synthesis and characterization of calcium phosphate/chitosan composites. *International Journal of Basic & Applied Sciences, 12*(1), 51–58.
60. Niekraszewicz, A., Kucharska, M., Wisniewska-Wrona, M., Cienchanska, D., Ratajska, M., & Haberko, K. (2020). Surgical bio composites with chitosan. *Progress on Chemistry and Application of Chitin and its Derivatives* (in press).

61. Wan, A. C. A., Khor, E., & Hastings, G. W. (1997). Hydroxyapatite modified chitin as potential hard tissue substitute material. *Journal of Biomedical Materials Research: Part B Applied Biomaterials, 38*(2), 235–244.
62. Yamaguchi, I., Tokuchi, K., Fukuzaki, H., Koyama, Y., Takakuda, K., Monma, H., & Tanak, J. (2001). Preparation and microstructure analysis of chitosan/hydroxyapatite nanocomposites. *Journal of Biomedical Materials Research, 55*(1), 20–28.

CHAPTER 7

Multifunctional Bio-Nanocomposite for Healthcare Application

ABHA KATHURIA[1] and SHRUTI GOEL[2]

[1]*Department of Chemistry, Ramjas College, University of Delhi, Delhi, India*

[2]*Department of Chemistry, IIT Roorkee, Roorkee, Uttarakhand, India*

ABSTRACT

Bio-nanocomposites have surfaced as a prominent field of research in nanotechnology over the past two decades. These are hybrid materials made up of naturally derived or biodegradable materials, along with fine nano-dimensional fillers. Being derived from natural resources, these bio-nano-composites are multifunctional with enhanced biocompatibility as well as reduced toxicity. This forms the foundation for their vast application, ranging from food packaging to biomedicines and healthcare. Bio-nanocomposites based on natural polymers such as starch, cellulose, chitosan, and many more, which are preferred due to their eco-friendly standpoint, are found to have exceptional activity in various regenerative medicines and biomedical applications. The healthcare applications of these multifunctional nanocom-posites are multitudinous, including wound healing and dressing, medical textiles, dental applications, osteoporosis, cancer therapy, drug delivery, and tissue engineering. Traditional biomedical processes such as wound dressing involve the use of antimicrobial chemical species. The incorporation of nano-scaled fillers with biomaterials eliminates the need for such species due to the exceedingly high antimicrobial activity of nanoparticles. Besides, bio-nanocomposites function as precursors for various scaffolds, biomedical devices, and diagnostics, and find applications in cosmetics as well.

Bioabsorbable Polymers for Drug Carriers and Fixation Devices. Arbind Prasad and Sougata Jana (Eds.)

This chapter discusses the utilization of various multifunctional bio-nanocomposites in biomedical and healthcare applications. It focuses on the nanocomposites based on different biomaterials and depicts the striking potential of these materials in the healthcare industry.

7.1 INTRODUCTION

Nanocomposites refer to composites having fillers of the nano size, i.e., up to 100 nm in size along at least one of the dimensions. Nanocomposites can be made up of various combinations of inorganic, organic, or natural substances, either of these forming one or both the components of a composite, i.e., matrix and fillers (Figure 7.1) [1]. The major advantage of incorporating nano-fillers is that it enhances the properties of a composite manyfold, leading to high efficacy in its application. The different types of matrices and fillers essentially affect the properties and consequently the applications of nanocomposites. The high flexibility and unusual properties rendered by the nanocomposites drive the attention of researchers exceedingly more in this discipline.

Bio-nanocomposite is one of the advancements in nanotechnology, which involves natural polymers or biodegradable materials as a component of the nanocomposite along with fine nano-fillers. These naturally derived polymers or compounds are biodegradable, less or negligibly toxic, and thus form a pathway to the greener utility of nanocomposites than the conventional ones. The term "green" here means that these bio-nanocomposites can be easily degraded or disposed of without any harm to the ecological system. These degrade naturally to form CO_2 and water, which do not have an adverse effect on the environment. Conventional nanocomposites, in this regard, are highly toxic as they are non-biodegradable, leading to harmful byproducts on decomposition. The bio-polymers have an edge over conventional inorganic/organic polymers as these are multifunctional.

7.2 CLASSIFICATION OF BIO-NANOCOMPOSITES

There are various classes of bio-nanocomposites that can be prepared based on the type of biopolymer used as well as the nanofillers. A change in either the biopolymer or the nanofiller helps in fine-tuning the desired properties for the expected application.

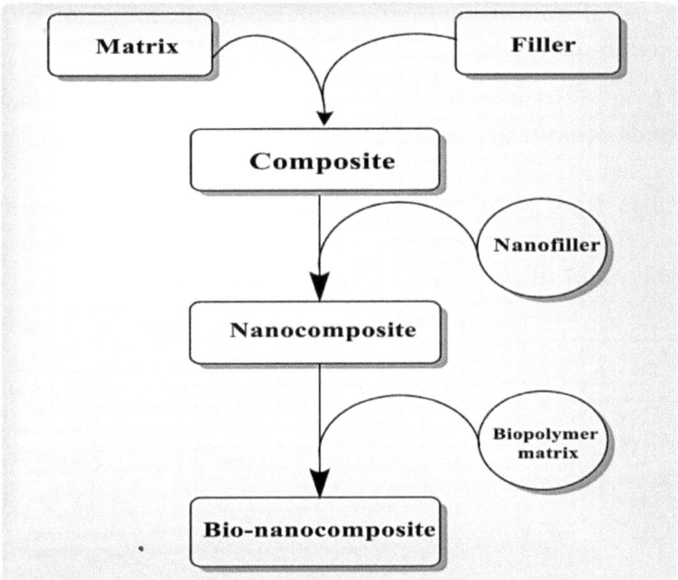

FIGURE 7.1 Schematic representation of composite, nanocomposite, and bio-nanocomposite.

It is interesting to note that the properties of bio-nanocomposites change not only by changing the components but also by changing the shape and size of the components. The effect of size is self-explanatory, as nano-sized fillers show drastic changes in properties. Besides, the shape of fillers also plays a crucial role in predicting the properties of bio-nanocomposites. Based on the size and shape of the reinforced nanoparticles, the bio-nanocomposites can be classified into three categories. (Figure 7.2) [2].

1. **Particulate Bio-Nanocomposite:** These bio-nanocomposites involve iso-dimensional particles, i.e., nano-sized particles along all dimensions as reinforcements. Due to the small size of these reinforcements, the aspect ratio, i.e., the length-to-diameter ratio, is small, leading to moderate to low variations in the properties. Such nanocomposites are inflammable and have a reduced cost of production.
2. **Elongated Bio-Nanocomposites:** These bio-nanocomposites comprise long 1D nanotubes, nanorods, etc., which, due to increased lengths, have good to remarkably high aspect ratios. A classic example of such nanocomposites includes carbon nanotubes, which have proved to be excellent fillers. Starch, cellulose fibers,

or cellulose whiskers form some bio-nanocomposites aiding several biocompatible properties.

3. **Layered-Structured Bio-Nanocomposites:** These may include several kinds of layering, including intercalated, flocculated, phase-separated, exfoliated, and sheet-like nanocomposites. The layers involved can range from platelets, microparticles, and sheets of different desired lengths as per the required property. The greater the length of the sheet or layer of fillers, the more would be the aspect ratio [3].

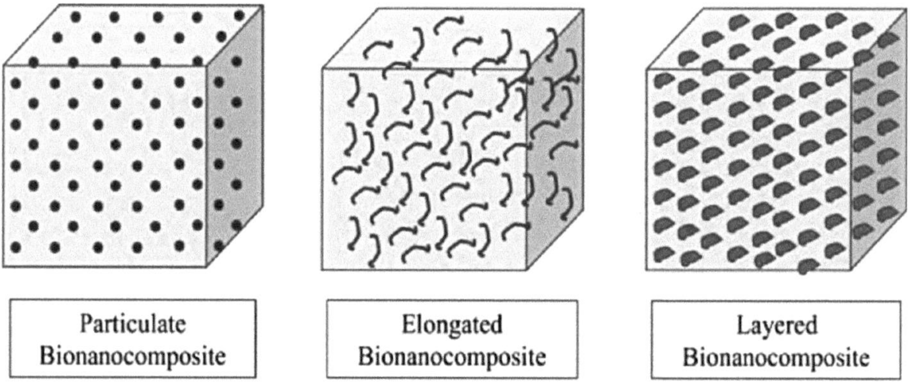

FIGURE 7.2 Different types of bio-nanocomposites based on the shape and size of reinforcements.

7.3 DIFFERENT BIOPOLYMERS IN BIO-NANOCOMPOSITES

Bio-nanocomposites can be structured by using diverse kinds of biopolymers, which may be available naturally or may be semi-synthetic. The naturally available biopolymers include proteins, polysaccharides, lipids, etc., while the synthetic or semi-synthetic biopolymers include polymers such as PLA (polylactic acid), PCL (polycaprolactone), PVA (polyvinyl alcohol), etc. However, due to the lack of renewability, several synthetic or semi-synthetic biopolymers are not considered suitable for forming bio-nanocomposites. Among the various biopolymers, it is found that polysaccharides form an important and widely studied class of biopolymers. The emerging trend of researchers in polysaccharide-based nanocomposites is primarily due to their large availability, low cost, and excellent biodegradable properties. Polysaccharide-based nanocomposites have also been found effective in absorbent properties owing to their hydrophilic nature. Some distinct types of polysaccharide-based bio-nanocomposites are cited below:

7.3.1 CELLULOSE-BASED BIO-NANOCOMPOSITES

Cellulose-based bio-nanocomposites have gained global attention due to their wide application and improved physicomechanical properties [4]. Cellulose fibers are made up of microfibrils that naturally orient and link to form cellulose fibers. These are naturally synthesized by several microorganisms and can also be obtained from a wide range of higher or power plant species [5].

7.3.2 STARCH-BASED BIO-NANOCOMPOSITES

Starch is another abundant natural polymer that primarily exists in two forms: amylose and amylopectin. Starch-based bio-nanocomposites have been found to be highly suitable for medical applications as a result of their high biocompatibility, nontoxicity, and biodegradability [6]. The various applications of starch-based nanocomposites are discussed later in the chapter.

7.3.3 CHITOSAN-BASED BIO-NANOCOMPOSITES

Chitosan is a natural cationic polymer that is extracted from chitin. Chitin can be found and extracted from the shells of crustaceans. Chitosan is found to have many amino ($-NH_2$) and hydroxyl functional groups, which leads to its high affinity for various biological polymers and constituents, including fats, proteins, tumor cells, and metal ions. Due to this, chitosan-based nanocomposites are widely used in drug delivery and other medical applications.

7.3.4 ALGINATE-BASED BIO-NANOCOMPOSITE

Alginate is a natural anionic polysaccharide composed of uronic acid residues, obtained from marine brown algae. It has been found that nano-alginate materials are more effective only in the presence of other polymers or additives [7]. The alginates are exceptionally useful in food and medical sectors as they are widely used in stabilization, gel and film formation, and in drug-delivery [8].

Apart from the above-cited polysaccharides, various proteins such as gelatin which is derived from collagen are also found and incorporated as polymers in bio-nanocomposites.

7.4 HEALTHCARE APPLICATIONS OF BIO-NANOCOMPOSITES

Through our discussion before, it is well-established that bio-nanocomposites have an edge over conventional composites in terms of thermal stability, flexibility, multifunctional characteristics, and specifically in their high biocompatibility and biodegradability. These properties of bio-nanocomposites make them a suitable partner for carrying out various applications, especially biomedical and healthcare applications. The utilization of different matrices and fillers in these bio-nanocomposites can help in achieving distinct health applications. Besides, bio-nanocomposites are also widely used in the cosmetic industry. The various healthcare applications include tissue engineering, regenerative tissues, wound healing, antidiabetic treatments, bio-adhesives, bio-imaging, burn dressing, etc. [9].

7.4.1 BIO-NANOCOMPOSITES IN DRUG-DELIVERY

Controlled and directed drug delivery is very crucial to harness the maximum therapeutic potential of any drug or medicine. Bio-nanocomposites can be used to serve this purpose due to safety concerns, high drug loading capacity, and targeted yet sustained drug delivery. Among the different biopolymers, alginate and chitosan-based bio-nanocomposites are widely used to form the drug delivery system. This wide application of alginate-based bio-nanocomposites in drug delivery systems is due to their ability to be structured as beads, films, sponges, or foams to serve different applications [10]. These bio-nanocomposites are generally hybrid materials with clay or other inorganic species, which aid in achieving higher precision in the targeted release of the encapsulated drug. Often, magnetic counterparts can be used in such drug delivery systems to enhance the process. It has been found that drug delivery can be tuned as per requirement by using such magnetic nanoparticles, which show variation in the amount of drug released based on the applied external magnetic field. An example of this is the release of Ibuprofen drug mediated using ALG/LDH–IBU/ MG. (Figure 7.3) [11].

7.4.2 BIO-NANOCOMPOSITES IN WOUND HEALING

Wound healing is a process involving tissue contraction, closure, and regeneration. The delayed process of wound healing often results in severe health conditions, and thus researchers have paid attention to this healthcare

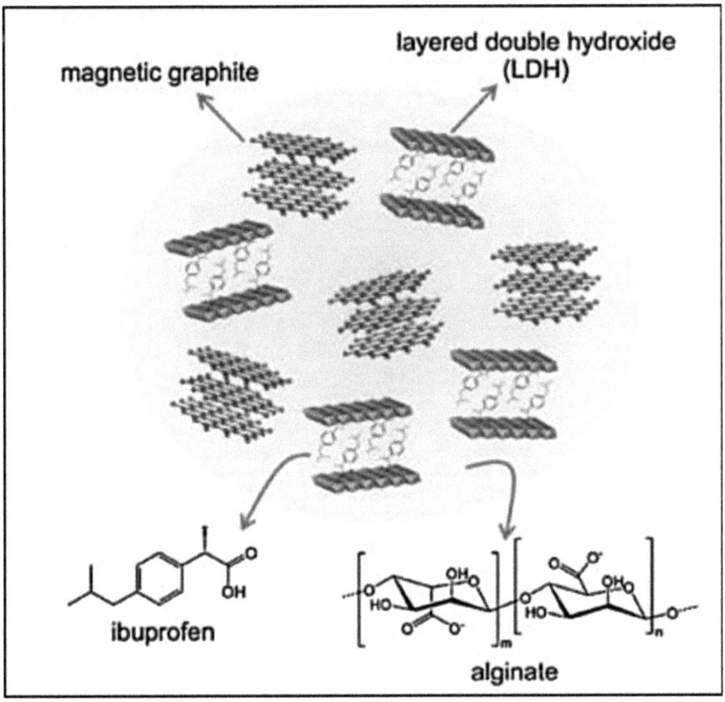

FIGURE 7.3 Schematic representation of a magnetic bio-nanocomposite for delivery of ibuprofen drug using alginate-magnetic graphite layer-LDH (ALG/LDH–IBU/MG).

Source: Reprinted with permission from Ref. [11]. Copyright © 2020 Elsevier Inc.

problem. Bio-nanocomposites have proven to be beneficial in several cases where they enhance and speed up the process of wound healing. Alginate-based bio-nanocomposites have shown significant efficacy in wound healing processes. The remarkable effectiveness of alginate-based bio-nanocomposites is due to their hydrophilicity, which ensures a moist environment at the site of injury. This moist condition facilitates the healing and tissue restoration process [12]. Besides, Chitosan-based bio-nanocomposites have also been reported [13]. Chitosan is found to accelerate the process of finding and treating the inflammatory cells that are affected by the injury. Thus, this bio-nanocomposite facilitates both the topical application as well as the speedy healing of the wounds. A chitosan-alginate-based nanocomposite loaded with curcumin was found to be effective in wound healing, as curcumin is a potent drug molecule for this purpose. The sponge-shaped bio-nanocomposite helped in increased loading of the drug, and the wound healing process was found to be more effective than the direct use of curcumin [15] (Figure 7.4).

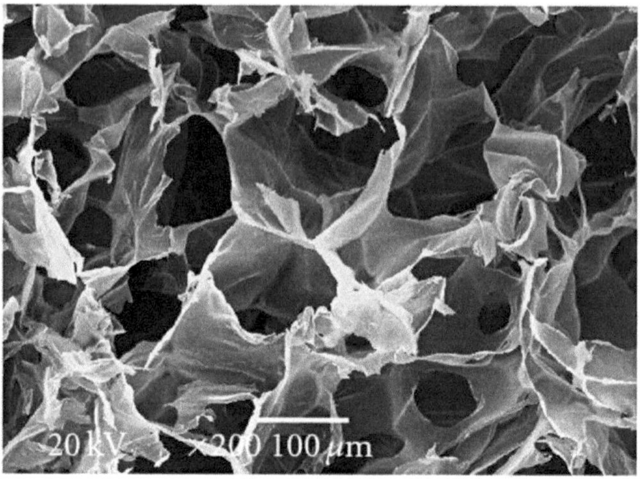

FIGURE 7.4 Chitosan–alginate sponge SEM images for curcumin delivery.

Source: Reprinted with permission from Ref. [14]

7.4.3 BIO-NANOCOMPOSITES IN ANTIMICROBIAL ACTIVITY

Antimicrobial agents are required to cease the development of harmful pathogens in biological systems. Bio-nanocomposites have rapidly made their mark in this healthcare application as well. Evidence for such cases can be found where bio-nanocomposites have helped in inhibiting microbial growth, exhibiting anti-tumor activity, and leading to significant pain reduction. Chitosan-based bio-nanocomposites have been found to be extremely effective in microbial growth inhibition owing to the biomedical and therapeutic properties of chitosan. The antimicrobial activities of such hybrids not only help in fighting microbes but also assist in wound healing, burn dressing, and regeneration of damaged cells. As per a study bio-nanocomposites have been found effective in fighting against *E. coli, Staphylococcus aureus,* and *Bacillus cereus* [15]. Besides, the antimicrobial characteristic of bio-nanocomposites facilitates there use in food packaging that helps in protection of food materials from pathogen damage.

7.4.4 DENTAL APPLICATION OF BIO-NANOCOMPOSITES

In addition to the flexibility, some bio-nanocomposites have been found to have excellent tensile strength, comparable to inorganic substituents. The mechanical strength of bio-nanocomposites can be adjusted based on the proportion of different fillers and matrices. The high tensile strength in some cases makes these bio-nanocomposites exceedingly supportive in dental applications such as enamel substitutes, crack-bridging, etc. An example of such a dental application is a PLA-silica-based nanocomposite, which shows high tensile strength. Besides, gelatin-based bio-nanocomposites have been found to be effective in the regeneration of the pulp-dentin complex (Figure 7.5).

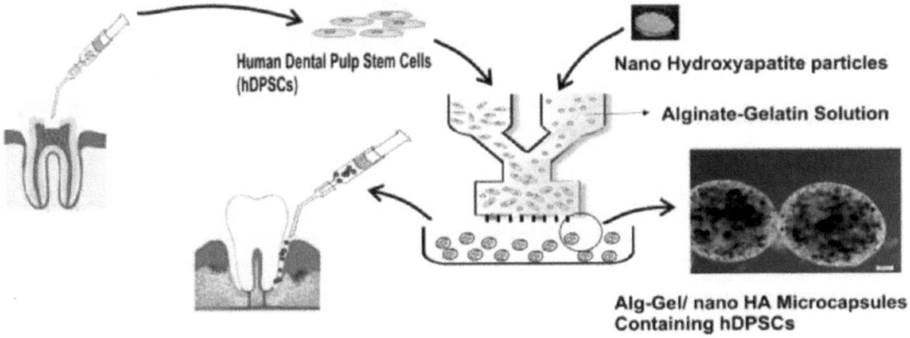

FIGURE 7.5 Schematic representation of use of ALG-gel/hydroxyapatite bio-nanocomposite for dental application.

Source: Reprinted with permission from Ref. [16]. https://creativecommons.org/licenses/by/4.0/

7.4.5 BIO-NANOCOMPOSITES IN OSTEOPOROSIS

One of the most common lifestyle disorders involves bone disorders. Poor dietary habits have been a major cause of bone disorders that lead to early fractures, cracks in bones, and osteoporosis. Osteoporosis is defined as a medical condition where the bone density decreases or there are deformations in the bone structure. Though numerous drugs are available for treating this disorder, most of them are found to have some side effects, predominantly the degradation of drugs is not so rapid. In such a scenario, bio-nanocomposites prove to be highly efficient. Chitosan-based bio-nanocomposites show high osteoconductivity and osteointegratability and are gradually biodegradable, which leads to their easy application in the treatment of osteoporosis. Chitosan also facilitates bone tissue regeneration, which helps in restoring bone density. Thus, chitosan-based bio-nanocomposites can be utilized for a healthier and more effective treatment [17] (Figure 7.6).

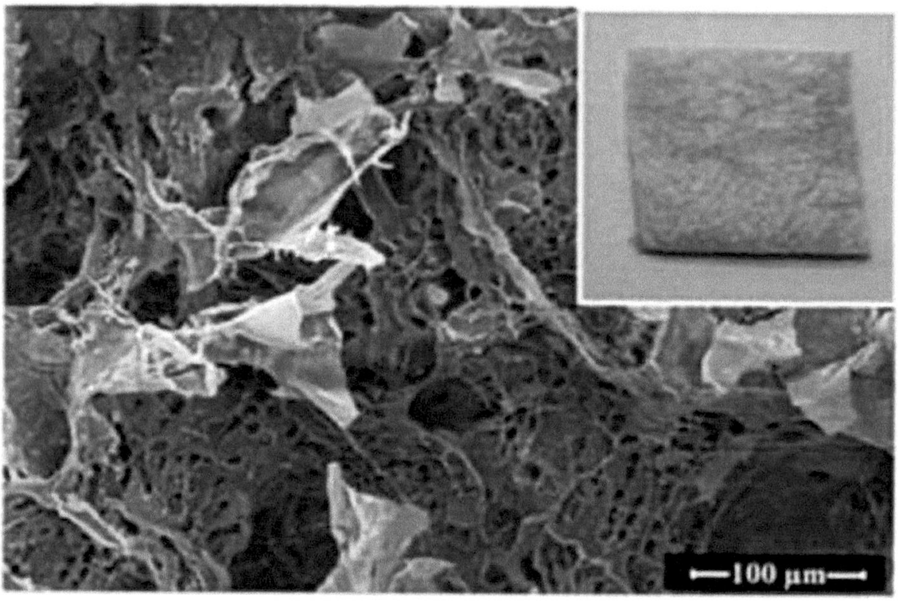

FIGURE 7.6 SEM images of chitosan/hydroxyapatite bio-nanocomposite.

Source: Reprinted from Ref. [18]. Copyright © 2021 by the authors. Licensee MDPI, Basel, Switzerland. http://creativecommons.org/licenses/by/4.0/

7.4.6 OTHER BIO-MEDICAL APPLICATIONS OF BIO-NANOCOMPOSITES

Besides the above-mentioned applications of bio-nanocomposites, they are also used in various other healthcare applications. Bio-imaging, for instance, is another crucial application of bio-nanocomposites. Chitosan nanocomposites, when hybridized with imaging materials such as Fe_3O_4, can be utilized in magnetic resonance imaging (MRI) [19]. Also, photoluminescence bioimaging can be performed using bio-nanocomposites [20]. Biosensors based on alginate-based nanocomposites can be helpful in detecting several diseases and can also be utilized to monitor glucose levels in the human body [21]. In addition, 3D-bioprinting and bone tissue engineering are some other applications of bio-nanocomposites.

7.5 CONCLUSION

This book chapter discusses the various kinds of bio-nanocomposites that are useful in healthcare and biomedical applications. The properties of these bio-nanocomposites are greatly influenced by the size and shape of the nanoparticles, based on which they can be classified. The presence of multiple functional groups in the biopolymer makes these bio-nanocomposites extremely useful for multiple applications. Bio-nanocomposites can be used for various healthcare applications such as drug delivery, wound healing, antimicrobial activity, osteoporosis, bio-imaging, 3D bioprinting, and dental applications. Besides, bio-nanocomposites are found to be useful in the cosmetic industry. Further advancements in this discipline would pave the way for more rapid, less toxic, and eco-friendly medical utilization. The threat generated by non-biocompatible and non-biodegradable medicines could be significantly reduced with the development of more bio-nanocomposites. The structure-activity relationships can be fine-tuned by varying and experimenting with the different shapes and assemblies of the biopolymers as well as the nanoparticles.

KEYWORDS

- **antimicrobial activity**
- **biocompatible medicines**
- **biomedicine**
- **bio-nanocomposite**
- **drug delivery**
- **nanoparticles**
- **tissue engineering**

REFERENCES

1. Esteves, A. C. C., Barros-Timmons, A., & Trindade, T. (2004). Polymer based nanocomposites: Synthetic strategies for hybrid materials. *Quimica Nova, 27*(6), 798–807.
2. Saini, R. K., Bajpai, A. K., & Jain, E. (2017). Fundamentals of bio nanocomposites. In *Biodegradable and Biocompatible Polymer Composites* (pp. 47–85). Springer.
3. Wani, S. D., & Mundada, A. S. (2021). A review: Emerging trends in bio nanocomposites. *International Journal of Pharmaceutical Research and Technology, 11*(1), 1–12.
4. Khairnar, Y., Hansora, D., Hazra, C., Kundu, D., Tayde, S., Tonde, S., Naik, J., & Chatterjee, A. (2021). Cellulose bio nanocomposites for sustainable planet and people:

A global snapshot of preparation, properties, and applications. *Carbohydrate Polymers: Technology and Applications, 267*, 100065.
5. Heux, L., Dinand, E., & Vignon, M. R. (1999). Structural aspects in ultrathin cellulose microfibrils followed by 13C CP-MAS NMR. *Carbohydrate Polymers, 39*(2), 115–121.
6. Arora, B., Bhatia, R., & Attri, P. (2018). Bio nanocomposites: Green materials for a sustainable future. In C. M. Hussain & A. K. Mishra (Eds.), *New Polymer Nanocomposites for Environmental Remediation* (pp. 699–724). Elsevier.
7. Zia, F., Salman, M., Ali, M., Iqbal, R., Rasul, A., Haq, M. N., Asgher, M., & Zia, K. M. (2020). Alginate-based bio nanocomposites. In K. M. Zia, F. Jabeen, M. N. Anjum, & S. Ikram (Eds.), *Bio Nanocomposites: Micro and Nano Technologies* (pp. 173–207). Elsevier.
8. Singha, K., Pandit, P., & Maity, S. (2021). Applications of alginate-based bio nanocomposites in drug delivery. In S. Ahmed (Ed.), *Bio Nanocomposites in Tissue Engineering and Regenerative Medicine* (pp. 399–426). Woodhead Publishing.
9. Idumah, C., & Hassan, A. (2016). Emerging trends in eco-compliant, synergistic, and hybrid assembling of multifunctional polymeric bio nanocomposites. *Reviews in Chemical Engineering, 32*(3).
10. Ribeiro, L. N. M., Alcântara, A. C. S., Darder, M., Aranda, P., Herrmann, P. S. P., Moreira, F. M. A., Hernández, M. G., & Hitzky, E. R. (2014). Bio nanocomposites containing magnetic graphite as potential systems for drug delivery. *International Journal of Pharmaceutics, 477*(1–2), 553–562.
11. Akbar, M. U., Athar, M. M., Bhatti, I. A., Bhatti, H. N., Khosa, M. K., Zia, K. M., Bokhari, T. H., & Ahmad, M. N. (2020). Biomedical applications of bio nanocomposites. In K. M. Zia, F. Jabeen, M. N. Anjum, & S. Ikram (Eds.), *Bio Nanocomposites: Micro and Nano Technologies* (pp. 457–486). Elsevier.
12. Qin, Y. (2008). Alginate fibers: An overview of the production processes and applications in wound management. *Polymer International, 57*(2), 171–180.
13. Ueno, H., Mori, T., & Fujinaga, T. (2001). Topical formulations and wound healing applications of chitosan. *Advanced Drug Delivery Reviews, 52*(2), 1052–1067.
14. Dai, M., Zheng, X. L., Xu, X. Y., Kong, X. Y., Li, X. Y., Guo, G., Luo, F., Zhao, X., Wei, Y. Q., & Qian, Z. (2009). Chitosan-alginate sponge: Preparation and application in curcumin delivery for dermal wound healing in rats. *BioMed Research International, 2009*(1110–7243), 595126.
15. Jayakumar, R., Radoor, S., Karayil, J., Nair, I. C., Siengchin, S., Parameswaranpillai, J., & Radhakrishnan, E. K. (2022). Antimicrobial properties of bio nanocomposites. In C. Muthukumar, S. M. K. Thiagamani, S. Krishnasamy, R. Nagarajan, & S. Siengchin (Eds.), *Polymer Based Bio-Nanocomposites* (pp. 189–213). Springer.
16. Alipour, M., Firouzi, N., Aghazadeh, M., Samiei, M., Montazersaheb, S., Khoshfetrat, A. B., & Aghazadeh, M. (2021). The osteogenic differentiation of human dental pulp stem cells in alginate-gelatin/Nano-hydroxyapatite microcapsules. *BMC Biotechnology, 21*(1), 40.
17. Niranjan, M. K., Baghel, K., & Azam, Z. (2021). Chitosan-based bio nanocomposites in osteoporosis. In S. Ahmed (Ed.), *Bio Nanocomposites in Tissue Engineering and Regenerative Medicine* (pp. 243–272). Woodhead Publishing.
18. Chaves, A. V., Freire, R. M., Feitosa, V. P., Ricardo, N. M. P. S., Denardin, J. C., Andrade Neto, D. M., & Fechine, P. B. A. (2021). Hydroxyapatite-based magnetic bio

nanocomposite as pharmaceuticals carriers in chitosan scaffold. *Journal of Composites Science, 5*(2), 37.

19. Ahmad, M., Manzoor, K., & Ikram, S. (2018). Chitosan-based nanocomposites for drug, gene delivery, and bioimaging applications. In I. Inamuddin, A. M. Asiri, & A. Mohammad (Eds.), *Applications of Nanocomposite Materials in Drug Delivery* (pp. 27–50). Woodhead Publishing.
20. Hari, K., Pichaimania, A., & Kumpati, G. (2013). Acridine orange tethered chitosan reduced gold nanoparticles: A dual functional probe for combined photodynamic and photothermal therapy. *RSC Advances, 3*(47), 20471–20479.
21. Buk, V., Emregul, E., & Emregul, K. C. (2017). Alginate copper oxide nano-bio composite as a novel material for amperometric glucose biosensing. *Materials Science and Engineering C, 74*, 307–314.

CHAPTER 8

Biomechanical Studies of Biocomposites for Bone Fixation Devices

NIPUN JAIN,[1] ARBIND PRASAD,[2] and SUDIPTO DATTA[1]

[1]Department of Materials Engineering, Indian Institute of Science, C.V. Raman Avenue, Bangalore, Karnataka, India

[2]Mechanical Engineering Department, Katihar Engineering College (Under Department of Science, Technology and Technical Education, Government of Bihar), Katihar, Bihar, India

ABSTRACT

The importance of the bone matrix to the human body has drawn attention due to its distinctive biophysical and mechanobiological assets. The bone matrix possesses tremendous toughness and substantial stiffness due to its unique structural anisotropy. The aforementioned mechanical characteristics reflect how bones work in the body and are strongly related to our daily activities. For fracture healing and long-term stability, the proper fixation design must be used; nevertheless, this is an intricate subject with many important considerations. The last few years have seen an interesting change in fracture therapy. This chapter presents some clinical and biomechanical findings related to cutting-edge implants. We conclude by highlighting the benefits of these novel implants in complex trauma scenarios.

8.1 INTRODUCTION

Bone is an essential body part that supports an individual's body mechanically, and the bone matrix plays a crucial role in this [1–3]. The overarching

Bioabsorbable Polymers for Drug Carriers and Fixation Devices. Arbind Prasad and Sougata Jana (Eds.)

function of the matrix associated with the bone and its distinct mechanical characteristics have long drawn significant interest from researchers worldwide [4–7]. Compared to synthetic materials, the bone matrix performs better mechanically and is obtained naturally. Bone replacement transplants, biomimetic materials, and scaffolds for repairing a patient's tissue will benefit from biomechanical characteristics, biological importance, structure, and arrangement [8–10]. Furthermore, before bone development and maintenance, the matrix can be influenced by various environmental factors, particularly mechanical stress [11–13]. Both strength and toughness are difficult for synthetic materials to accomplish; as a result, materials with high strength typically exhibit poor toughness, whereas those with high toughness show an inverse relationship [4, 14]. Most of the bone-associated matrices are made up of hydroxyapatite and collagen. Collagen makes up 55% to 60% of the bone matrix's size, whereas hydroxyapatite makes up 40% to 45%. Hydroxyapatite provides high strength features, while collagen fibers exhibit considerable toughness [14]. The intricate matrix structure consists of multiple levels ranging in size from nano to macro scale and offers strength and durability as an organic biomaterial. This detailed, multifaceted matrix structure and biomechanical characteristics are a template for creating novel composite biomaterials. Nowadays, various researchers are conducting research on biobased resorbable composites for scaffold fabrication, bone implants, internal fixation devices, and using naturally sourced materials to fabricate the composite more efficiently [43–47]. The advantages associated with resorbable composites are that the patient does not need to undergo resurgery for implant removal, resorbable implants are lightweight, prevent stress shielding, prevent corrosion, and do not cause underlying bone damage. These advantages make resorbable composites a more valuable and promising solution for bone-related issues. The challenges associated with biobased resorbable composites include the mechanical strength and degradation rate of the fabricated implants [48–53]. Numerous elements of the environment have an impact on the development, perpetuation, and restoration of human bones. One of the most crucial environmental elements is mechanical stimulation [11, 13, 15]. Running, jumping, swimming, and bungee jumping are only a few examples of daily human activities that drastically alter the physical conditions surrounding the bone matrix. Mechanical stimulation will significantly change the relationship between the bone-constituted elements and the cells that comprise the whole structure [11, 13, 15]. Compressive, tensile, and fluid shear stress are the three basic types of mechanical stimuli experienced by humans [15]. Among them, fluid shear stress (FSS) significantly affects the cells and elements of the bone matrix [11, 13, 16].

Fluid shear stress primarily affects the endosteal surface, cell membranes, and surfaces of lacunar-canalicular walls *in vivo*. Additionally, the collagen (Col) coating on the surface of the bone and that of freshly produced osteoid could be exposed to fluid flow. New surgical techniques and unique implants are currently in development due to the challenges caused by complex peri-articular cracks and multiple impediments after using traditional plates and gap reduction procedures. A new generation of implants has been created by combining three essential criteria for treating fractures: anatomically reduced articular surfaces, minimized soft tissue damage during percutaneous insertion, and mechanical resilience. The goal of this chapter is to outline the benefits of cutting-edge traumatology implants, such as the advantages possessed by the dynamic condylar screw over the condylar blade plate for treating persistent femur and humeral fractures, the XS nail for treating ankle and patella fractures, the gliding nail for treating trochanteric injuries, and bone plates to provide axial stability.

8.2 BIOMECHANICAL PROPERTIES OF THE BONE MATRIX

Human beings rely on the skeleton as one of their primary supporting load tissues; the bone matrix is one of its main constituents. Because of its remarkable mechanical qualities, intricate multistage structure, and biological significance, it has attracted a lot of research over the years. This study investigates how the chemical makeup and the arrangement of different elements influence the physical characteristics of the bone structure constituent. The mechanical characteristics of this associated structure are governed by an anisotropic structure in which elevated strength and overhead toughness are major biomechanical characteristics that have drawn much interest [4, 6, 14]. These traits result from extensive natural evolution and are fundamental to everyday human activity. Clarifying the mechanical characteristics advances the knowledge of this constituent bone matrix and guides the creation of scaffolds and bone replacement devices for tissue engineering. Cortical bone has a Young's modulus of 15 to 25 GPa, substantially greater than its transverse section. Thus, the associated biomechanical characteristics have garnered much interest and are currently used to create scaffolds. To create wood-based gel systems that exhibit structural anisotropy, Wang, for instance, combined alginate into delignified wood and later submerged it successively into solutions of K_2HPO_4, $CaCl_2$, $NH_3 \cdot H_2O$, and PBS. Artificial compounds struggle to achieve high strength and good toughness simultaneously [4, 14]. The ordinary organic biomaterial bone matrix can concurrently exhibit both properties and fails to achieve both properties. The properties exhibited by the bone matrix serve as the ideal reference for creating artificial materials.

8.3 A MECHANICAL COMPARISON OF DCS AND CBP IN CONVOLUTED SUPRACONDYLAR FEMORAL INJURIES

Orthopedic surgeons face a problem when treating distal femoral fractures, and despite several biomechanical studies, the best prosthetic transplant remains debatable [1–4]. Yet, before the invention of these cutting-edge implants, CBP and DCS were considered popular substitutes, even though plates providing angular consistency and interlocked nails have become other alternative options in therapy [5]. In another biomechanical study, the stiffness of the implanted composite was examined in more convoluted supracondylar femoral injuries [5, 6]. Six pairs of DCS and CBP were utilized to fix the distal portions of prosthetic femoral bones. Later, a 1.5 cm bone defect was created using osteotomy to mimic a supracondylar fracture (Figure 8.1). Distal halves of the bones were halved, and proximal portions were fixed in a metal adaptor sleeve.

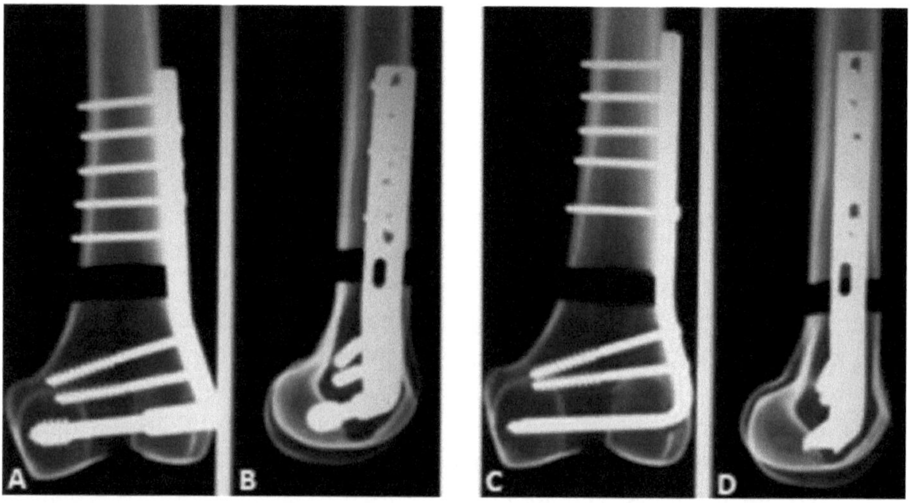

FIGURE 8.1 (a) and (b) DCS fixed synthetic composite femur radiographic aspect; (c) and (d) CBP fixed synthetic composite femur radiographic aspect.

Source: Reprinted from Ref. [42]. https://creativecommons.org/licenses/by/3.0/

Seven different forms of loading were investigated on the bone-implant constructions: (i) internal compression; (ii) external compression; (iii) anterior compression; (iv) posterior compression; (v) axial compression; (vi) external torsion; and (vii) internal torsion. Compressive and torsional trials were conducted six times to determine the dispersion statistically. Every DCS measurement was carried out either with or without a compaction screw. An M221B04 (PCB Piezotronics force transducer) was used to determine loading forces, and a set of inductive transducers was used to measure the deformation values during frontal and sagittal axes, respectively. A laptop-connected automated approach was used for data acquisition. The following research illustrated hysteresis cycles by relating the load forces with transducer movement. The authors' preliminary findings about DCS versus CBP were determined by examining these measurements and diagrams, and these findings calculated the average stiffness and "p" value for the statistical evaluation. A considerable distinction exists between the two implants' stiffnesses for p-value <0.05 (95% reliability). The DCS construct was found to possess higher stability in the compression tests except for the posterior and axial ones, while CBP appears less susceptible in the TD2 transducer after interpretation. One report on artificial femurs indicates the better performance of DCS over CBP in the loading trials and enhances the structure's durability. In contrast to Jaakkola et al.'s [5] finding from 2002, CBP has no mechanical edge over DCS regarding plastic bones, and the DCS appears superior in most loading tests.

8.4 BIOMECHANICAL EVALUATION OF FOUR VARIOUS IMPLANTS FOR HUMERAL SHAFT INJURIES

Likewise, the "nailers" maintain a near intramedullary method despite a higher chance of shoulder pain. The surgical governance of humeral shaft injury is still in dispute; "platers" highlight the benefits of reduction internal fixation, and this procedure shows no shoulder injury [7, 8]. For lower limb-related injuries, certain research investigations in scientific journals highlight the biomechanical benefits of medullary nails [9]. In contrast, another group highlights the benefits of load-bearing properties in fixing plates [10]. An evaluation of the biomechanical importance of different implants used to repair shafts was conducted in a recent investigation [11]. The researchers removed a 38-mm thick fragment from each artificial compound to represent a trample in the diaphysis. Different types of implants were used to instrument the fractures after the bones were divided into four groups: (i) locked compression plate (LCP; Synthes®); (ii) intramedullary static locked (Medimetal®) nail; (iii) long monoaxial locked plate (Stryker®); and (iv) long dynamic compression plate (DCP) Figure 8.2. The biomechanical testing was carried out using an LLOYD LRX 5kN loading machine that enables compression tests up to 5,000 N at varied speeds with a minimum precision of 0.2%. The machine's force cell was used to determine the compression forces with an accuracy of 0.01% and a resolution of 0.1 microns for deformations. The software that Nexygen and Ondio producers supplied was utilized for the testing experiments. Structures were subjected to torsion essay rotations to generate the same torque [11]. Based on the measured data, illustrations of load deformation were acquired for the two forms of torsion loading and various implants. The load-deformation diagrams have been contrasted and examined for every kind of implant. The reduced LCP was the stiffest for multiple loading essays, with the greatest mean loading values across the board. However, the implant is rigid, having a small transverse plate and a limited working length in which stresses are concentrated at contacts. The medullary locking nail proved to be the least rigid in torsion and highly elastic in different loading types. The biomechanical force acting between the bone and screws lowers; stress caused by rotation is spread uniformly down the length, and the whole design turns elastic by employing longer plates with fewer screws placed. This result relates to using long-length plates with fewer screws working at a longer working site.

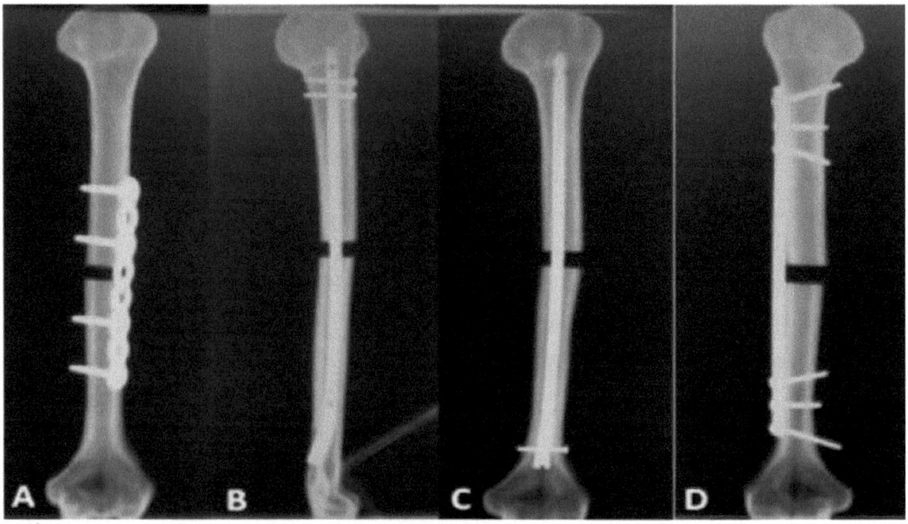

FIGURE 8.2 (a) Locked plate type; (b) and (c) locked nail type; and (d) DCP-buttress plate.

Source: Reprinted from Ref. [42]. https://creativecommons.org/licenses/by/3.0/

8.5 MEDICINAL AND INVESTIGATIVE RESEARCH ON GLIDING NAILS FOR TROCHANTERIC FRACTURES STABILIZATION

The trochanteric area is a frequent fracture site due to the increased prevalence of osteoporosis in the senior community and significant stress on the proximal femur. Designing an implant that may be used globally is challenging due to the various fracture patterns and their specific properties. Different factors, including bone quality, splinter shape, fracture reduction, prosthetic design, and the site, affect the fixation stability for a pertrochanteric injury [12]. Multiple investigations have demonstrated that the implant type and its placement are crucial for a successful outcome [13–15]. Extramedullary or intramedullary implants can be implemented based on location. In pertrochanteric fractures, the hip screw and plate are often utilized. They are more susceptible to fatigue injuries or cutting than medullary implants because of increased arm length exposure to greater stretching forces. Furthermore, placing such an implant necessitates extensive incisions that cause soft tissue injury and deterioration. These circumstances severely decrease local vascularization, increasing the likelihood of local complications. Additionally, given the average age of the patients, it is crucial to note that quick rehabilitation is not always feasible. Intramedullary implants have been used since the Y-profile Küntscher nail was created. These possess a lower bending force than medullary implants because of their slightly different placement. The medical procedure also minimizes nearby tissue harm [16]. The proximal femoral nail (PFN) and the gamma nail are the two most popular in this category. Due to considerable clinical and experimental research, an intramedullary gliding nail (GN) was created in Germany in 1994. The double-angle shape of the gliding system, combined with the mechanical benefits of an intramedullary implant, results in greater resistance [17] (Figure 8.3). The stable rotation and decreased risk of injury give the double-T profile its rigidity. The site of the entrance at the trochanter's end is made possible by the nail's 6? frontal plane curvature and straight plane, which reduces the likelihood of femoral head circulation problems compared to accessing the piriformis fossa.

The gliding nail system produced superior intraoperative and postoperative results compared to the gamma nail, according to the initial study in 1996 [18], which compared the two methods. Intraoperative complications were 2.7% for the gliding nail, ranging from 17.2% to 42.2% for the gamma nail. The extended findings showed that the gliding nail has a 4% rate of problems, while the gamma nail has 6–15%, demonstrating the difference in the outcome [18]. A biomechanical investigation in 1998 confirmed the positive findings by showing the significance of blade shape for proper fixation

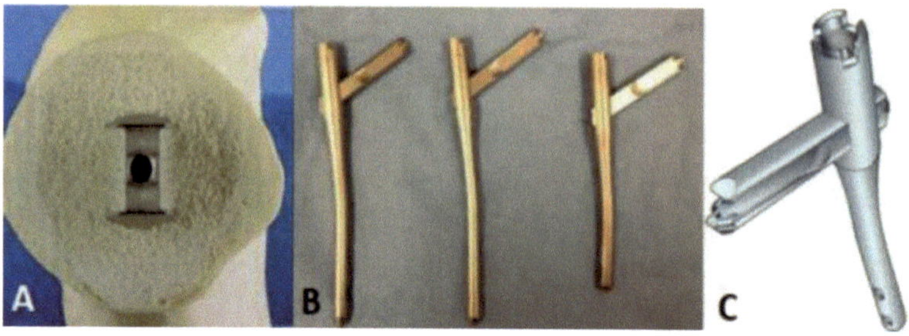

FIGURE 8.3 (a) Double-T blade profile inside the femoral head (axial view of sawbone); (b) GN of three different sizes (lateral view); and (c) gliding nail (3D view).

Source: Reprinted from Ref. [42]. https://creativecommons.org/licenses/by/3.0/

in femoral injuries. The Sawbone femoral heads' alternate load tests after 1,00,000 cycles at a load of 2,000 N showed no implant instability. After 1,000 cycles at 1,500 N, the double-T blade displaced 1–4 mm, whereas the gamma nail's 10 mm screw displaced 4–8 mm [19] (Figure 8.4). The gliding nail was used in a Garden IV femoral neck fracture with closed reduction and osteosynthesis. Friedl et al. reported a positive result with reduced complications, particularly for intraoperative and local problems, in an investigation conducted on over 186 patients with pertrochanteric injuries [20]. The authors underlined the advantages of gliding nails over DHS through multiple experiments. The most current trial included 501 people reporting trochanteric injuries treated solely, and subsequent load bearing was conducted over five years. The findings showed that the gliding nail technology could prevent local consequences of these complex fractures, such as cutting or severe impaction [21].

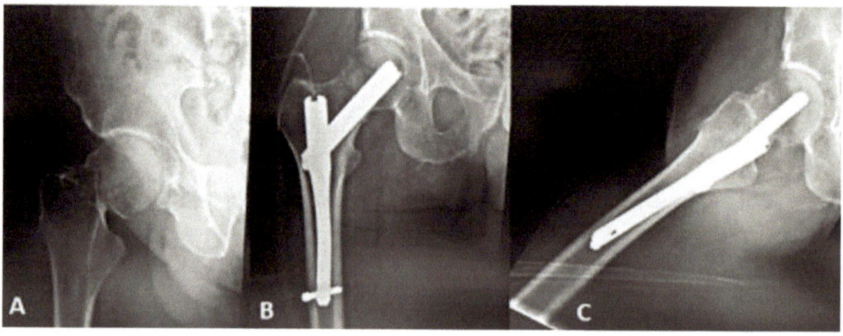

FIGURE 8.4 (a) Garden IV femoral neck fracture; and (b) and (c) closed reduction and osteosynthesis with gliding nail.

Source: Reprinted from Ref. [42]. https://creativecommons.org/licenses/by/3.0/

8.6 THE PATELLA AND OLECRANON FRACTURE TREATMENT WITH XS NAIL

The medical procedure using the tension band synthesis method is currently a gold standard for treating patella fractures. However, the long-term outcomes are not always favorable. Around 20% to 50% of instances may involve dislocation and functional impairment (restricted movement) [22]. A possible reason is that the aperture between band wires and the bone is caused by inserting the tendons, and the presence of a retinaculum prevents tight fixation, which is why loosening occurs after loading [23]. Additionally, because the tension band is attached to the anterior portion of the patella, the injury position on the articular side is distracted, resulting in fracture gaps, dislocations, and, ultimately, device collapse. A system that enables compression of the whole surface is required. A Tension Band Compression Nail (TCN) is an implant designed and positioned locally on the patella for even compression distribution by distracting the muscles [23]. In a biomechanical investigation, the authors classified the four types of fractures in 30 sawbone patellas. Osteotomy was used to create proximal and distal thirds with Y-shaped fractures. One or two XS nails and a tension band are used for osteosynthesis. The AO tension band group used an extra circular wire system (cerclage) to treat three-part Y-pattern fractures. The sawbone patellas, when subjected to 250 and 500 N, exhibited plastic and complete deformations. The batch that contains XS nails establishes the lot's lowest value. The AO tension band group underwent the most distortion over a significant distance among pieces. There was zero space in XS nails. On the backbone of the band group's addition, minor changes were found within the Y-pattern group based on the round wire's ability to withstand when close to a bone. It should be noted that this is not achievable because of the positioning of nearby tissues in actual clinical circumstances. The effective fixing and lower degree of deformation during physiological stress demonstrate that the XS nails are a competitive replacement for the tension band. Due to the features associated with this implant, patients will heal more quickly and experience better long-term outcomes. Since 1963, tension band wire has been the recommended treatment for olecranon fractures. However, in up to 80% of the cases, relocation of Kirschner wire and cerclage collapse is documented [24]. High von Mises stresses could be felt along the connection between segments through the Kirschner wire, as demonstrated by a computer simulation [25]. The alternative to plate osteosynthesis, which typically results from direct trauma, may exacerbate a faint lesion. Centrally inserting the implant and intramedullary XS nail enables homogeneous compression. Moreover, securing threaded wires along the nail can achieve greater fixation in the cortical bone. The intramedullary position makes the surgical procedure simple and protects soft tissue. In clinical research from 2006, XS nail osteosynthesis was used to treat 80 olecranon fractures, and the outcomes were favorable at 93.2% [26]. The XS nail is a potential advancement in treating olecranon fractures, particularly in older populations with poor bone quality.

8.7 PRECLINICAL RESEARCH ON POLYAXIAL STABLE PLATES FOR PROXIMAL HUMERUS AND DISTAL RADIAL FRACTURES

Distal radial fractures follow hip injuries in frequency among the elderly population. A variety of fracture patterns were presented by Mauck et al. [27]. The most common treatments for dorsal and metaphyseal radius fractures include fastened reduction, immobilization, or fixation. The associated fracture is found to be frequently non-stable. Thus, surgical treatment is required for any unstable articular fractures. Based on the fracture type and the ordinary plates' lack of stability, an additional fixation step ventrally or dorsally with higher intricacy is required during osteosynthesis. Studies revealed a substantial risk of subsequent dislocation or angulation and problems associated with tendon lesions with this kind of osteosynthesis. Plates with angular stability have become more popular for treating distal radius fractures since the 1990s. Depending on the fracture pattern and primarily employed in metaphyseal fractures, the angular plates were utilized in complex fractures to provide stability. Many particular pieces that needed to be repaired required specialized screw types. It was also necessary to avoid placing the screws in the articular plane, which could lead to certain stability problems [28]. As a result, multidisciplinary plates with various angular formations were created. It is possible to implant the screws at plate level at locations extremely close to the articular surface by inserting them perpendicular or at an angle concerning the plate surface. Fixing the fractured pieces in the proper place depends on the bone's structural arrangement and various fracture courses. A new kind of implant was created since existing implants require significant incisions that cause soft tissue injury and deterioration [29]. Using an XS nail and stable angular plate, the authors have tested the osteosynthesis on sawbones, specifically 16 osteotomized sawbones, which resemble distal radius AO/A3 fractures (Figure 8.5). The XS radius nail is established after drilling into the medullary canal and placing a guide wire. After that, it is fastened in three separate directions using threaded wires.

No consensus exists on treating proximal humerus fractures [30]. Surgery is frequently needed to correct instability and fragment displacement for a higher quality of life. Most osteosynthesis procedures can cure fractures using multifaceted angle stability plates or other types, but severely pulverized injuries require shoulder arthroplasty.

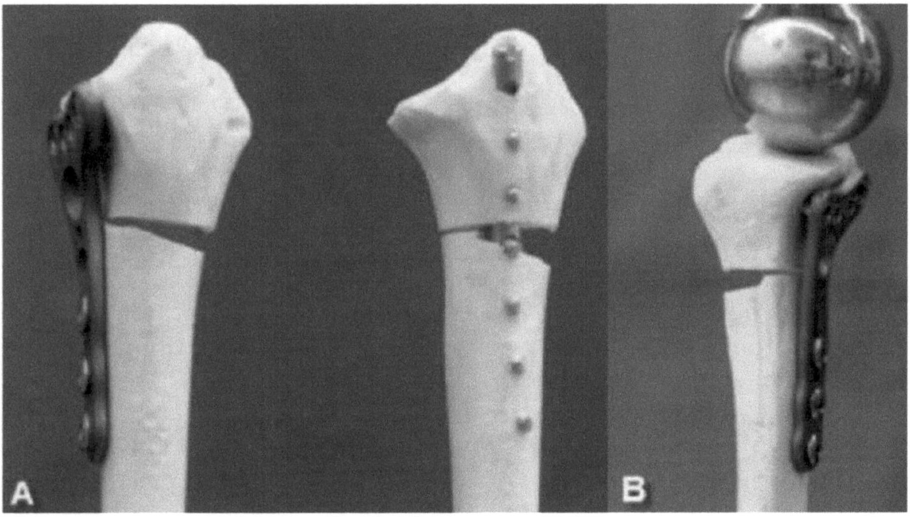

FIGURE 8.5 (a) Angular stable plate and XS nail osteosynthesis; and (b) alternating load test. *Source*: Reprinted from Ref. [42]. https://creativecommons.org/licenses/by/3.0/

8.8 CLINICAL OUTCOMES WITH THE LOCKED INTRAMEDULLARY XS NAIL FOR ANKLE AND PILON FRACTURES

The purpose of the therapy for frequent ankle fractures is to restore the anatomy using reliable and minimally invasive procedures [31, 32] and to avoid soft tissue injury in an area of anatomical abnormality: thin and almost non-existent skin excess is an extremely poor representation of soft tissue with inadequate blood availability [33, 34]. The "gold standard" treatment for distal fibula and lower leg fractures is plate osteosynthesis. Still, Zaghloul et al. found that 21.5% of problems overall consisted of infections and surgical re-evaluations [35]. Due to the fragile soft tissue envelope and severe wound complications from an extramedullary implant, the plate must be removed, and supplementary remodeled infusions such as thin skin transplants and distinct flaps are utilized. These conditions include arterial occlusive diseases, diabetes, and post-thrombotic sequelae [36–38]. The skin grafts are frequently impractical in certain cases of soft tissue abnormalities of the ankle that are largely caused by tendon exposure. Negative pressure therapy has recently emerged as a viable option to establish a healthy, vascularized bed that will enable the same. The medullary devices outperformed the plates biomechanically by lowering the lever arm and boosting the construct's sustainability [36, 39]. Clinicians eventually turned to search for an alternate osteosynthesis technique because there was no length preservation or rotation possible with bare wires, medullary pins, and interlocked nails. The most important criteria comprised fewer incisions with good biomechanical resilience and no impact on the surrounding tissue. Excision and split skin grafting are necessary for treatment because there isn't an implant in which a soft tissue problem does not arise. A unique medullary-locked nail with a minimum diameter used for osteosynthetic state progression that was intended for fracture reception was first used by several German researchers in 1999 [36, 39]. The length of the device was increased to meet the requirements for osteosynthesis. The included benefits were suitable for treating fibula and pilon fractures. The XS(L) nail, used to repair malleolar injuries, has a round shape and a diameter of 4.5 to 3.5 mm [36, 37, 39]. The total locking holes required depend on the fracture type. Two nearby holes are aligned longitudinally oval for fixation [28]. Experimental experiments were carried out before the clinical use of this novel implant, contrasting conventional plate and screw osteotomies [36, 40]. Based on these encouraging outcomes, the clinicians used the unknown XS nail to treat ankle joint fractures [36, 39]. The resulting consequence (based on the Olerud score) was positive, with only one non-union and an excellent outcome rate of 58.6%, a good outcome rate of 33.3%, a fair outcome rate of 5.5%, and a disagreeable rate of 2.5%. The nail is inserted following a surgical break in displaced ankle fractures, whereas the nail is implanted percutaneously in lower leg fractures [36, 37, 39]. Preoperative planning is essential and includes assessing the medullary canal's diameter up to the ideal degree with maximum stability.

In rare instances where the channel is too small, the XS nail is not recommended; instead, the XXS nail should be utilized for extremely narrow medullary spaces. The medullary canal must be a minimum of 3 mm in diameter for osteosynthesis [36, 37, 39]. The stretching from the peroneal tendons and separation of the retinaculum distal is necessary for nail insertion. After compression with reduction forceps and open reduction of the distal fibular fracture, a wire (1.6–2 mm thick) is introduced into the medullary canal as guidance while continuously being monitored by a fluoroscope. Two radiological images confirm the wire's location, and the same diameter is drilled into the nail to obtain the desired length. Inserting a nail at a minimum distance of 2.7 cm from the fracture point provides the most stability. To achieve syndesmosis stability without a fibulotibial set screw, select the largest nail diameter that will fit into the medullary canal [36, 37]. The XS nail's least disruptive osteosynthetic fracture and lack of plates on the surface of the bone considerably lower the rate of complications and healing issues for these challenging fractures [41]. XS and XXS nails are significant substitutes for primary plate-based fracture healing to avoid firm tissue problems and ensure stable fixation with a high tolerance to bear weight.

8.9 CONCLUSION

The benefits of novel implant devices for medically injured patients are highlighted in this article. Most loading tests show that DCS is superior to CBP for simulating supracondylar fractures on composite bones. In severe humeral fractures, the medullary nail proved to be an especially flexible device, while the more compact lock plate (LCP-Synthes) appeared to be the hardest. The shorter locked plate (DCP) provides unexpected additional torsion forces similar to long leaves. Surgical and mechanical investigations showed that the intramedullary gliding nail's double-T blade profile made it superior to DHS and gamma nails. The XS nail is a reliable fixing method for ankle and pilon injuries as it significantly outperforms plate fixation and overcomes nearby tissue injury. It also eliminates the drawbacks of the AO tension band and enables uniform compression of the fracture surface in patella fractures. Moreover, it is stronger than the plates due to the customizable trajectory of the screws; the above testing demonstrated the advantage of locking plates in injuries of the proximal humerus and distal radius.

KEYWORDS

- **biocomposite**
- **biomaterials**
- **bone**
- **bone implants**
- **distal radius**
- **fracture**
- **nail insertion**

REFERENCES

1. Koval, K. J., Hoehl, J. J., Kummer, F. J., & Simon, J. A. (1997). Distal femoral fixation: A biomechanical comparison of the standard condylar buttress plate, a locked buttress plate, and the 95-degree blade plate. *Journal of Orthopedic Trauma, 11*(7), 521–524. https://doi.org/10.1097/00005131-199710000-00010.
2. Marty, A., Fankhauser, C., Frenk, A., Cordey, J., & Gasser, B. (2001). Biomechanical evaluation of the less invasive stabilization system for the internal fixation of distal femur fractures. *Journal of Orthopedic Trauma, 15*(7), 482–487. https://doi.org/10.1097/00005131-200109000-00004.
3. Higgins, T. F., Pittman, G., Hines, J., & Bachus, K. (2007). Biomechanical analysis of distal femur fracture fixation: Fixed-angle screw-plate construct versus condylar blade plate. *Journal of Orthopedic Trauma, 21*, 43–46. https://doi.org/10.1097/BOT.0b013e31802bb372.
4. Heiney, J., Barnett, M., Vrabec, G., Schoenfeld, A., Baji, A., & Njus, G. (2009). Distal femoral fixation: A biomechanical comparison of trigen retrograde intramedullary (IM) nail, dynamic condylar screw (DCS), and locking compression plate (LCP) condylar plate. *The Journal of Trauma, 66*, 443–449. https://doi.org/10.1097/TA.0b013e31815edeb8.
5. Jaakkola, J. I., Lundy, D. W., Moore, T., Jones, B., Ganey, T. M., & Hutton, W. C. (2002). Supracondylar femur fixation: Mechanical comparison of the 95° condylar side plate and screw versus 95° angled blade plate. *Acta Orthopaedica Scandinavica, 73*(1), 72–76. https://doi.org/10.1080/000164702317281440.
6. Sirbu, P. D., Carata, E., Petreus, T., Munteanu, F., Popescu, C., Asaftei, R., et al. (2009). Dynamic condylar screw (DCS) versus condylar blade plate (CBP) in complex supracondylar femoral fractures–a biomechanical study. In *IFMBE Proceedings, International Conference on Advancements of Medicine and Health Care through Technology* (Vol. 26, pp. 409–412). https://doi.org/10.1007/978-3-642-04292-8_90.
7. Jeffrey, K., Booth, G., & Day, R. (2007). A biomechanical comparison of locking plate and locking nail implants used for fractures of the proximal humerus. *Journal of Bone and Joint Surgery, 16*, 362–366. https://doi.org/10.1016/j.jse.2006.01.019.
8. Sanders, B. S., Bullington, A. B., McGilivary, G. R., & Hutton, W. C. (2007). Biomechanical evaluation of locked plating in proximal humeral fractures. *Journal of Bone and Joint Surgery, 16*, 229–234. https://doi.org/10.1016/j.jse.2006.03.013.
9. Dunlap, J. T., Chong, A. C., Lucas, G. L., & Cooke, F. W. (2008). Structural properties of a novel design of composite analogue humeri models. *Annals of Biomedical Engineering, 36*(11), 1922–1926. https://doi.org/10.1007/s10439-008-9568-y.
10. Ulian, V., Mazzer, N., Barbieri, C., Moro, C. A., & Oliveira, L. A. (2008). Primary stabilization of humeral shaft fractures: An experimental study of different osteosynthesis methods. *Acta Orthopedic Brasileira, 16*, 8–12. https://doi.org/10.1590/S1413-78522008000100001.
11. Asaftei, R., Sîrbu, P. D., Carata, E., Bar, M., & Botez, P. (2010). Biomechanical analysis of three different types of implants in humeral diaphysis fractures. In *Proceedings at Equal: Advanced Technologies for Enhanced Quality of Life* (pp. 14–17). IEEE. https://doi.org/10.1109/ATEQUAL.2010.35.
12. Kaufer, H. (1980). Mechanics of the treatment of hip injuries. *Clinical Orthopedics and Related Research, 146*, 53–61.

13. Kyle, R. F., Gustilo, R. B., & Premer, R. F. (1979). Analysis of six hundred and twenty-two intertrochanteric hip fractures. *The Journal of Bone and Joint Surgery, American Volume, 61*, 216–221.
14. Baumgaertner, M., Custin, S., Lindskog, D., & Keggi, J. (1995). The value of the tip-apex distance in predicting failure of fixation of peri trochanteric fracture of the hip. *Journal of Bone and Joint Surgery, 77*, 1058–1064.
15. Baumgaertner, M. R., & Solberg, B. D. (1997). Awareness of the tip-apex distance reduces failure of fixation of trochanteric fractures of the hip. *Journal of Bone and Joint Surgery, British Volume (London), 79*, 969–971.
16. Suckel, A., Helwig, P., Schirmer, A., et al. (2003). Komplikationsraten beider Versorgung von der per-und subtrochanteren Femurfrakturen mit zwei intramedullaren Osteosynthesenverfahren. Vergleich eines konventionellen Nagelsystems mit einem rotationsstabilen Verfahren im Kopf-Hals-Fragment, Gammanagel und Gleitnagel. *Zentralblatt für Chirurgie, 128*(3), 212–217. https://doi.org/10.1055/s-2003-38535.
17. Gehr, J., Arnold, T., Hilsenbeck, F., et al. (2006). The gliding nail, a universal implant in the treatment of proximal femur fractures. *European Journal of Trauma, 32*, 562–569. https://doi.org/10.1007/s00068-006-5117-2.
18. Friedl, W. (1996). The gliding nail. A new implant for complication-free primary load-bearing management of per and subtrochanteric femoral fractures. *Langenbecks Archiv für Chirurgie, Supplement. Kongressband, 113*, 970–973.
19. Friedl, W., Anthoni, C., Fritz, T., Schmotzer, H., & Wipf, M. (1998). Importance of blade geometry for stability of fixation with short intramedullary nailing systems for the proximal end of the femur (gliding nail). *Langenbeck Archiv für Chirurgie, Supplement. Kongressband, 115*, 1224–1226.
20. Friedl, W., Göhring, U., Fritz, T., et al. (1998). Die Gleitnagelosteosynthese: Ein neues universell einsetzbares Implantat zur Versorgung per- und subtrochanterer Femurfrakturen. *Der Chirurg, 69*, 191–197. https://doi.org/10.1007/s001040050395.
21. Friedl, W., Hilsenbeck, F., & Sturzenhofecker, P. (2009). The gliding nail (GN). A universal implant for immediate weight bearing restoration in all per- and subtrochanteric femur fractures: Evaluation of 501 patients. In *Advanced Technologies for Enhanced Quality of Life* (p. 61). https://doi.org/10.1109/AT-EQUAL.2009.41.
22. Klute, I., & Meenen, N. M. (1998). *Die Fraktur der Kniescheibe*. Heidelberg & New York: Springer.
23. Friedl, W., & Clausen, J. (2000). Experimental examination of a tension-compression-nail (XS) in the osteosynthesis of patella fractures. *Osteosynthese International, 8*, 252–260.
24. Finsen, V., et al. (2000). AO tension band osteosynthesis of displaced olecranon fractures. *Orthopedics, 23*, 1069–1071.
25. Greenfield, J. R. F., et al. (2016). A numerical model of the tension band wiring technique for olecranon fracture reduction. *Applied Mathematics and Computation, 297*, 31–38. https://doi.org/10.1016/j.amc.2016.10.016.
26. Gehr, J., & Friedl, W. (2006). Intramedullary locking compression nail for the treatment of an olecranon fracture. *Operative Orthopädie und Traumatologie, 3*, 199–213.
27. Mauck, B. M., & Swigler, C. W. (2018). Evidence-based review of distal radius fractures. *Orthopedic Clinics of North America, 49*(2), 211–222. https://doi.org/10.1016/j.ocl.2017.12.001.

28. Sirbu, P. D., Friedl, W., Botez, P., Stratan, L., Hopulele, S., & Asaftei, R. (2008). *Minimally Invasive Plate Osteosynthesis–Internal Fixators*. Iasi: Casa deeditura Venus.
29. Friedl, W., Rinner, M., Simnacher, M., & Mathieu, C. (2010). Angle stable plate or angle stable locked nail fixation in distal radius fractures: An experimental examination and phase I clinical study. In *Advanced Technologies for Enhancing Quality of Life* (pp. 14–17). IEEE. https://doi.org/10.1109/ATEQUAL.2010.26.
30. Klug, A., Wincheringer, D., Harth, J., Schmidt-Horlohé, K., Hoffmann, R., & Gramlich, Y. (2019). Complications after surgical treatment of proximal humerus fractures in the elderly: An analysis of complication patterns and risk factors for reverse shoulder arthroplasty and angular-stable plating. *Journal of Shoulder and Elbow Surgery, 28*(9), 1674–1684. https://doi.org/10.1016/j.jse.2019.02.017.
31. Phillips, W. A., Schwartz, H. S., & Keller, C. S. (1985). A prospective, randomized study of the management of severe ankle fractures. *Journal of Bone and Joint Surgery, American Volume, 67*, 67–78. https://doi.org/10.2106/00004623-198567010-00010.
32. Collinge, C. A., & Heier, K. (2007). Ankle fractures and dislocations. In J. P. Stannard, A. H. Schmidt, & P. J. Kregor (Eds.), *Surgical Treatment of Orthopedic Trauma* (pp. 792–814). Germany: Thieme.
33. Batten, T. J., Scott-Davies, C., Butler, M., Parsons, S. W., & Walter, R. P. (2018). Percutaneous screw fixation for painful non-union of lateral malleolus ankle fractures. *Injury, 49*(10), 1936–1941. https://doi.org/10.1016/j.injury.2018.08.010.
34. Chiang, C. C., Tzeng, Y. H., Lin, C. C., Huang, C. K., & Chang, M. C. (2016). Minimally invasive versus open distal fibular plating for AO/OTA 44-B ankle fractures. *Foot & Ankle International, 37*(6), 611–619. https://doi.org/10.1177/1071100715625292.
35. Zaghloul, A., Haddad, B., Bakersfield, R., & Davis, B. (2014). Early complications of surgery in operative treatment of ankle fractures in those over 60: A review of 186 cases. *Injury, 45*, 780–783. https://doi.org/10.1016/j.injury.2013.11.008.
36. Gehr, J., Neber, W., Hilsenbeck, F., & Friedl, W. (2004). New concepts in the treatment of ankle joint fractures: The IP-XS (XSL) and IP-XXS (XXSL) nail in the treatment of ankle joint fractures. *Archives of Orthopedic and Trauma Surgery, 124*, 96–103. https://doi.org/10.1007/s00402-003-0606-9.
37. Sirbu, P. D., Tudor, R., Scripcaru, A., Veringa, V., Sirbu, M. T., Forna, N., & Pertea, M. (2019). Locked intramedullary XS nail for ankle fractures: Design, biomechanics, and preliminary results. In *E-Health and Bioengineering Conference (EHB)* (pp. 1–4). https://doi.org/10.1109/EHB47216.2019.8969958.
38. Mb, O., Aksan, T., Ertekin, C., & Tezcan, M. (2019). Coverage of exposed bone and hardware of the medial malleolus with tibialis posterior artery perforator flap after ankle fracture surgery complications. *International Wound Journal, 16*(2), 429–435. https://doi.org/10.1111/iwj.13289.
39. Gehr, J., & Friedl, W. (2006). Intramedullary locked fixation and compression nail (XS nail) in the treatment of ankle fractures. *Open Orthop Traumatol*, 155–170. https://doi.org/10.1007/s00064-006-1168-0.
40. Gehr, J., & Friedl, W. (2002). New concept in the treatment of distal metaphyseal and little dislocated pilon fractures with soft tissue damage. *Unfallchirurg, 2*, 520–532. https://doi.org/10.1007/s00113-001-0395-y.
41. Friedl, W., & Gehr, J. (2010). Intramedullary/intraosseous osteosynthesis of pilon and ankle fractures. In *Advanced Technologies for Enhancing Quality of Life* (pp. 3–5). https://doi.org/10.1109/ATEQUAL.2010.25.

42. Sirbu, P. D., Friedl, W., Mihailescu, D., Savin, L., Scripcaru, A., Forna, N., Sirbu, M. T., Pertea, M., & Tudor, R. C. (2020). Clinical and experimental biomechanical studies regarding innovative implants in traumatology. In *Recent Advances in Biomechanics* (pp. 1–16). InTech Open. https://doi.org/10.5772/intechopen.91728.
43. Katiyar, V., Prasad, A., Sankar, M. R., & Bhasney, S. M. (2022). Process for the preparation of polymer composite-based cancellous screw and pins (Indian Patent No. 401811).
44. Prasad, A., Bhasney, S. M., Prasannavenkadesan, V., et al. (2023). Polylactic acid reinforced with nano-hydroxyapatite bioabsorbable cortical screws for bone fracture treatment. *Journal of Polymer Research, 30*(177). https://doi.org/10.1007/s10965-023-02995-5.
45. Sarkar, K., Dutta, K., Chatterjee, A., Sarkar, J., Das, D., Prasad, A., Chattopadhyay, D., Acharya, K., Das, M., Verma, S. K., & De, S. (2023). Nanotherapeutic potential of antibacterial folic acid-functionalized nanoceria for wound-healing applications. *Nanomedicine, 18*(2). https://doi.org/10.2217/nnm-2022-0233.
46. Prasad, A. (2022). Biomaterial-based nanofibers scaffolds in tissue engineering applications. In *Functional Biomaterials* (pp. 245–264). Springer. https://doi.org/10.1007/978-981-16-7315-8_11.
47. Prasad, A., Chakraborty, G., & Kumar, A. (2022). Bio-based environmentally benign polymeric resorbable materials for orthopedic fixation applications. In *Advanced Materials for Biomedical Applications* (pp. 251–266). CRC Press. https://doi.org/10.1201/9780429279548-17.
48. Prasad, A., Sankar, M. R., & Katiyar, V. (2017). State of the art on solvent casting particulate leaching method for orthopedic scaffolds fabrication. *Materials Today: Proceedings, 4*(2), 898–907. https://doi.org/10.1016/j.matpr.2017.01.101.
49. Prasad, A., Bhasney, S. M., Katiyar, V., & Sankar, M. R. (2017). Biowastes processed hydroxyapatite filled poly (lactic acid) bio-composite for open reduction internal fixation of small bones. *Materials Today: Proceedings, 4*(9), 10153–10157. https://doi.org/10.1016/j.matpr.2017.06.158.
50. Prasad, A., Devendar, B., Sankar, M. R., & Robi, P. S. (2015). Micro-scratch based tribological characterization of hydroxyapatite (HAp) fabricated through fish scales. *Materials Today: Proceedings, 2*(4–5), 1216–1224. https://doi.org/10.1016/j.matpr.2015.02.013.
51. Gupta, A., et al. (2017). Multifunctional nanohydroxyapatite-promoted toughened high-molecular-weight stereo complex poly (lactic acid)-based bio nanocomposite for both 3D-printed orthopedic implants and high-temperature engineering applications. *ACS Omega, 2*(7), 4039–4052. https://doi.org/10.1021/acsomega.7b00588.
52. Prasad, A. (2021a). Bioabsorbable polymeric materials for biofilms and other biomedical applications: Recent and future trends. *Materials Today: Proceedings, 44*, 2447–2453. https://doi.org/10.1016/j.matpr.2020.12.489.
53. Prasad, A. (2021b). State of the art review on bioabsorbable polymeric scaffolds for bone tissue engineering. *Materials Today: Proceedings, 44*, 1391–1400. https://doi.org/10.1016/j.matpr.2020.11.622.

CHAPTER 9

Biocomposites in Craniofacial Fixations and Applications in Maxillofacial Fixations

HEMANT KUMAR,[1] PURNIMA JUSTA,[2] NANCY JASWAL,[2] REENU GANGWAR,[3] SUNDAR SINGH,[4] BALARAM PANI,[5] and PRAMOD KUMAR[2]

[1]*Department of Chemistry, Ramjas College, University of Delhi, Delhi, India*

[2]*Department of Chemistry and Chemical Science, School of Physical and Material Sciences, Central University of Himachal Pradesh, Dharamshala, Himachal Pradesh, India*

[3]*Institute of Dental Sciences, Bareilly International University, Bareilly, Uttar Pradesh, India*

[4]*Department of Physics, Bareilly College Bareilly, Bareilly, Uttar Pradesh, India*

[5]*Bhaskaracharya College of Applied Sciences, Department of Chemistry, University of Delhi, Delhi, India*

ABSTRACT

Jaw-and-mouth reconstruction may correct several cranial bone malformations, most notably severe maxillary and mandibular bone shortages. Craniofacial reconstruction is difficult due to the variety of tissues involved and the number of defects caused by accidents, violence, tumors, or atrophy. Rebuilding bones and surrounding tissues that look and feel like the patient

Bioabsorbable Polymers for Drug Carriers and Fixation Devices. Arbind Prasad and Sougata Jana (Eds.)

is necessary to address the physical and psychological impact of these difficulties on a patient's quality of life. Early bone grafting may benefit people with cleft palates. The effectiveness of alveolar bone grafting in children with cleft lips and palates depends on the timing of the procedure. Poorer results should be anticipated as people age. Recent studies have looked at the need for bone grafting prior to dental implants. The bones and cartilage of the cranium support the muscles, ligaments, glands, layers of skin, and tissue under the skin. These components are linked by the body's most complicated neurovascular network, which provides them with function and sensation. Titanium alloys (Ti) are commonly utilized to repair maxillofacial and cranial fractures (miniplates and mesh). Cranial materials are composed of PMMA and titanium alloys. Adding bioactive materials, osteoconductive materials, or bioactive glass fibers to implants has been suggested by several authors to improve osseointegration and angiogenesis. These bioinert alloys offer exceptional mechanical strength, osseointegration, and bioactivity. Metals in craniofacial implants are used following tumor excision. Injectable platelet-rich fibrin (I-PRF) has attracted interest in bone tissue engineering. I-PRF is a promising frontline alternative because it has antibacterial, anti-inflammatory, and healing properties. It also has a lot of physiologically active chemicals. Modern advanced composites inspired by biology are strong, robust, and impact-resistant. The study of artificial materials that imitate biological materials has gained popularity. Meta-biomaterials may be created using bio-inspired materials. Craniofacial bone regeneration is crucial for regaining the form and functionality of essential components. This is challenging due to physicochemical and biological requirements. Utilizing magnesium aluminate ($MgAl_2O_4$) spinel, tricalcium phosphate (TCP), poly lactic-co-glycolic acid (PLGA), or polycaprolactone (PCL), two types of polyphasic composite scaffolds were created. Given that bone shows fracture deflection, crack bridging, and microcracking, synthetic biomaterials that mimic bone structures should provide appealing toughening processes, especially in bone-related applications. In medicine, the mechanical compliance of craniofacial implants is essential because the brain must be shielded after neurosurgery or trauma. Innovative cranial implants were made by combining bioactive ceramic powders with metallic scaffolds. The combination of powder bed fusion and powder metallurgy created scaffolding. Porous tantalum bone plates are also mentioned in this chapter as innovative internal fracture-mending implants. This chapter also talks about how bioactive glass polyester composites are made and used in orthopedics, craniomaxillofacial surgery, dentistry, and bone tissue engineering. The combination of these compounds optimizes the breakdown of bone replacement, mechanical characteristics, cell response, and osteo-stimulation. Reducing stress shielding speeds fracture healing. Biodegradable metals might prevent a second implant removal surgery. Biometals and their design for orthopedic bone plates will enhance bone fracture therapy, particularly for refractory fractures.

9.1 INTRODUCTION

The bones and cartilage that make up the craniofacial area serve as a framework for the muscles, ligaments, glands, several layers of skin, and subcutaneous tissues. All these parts are connected by the most complex neurovascular network in the body, which gives them function and sensory abilities [1]. Traumatic injuries can cause bone fractures. Fracture repair involves a cascade of biological and biomechanical processes. Around 5% to 10% of bone fractures do not heal properly, causing delayed healing or non-union. Stabilization is necessary for broken bones so that healing may take place. Internal fracture fixation plates are necessary for complicated fractures and in anatomical regions where external fixing is not possible. Currently, titanium alloys are the most popular materials utilized for these plates since they are strong and rigid enough to protect the broken bone during healing. However, once the healing is complete, these strong mechanical characteristics can cause problems, especially if they interfere with the regular remodeling processes of the bone. This results in a decline in bone quality underneath the plates, a condition known as stress shielding. In fact, stress shielding may become so severe that removing the fracture plates requires a substantial number of revision surgeries each year, resulting in expenses for healthcare payers and patient health hazards [2]. Primary healing and secondary healing are the two types of bone fracture healing. Primary healing is the cortex's immediate effort to reestablish itself after being interrupted. Primary healing only occurs with the anatomical repair of fracture pieces by rigid internal fixation and micrometric interfragmentary strain. Most fractures are mended by secondary healing, which includes periosteum and soft tissue reactions and callus formation. This sort of healing benefits from micromotion, whereas tight immobilization suppresses it. Secondary healing includes intramembranous and endochondral ossification, with at least five healing steps [3–6].

Because of their mechanical performance and long-term durability, these biomedical materials are commonly used for permanent orthopedic implants. Research on the topic focuses on wear, fatigue fracture, and post-operative infection. The greater stiffness of metals and ceramics relative to the bone causes stress shielding, a shift in stress distribution between the implant and bone that may lead to bone degeneration and aseptic loosening. Professor Larry Hench started studying bioactive glass (BG) systematically in the late 1960s [7]. He found that inorganic materials could actively catch the desired response *in vivo*. This led to a strong bond between bone and synthetic material, which was caused by chemical and biological reactions at the surface of the BG [8]. BGs were first employed in medical applications as monoliths (e.g., middle ear implants) and in the form of granules (i.e., to fill bone defects). According to a later study, BGs enhance bone repair. BGs were suggested for bone tissue engineering. BGs have been created with customized physicochemical and biological characteristics. BGs are too brittle to withstand the majority of the bone's load. Bioactive glass shaping (e.g., 3D scaffolds) is challenging and dependent.

Jaw and mouth reconstruction techniques treat cranial bone deficiencies (particularly major maxillary and mandibular bone deformities). Craniofacial reconstruction is difficult owing to the diversity of tissues involved and the number of abnormalities caused by accidents, violence, tumors, or atrophy. A rebuilding technique that mimics native bone and surrounding tissues is necessary due to the physical and psychological effects these inadequacies have on the quality of the patient's life. Early bone grafting can benefit individuals with cleft palates. The success of alveolar bone grafting in children with cleft lips and palates is influenced by the timing of the procedure, with poorer outcomes expected as patients age. Recent studies have examined the necessity of bone grafting before dental implants. Alveolar bone grafts were sought by 55.6% of patients in their 60s. Due to health problems, fewer bone transplants are used in people over 70 years of age. Tissue engineering combines biological sciences and engineering for reconstructive dentistry. The basic goal of tissue engineering is to restore, preserve, or improve the function of natural tissues or organs. Later, tissue regeneration became a research tool for studying tissue development to generate more natural-looking tissue substitutes for dental and craniofacial procedures. Biological materials, organic biomaterials, and alloplastic grafts are used in oral and craniofacial reconstruction. The biological materials might be autologous grafts, allogeneic grafts, or xenogenic transplants. The recipient's own body provides the autologous bone transplant. Allografts are acquired from a donor of the same species. Heterologous bone transplants are from a distinct species from the recipient. The alloplastic grafts are synthetic materials not covered by Bratt Strom et al. [9]. After biological materials, organic biomaterials are the most popular for creating natural matrices for tissue regeneration. The removal of skin, tendons, and cartilage provides organic biomaterials. Despite this method's potential future, no successful decellularization of bone has been documented. Finding an appropriate bone graft or bone regeneration matrix is expected to be a huge worldwide business. Bone grafting cost US $3.02 billion (about $9 per person in the US) in 2014 and is expected to climb 15% by 2023 [10].

A potential scaffolding material for bone regeneration is organic, nature-derived biopolymers because of their biocompatibility, biodegradability, and affinity for bone morphogenetic proteins (BMPs). Some studies have mixed hyaluronic acid and beta-tricalcium phosphate (β-TCP) with these organic compounds (HA). The best-studied and most advertised natural polymer for periodontal bone healing is collagen. In the future, scientists will focus on making organic composite polymers that are completely biodegradable and made from non-immunogenic organic materials like collagen, chitosan, and alginate [11]. These composite polymers' constituent parts may be created synthetically, producing materials that are resorbable and have adjustable chemical and molecular compositions. Traditional oral procedures use non-resorbable synthetic membranes as guided bone regeneration (GBR) to help guide bone regeneration in the right direction. This study focuses on biological and natural organic materials that could be used as scaffolding in the regeneration of orofacial and craniofacial bones to cure bone abnormalities [12].

The worldwide market for fracture fixation devices is expected to be worth $5.5 billion (about $17 per person in the US). The medical equipment used to treat fractures includes plates, intramedullary nails, wires, screws, pins, etc. Different internal fixation techniques should typically be used to treat different fracture locations. Oral and maxillofacial structures are some of the most useful and aesthetically valuable parts of the body. Maxillofacial osteosynthesis operations need solid anchoring for optimum bone recovery. Maxillofacial and cranial injuries are serious. Once injured, it is hard to fix. Vehicle accidents are a significant cause of 45% of all facial trauma; nasal bones, alveolar processes, and zygomatic bones often fracture. In many nations, maxillofacial injuries are a major health issue. Bone substitutes, such as autograft, allograft, xenograft, and artificial materials, are used to fix the mouth and face. Biomaterials have traditionally been classified into four generations (1st generation – *bioinert*; 2nd generation – *bioactivity*; 3rd generation – *bioactive and bioresorbable*; and 4th generation – *biomimetic*). The first generation of biomaterials, sometimes known as "conventional materials," contained inert and tolerant biomaterials that were designed to resist physiological stress without inducing any biological reactions [13, 14]. Even though these materials were stable over time, the body was not able to adapt to them, which meant there was a high chance of failure.

As a result, focus switched away from first-generation biomaterials that were "tolerant" and "inert" and toward second-generation biomaterials that were "responsive" and able to elicit biological reactions. Particularly, a great deal of focus has been given to synthetic biomaterials with bioactive properties, osteointegration, and osteoconductive properties. To make a direct link between the synthetic material and bone, the material must have bioactive properties, such as the ability to push bone-forming tissue onto a surface or into pores. The focus of biomaterials has shifted from bioinert tissue response to the generation of bioactive components capable of eliciting a regulated action and reaction in the physiological environment. Bioactive glasses (Na_2O, CaO, P_2O_5, and SiO_2) link to live tissue in 11 stages. The first five processes took place on the material's surface and involved rapid ion exchange of Na^+ with H^+ and H_3O^+. This was followed by a polycondensation reaction of surface silanols to produce a high-surface-area silica gel, which provided numerous sites for heterogeneous nucleation and crystallization of a physiologically reactive layer of hydroxy-carbonate apatite (HCA), which is similar to the inorganic mineral phase of bone. With a close connection to the implant surface, the forming HCA layer on the material's surface provided an ideal environment for six biological response steps, such as osteoblast colonization, proliferation, and differentiation to produce new bone [15].

Controlled chemical breakdown and resorption were features of second-generation biomaterials. The interface problem is eliminated since the foreign material is replaced by regenerated tissues, and there is no obvious difference seen between the implant site and the host tissue. Biodegradable seams made of polyglycolic acids (PGA) and polylactic acids (PLA) hydrolyze into H_2O and CO_2. At the end of 1984, resorbable sutures were standard. Orthopedic resorbable fracture plates and screws, as well as drug-delivery devices, were new.

Orthopedic implants include non-bioactive metals. However, there are two ways to achieve bioactivity. The first step is to cover the implant's surface with a bioactive ceramic, such as HA, or hydroxyapatite. The second method involves chemically modifying the metal surface to encourage protein and cell attachment, as well as other interactions with tissues or materials. The most used coating technique is HA plasma spraying, in which HA is projected onto a cool metal surface while in the plasma state. The biodegradable metals are zinc, magnesium, and iron. Table 9.1 describes how bone and bone substitute material interacts biologically.

TABLE 9.1 Biological Interaction of Bone and Bone Substitute Material

Substitution	Complete resorption and autologous bone material replace the implant. In cases of excessive resorption, an (unwanted) fibrous interlayer may form.
Osteoinduction	Explains how mesenchymal precursor cells become osteoprogenitor cells, which then cause endochondral ossification.
Osteostimulation	Bone metabolism is stimulated and differentiated bone cells are activated.
Osteoconduction	This explains the material's ability to control the formation of bone tissue because of its geometric design. A scaffolding over which the osteoblasts may move into the defect is required for bone regeneration. According to the evidence, the best interconnecting pores for that are those between 150 and 450 nm. For instance, bio glass and calcium phosphate both have advantageous osteoconductive characteristics [16].

Table 9.2 shows the materials and methods used for oral and maxillofacial reconstructions.

9.2 FIRST GENERATION (INERT BIOMATERIALS)

The choice of material for an engineering design that matches the appropriate application determines which materials have the necessary characteristics for this application. Biomaterials are made of biological materials. The usual ones must be supplemented with specific needs (chemical, physical, and mechanical). Consequently, concepts such as foreign body response (especially stress shielding, biocompatibility, and wear debris) and, more recently, osteoinduction and bioactivity were eventually implemented as prerequisites for implantable device design using biomaterials. The sole prerequisite for the first use of synthetic materials in biological applications was to "achieve an acceptable set of physical characteristics to match those of the substituted tissue with a low-hazard reaction from the host" [17]. They were the ones to whom Hench's classification of "first-generation biomaterials" was meant to minimize the foreign body reaction and the immunological response.

TABLE 9.2 The Current Materials as well as Methods That are Used for Oral as well as Maxillofacial Reconstructions [52]

Source	Methods and Materials
Allogenic	**Hard Tissue Type:** • Allogeneic mineralized bone is offered through tissue banks. • Coupled with a variety of carriers, demineralized bone matrix: ▪ w/calcium sulfate ▪ w/glycerol ▪ w/poloxamer ▪ w/hyaluronic acid **Soft Tissue Type:** • Short-term skin allografts • Freeze-dried acellular de-epithelialized dermal transplant
Synthetic	**Hard Tissue Type:** • **Ceramics:** ▪ Bovine bone ▪ Hydroxyapatite of natural origin ▪ Synthetic unsintered calcium deficient apatite ▪ Synthetic biphasic calcium phosphate ▪ Coral sources ▪ Calcium phosphate cement ▪ Recombinant growth factors ▪ Growth factor from platelets in a b-tricalcium phosphate carrier ▪ An absorbable collagen sponge containing bone morphogenetic protein-2 • **Polymers:** ▪ Polylactic acid, polyglycolic acid ▪ Resorbable fixation plates and screws, as well as resorbable membranes, are typical applications. **Soft Tissue Type:** • **Dermal fillers** **Composite Tissue:** • Polymeric prosthesis materials • Techniques used are tissue engineering.
Autologos	**Hard Tissue Type:** • Bone grafts from the iliac crest, tibia, skull, and mandible that are nonvascularized. **Soft Tissue Type:** • Skin grafts that have full and partial thickness • Microfat grafting • Vascularized free flaps **Composite Tissue:** • Vascularized osseo-fascio-cutaneous free flaps from the fibula, iliac crest, deltoid, and scapula, as well as the radial forearm.

TABLE 9.2 *(Continued)*

Source	Methods and Materials
Xenogeneic	**Hard Type Tissue:** • Hydroxyapatite-coated crosslinked bovine collagen I • Porcine collagen I and III membrane that is resorbable **Soft Type Tissue:** • Bovine collagen fibrillar types I and II • Derivatives of crosslinked hyaluronic acid.

9.2.1 METALLIC MATERIALS

The first metals used in orthopedics were stainless steel and cobalt chrome alloys. The 1940s brought titanium and titanium alloys. Nickel-titanium shape memory alloys were first made in the 1960s. Due to their unusual mechanical behavior, they were thought to have a wide range of uses, but nickel's allergenic effect has limited their use. Charnley's complete hip prosthesis was the first successful artificial joint [18]. This was a stainless steel-stemmed, cemented prosthesis.

9.2.1.1 COBALT-BASED ALLOYS

An iron-free molybdenum cast alloy on a chrome and cobalt base was produced in the 20th century because of new breakthroughs in the metalworking sector. Drs. Reiner Erdle and Prange (Stryker Howmedica, formerly Austenal Laboratories) launched them under the brand name Vitallium®, initially primarily for dental use. After that, Vitallium® was used in a few indications for endoprosthesis and osteosynthesis as a particularly corrosion-resistant material. The Luhr® Modular Craniomaxillofacial/Mandibular Fixation System, Leibinger Co., is the first system for craniofacial mini-osteosynthesis based on Vitallium. Cobalt alloys, like stainless steel, may have undesirable side effects because of corrosion. This includes a rise in the level of metal ions in the blood and potentially their buildup. Given the substantial number of implants around the world, which is the reason the systems are so popular today, these rare side effects are not that big of a deal [19, 20].

9.2.1.2 TITANIUM ALLOYS

Titanium (Ti) and its alloys can be processed by 3D printing or molding metal injections. Medical equipment manufacturers are focusing more on this subject. Advanced manufacturing processes might replace machining or casting metal alloys in device production due to design flexibility, decreased processing costs, reduced waste, and the ability to make complicated or custom-shaped implants more readily. Metal injection molding and additive layer manufacturing are gaining interest in the implant fabrication sector because they potentially solve some of the challenges of existing methods like titanium casting. Advanced manufacturing may build more complicated porous materials with higher mechanical performance, matching bone's elasticity. Advanced manufacturing offers strong economic and technical possibilities for musculoskeletal implants, but its influence on biocompatibility is less evident. In this research, modern powder manufacturing techniques are evaluated for their ability to produce biomedical implant components with appropriate surface finishes and porosity architectures. Biocompatibility and how the host bone response is important for clinical success, so both *in vitro* (in a test tube) and *in vivo* (in a living animal) tests were carefully done. Commercially pure titanium (CP-Ti) and the titanium alloy Ti_6Al_4V are the two most popular alloys for making titanium implants (Ti-64). Due to a permanent and inert oxide layer that develops on its surface when exposed to oxidizing solutions, CP-Ti has superior resistance to corrosion and is recognized as the most biocompatible metal. Due to the groundbreaking work of Brånemark and his team, CP-Ti is used in all-per-mucosal dental implants that are now on the market [21, 22].

9.2.2 CERAMIC BIOMATERIALS

The invention of bone cement and various metallic alloys are two great instances of how the materials utilized in clinical applications were first created for different objectives, as is the case with many biomedical implants. In recent years, however, people have been paying more attention to the advantages of ceramics, such as their high chemical resistance, compressive strength, and wear resistance.

9.2.2.1 BIOGLASS

Professor Larry Hench invented bioglass in 1967 after learning about the high expense of amputations for Vietnam War wounds. It is necessary for materials that will help repair tissues by forming a direct link with them rather than the interfacial scar tissue that currently surrounds metal and polymer implants [23].

The bio glass, known as 45S5, has a weight percentage of 45% silica, 24.5% Na_2O, 24.5% CaO, and 6% P_2O_5. All these oxides are combined and melted at around 1,350°C to produce a glass with a uniform silica network. When implanted in live tissue, bioglass exhibits a rapid biological reaction and rapid bioactivity. Since it was discovered over 35 years ago that the bioglass composition could chemically link to bone, there has been a lot of activity around bioactive glasses research and development. Tens of thousands of papers on bioactive glasses have been published. But so far, bioglass is the only bioactive glass that has been shown to react more quickly with living things [8, 24, 25].

Since then, several glasses have been created and documented in the literature. These substances often have the same foundation as Hench's original composition. Although many good studies have been published (for instance, by Hatton, Hoeland, Andersson, and Knowles and their respective coworkers), the scope of this study does not allow for a comprehensive examination of all the work done in this field.

9.2.3 BIOCERAMICS

As an alternative to metallic implants, bioceramics—either synthetic or natural in origin—have begun to gain popularity. Metal and metalloid oxides, nitrides, sulfides, and carbides are referred to as ceramics [26]. Because they have excellent and compatible physiochemical qualities with human body components, they are significant in the biomedical sector. In terms of mechanical properties, limited plasticity, poor degradability, high melting temperature, and non-corrosiveness, bioceramic materials perform better than metal-based biomaterials. Bioceramics are harder and more brittle than bone, have a lower elastic modulus, and have worse fracture toughness. Dental work, orthopedics, calcified tissues, implants, coatings, medical sensors, and many more fields make use of bioactive glasses or glass ceramics (Figure 9.1). Alumina, zirconia, titania, and porous Ca-P-based materials are some of these materials [27]. In terms of soft tissue repair and regeneration, bio-ceramics opens new possibilities.

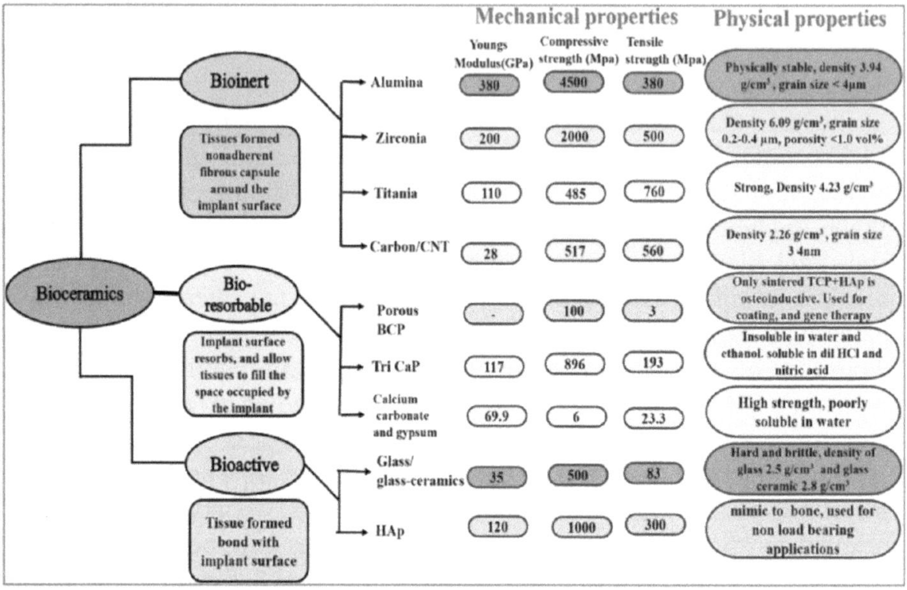

FIGURE 9.1 Bio-ceramic materials are put into distinct categories based on how they interact with body tissues and implants in a physiological environment.

9.3 SECOND-GENERATION BIOMATERIALS

As a result, the focus changed from "tolerant" and "inert" first-generation biomaterials to "responsive" second-generation biomaterials that may trigger biological reactions. Particularly, a great deal of focus has been given to synthetic biomaterials with bioactive properties, osteointegration, and osteoconductive properties. To create a direct link between the artificial material and bone, bioactive characteristics relate to active interactions with surrounding bone tissue (i.e., the capacity to guide bone-forming tissue on a surface or down into pores). The development of biodegradable polymers was another big step forward for these second-generation biomaterials. These polymers allow bone tissue to slowly replace a bone substitute material without stopping the healing process.

The development of bioactive materials' ability to interact with the biological environment to enhance the biological response and the bonding between the tissue and the surface, as well as the development of bioabsorbable materials' ability to undergo gradual degradation while new tissue regenerates and heals, were the defining features of the second generation of biomaterials, which should be regarded as having emerged between 1980 and 2000. The word "bioactivity" refers to any interaction or impact a drug has on a cell with the intention of causing it to behave or respond in a certain manner. The mineralization and binding of the bone tissue to the implant is one of the best-known processes for enhancing bioactivity in applications for bone repair and fixation. The bioactive biomaterials developed for bone fixation, repair, and regeneration were what prompted the *in vivo* deposition of a layer of HA at the material surface. These bioactive materials, which comprised a few bioactive glasses (BGs), ceramics, glass-ceramics, and composites, had been used in a few orthopedic and dental applications by the middle of the 1980s. But there are other methods to increase biological activity. These methods focus on changing surfaces with proteins that stick to them, polymers that adhere to them, and biomolecules that, depending on the application, make cells respond in certain ways.

9.4 THIRD-GENERATION BIOMATERIALS

Third-generation biomaterials are intended to be innovative substances that may molecularly trigger certain biological responses. The ideas of bioactivity and biodegradability are merged for these biomaterials, transforming bioabsorbable substances into bioactive substances and vice versa. These materials' properties need to be compatible with their ability to signal and promote certain cellular behavior and activity. In addition to temporary three-dimensional porous structures that promote cell invasion, adhesion, and proliferation, functionalized surfaces with peptide sequences mimicking ECM components are being developed. Delivery of biological components and medications, as well as the use of mechanotransduction to regulate how cells behave, are some of the topics of interest [28].

Third-generation biomaterials are being developed to molecularly activate certain biological responses. Bioactive materials are rendered resorbable, while resorbable polymers are converted into bioactive materials, merging the previously distinct notions of bioactive materials and resorbable materials. Resorbable polymer systems that have undergone molecular changes cause interactions with cell integrins that control extracellular matrix synthesis and structure, as well as cell proliferation and differentiation. To activate the genes that promote the regeneration of living tissues, third-generation bioactive glasses and macroporous foams are being developed. The use of these customized biomaterials has opened two more paths for repair.

9.5 FOURTH-GENERATION BIOMATERIALS

Biomimicry is an interdisciplinary approach that assimilates biotechnology, bioengineering, medicine, and computational sciences to give new heights to medicinal research [29]. It includes bioengineering strategies for the regeneration of craniofacial bone [30–32]. Building biomimetic matrices to replicate biological structures is the emerging approach in tissue engineering and regenerative medicine. It mimics nature's simple and hierarchical structural assemblages, which are present in all genera and species [33, 34]. Fourth-generation biomaterials consist of biomimetic scaffolds that not only reproduce the environment of the extracellular matrix of the tissue of interest but also deliver growth factors to the site of regeneration [35]. The use of biomimetic agents represents a widely growing field of research in implant dentistry to achieve rapid osseointegration and expedite the overall treatment process. Biomimetics investigates the addition of bioactive agents to an implant surface to hasten the healing events. They are designed in a way to replace or imitate a body structure (anatomy) and/or function (physiology). Various bioactive agents that may be applied to coat the implant surface are (Figure 9.2) bioactive proteins, biocompatible ceramics, bone morphogenetic proteins, growth factors, RGD peptide, fluoride, chitosan, etc. Some of these are also commercially available [36, 37]. Characteristic features of various biomimetic agents are illustrated in Table 9.3. The biomimetic coating based on cytokines overcomes the drawbacks of autografts and allografts for treating critical size bone defects.

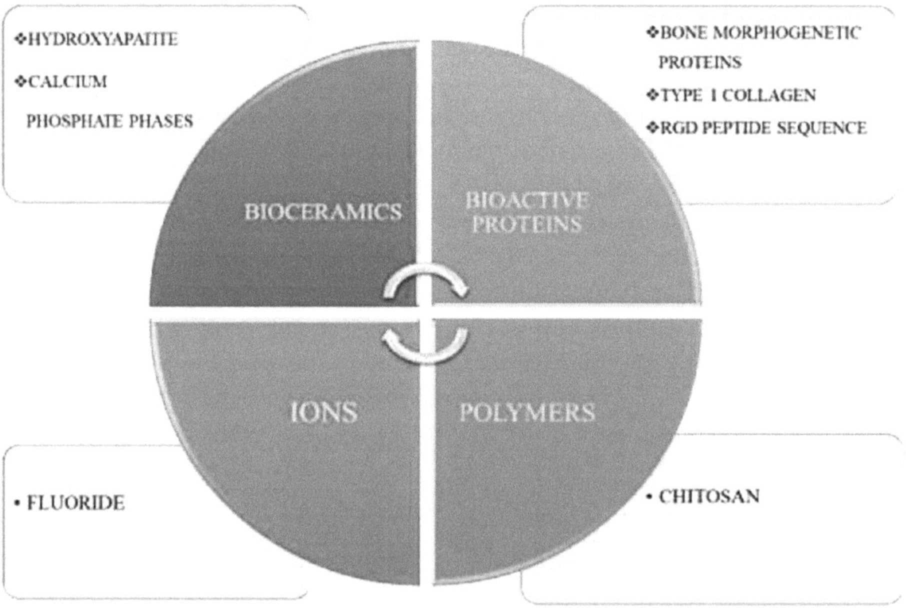

FIGURE 9.2 Image depicts the agents that could be used for biomimetic activities.

TABLE 9.3 The Characteristic Features of the Biomimetic Agents

Agents	Cost	Immune Reaction Risk	Stability	Osteo-Inductive Characteristics	Osteo-Conductive Characteristics	Quickly Synthesized	Quickly Absorbed
Hidroxyapatite	Less	×	✓	×	✓	✓	×
Calcium phosphate phases	Average	×	✓	×	✓	✓	✓
Bone morphogenetic proteins	High	×	✓	✓	×	×	✓
Type 1 Collagen	less	✓	✓	×	✓	✓	✓
RGD peptide sequence	Moderate	×	✓	✓	✓	✓	✓
Growth factors	less	×	×	✓	×	✓	✓
Fluoride	less	×	✓	✓	×	✓	✓
Chitosan	less	×	✓	×	✓	✓	✓

Nanoparticle composite scaffolds not only enhance mechanical strength for bone grafts but also act as a medium for the novel delivery and targeting of genetic material encoding osteogenic growth factors [38, 39]. Nanocomposite biomimetic scaffold nano-hydroxyapatite/polyamide 6 seeded with allogenic bone marrow-derived stem cells were found to exhibit good biocompatibility and osteoconductivity, thus acting as a potential matrix for bone tissue engineering [40]. Grafting the post-extraction socket with a biomimetic nanostructured matrix composed of equine collagen I and Mg-hydroxyapatite was found to exhibit excellent biocompatibility and enhance the healing rate by accelerating socket closure and tissue maturation [41]. Lyophilized Platelet-Rich Fibrin (PRF) works as a proficient biomimetic scaffold for craniofacial bone regeneration and mineralized tissue engineering [42]. Biomimetic matrices seeded with stem cells show widespread potential in craniofacial and other reconstructive surgical therapies [43]. The durability of these implanted stem cells can be enhanced by vascularization [44, 45]. Biomimetic composites composed of collagen/β-tricalcium phosphate incorporating bone morphogenetic protein-2 were found to improve tissue growth in bone grafting applications [46]. Three-dimensional technologies have found widespread applications in orthodontics and maxillofacial surgery, as these technologies provide tri-dimensional anatomy accuracy [47]. 3D bioprinting is a less invasive technique that promotes the chances of constructing patient-tailored bioactive tissue for craniofacial reconstruction [48–50]. To get the best results from 3D printing, it is suggested to collaborate laser-powder bed fusion with traditional methods [51].

9.6 CONCLUSION

Examining recent trends in injectable biomaterials for tissue engineering in the difficult but instructive setting of complicated tissue engineering inside the craniofacial complex is the goal of this study. Current methods and biomaterials for craniofacial augmentation and repair were presented to establish the current end-stage state of the art in a domain that has a large demand for better biomaterials and tissue engineering techniques. An introduction to injectable material technologies and the challenges of designing complicated tissues was given, followed by a description of the wide range of craniofacial tissues and advancements in tissue engineering. The major difficulties and anticipated future requirements and directions in resolving the identified challenges were then highlighted. There are several potential injectable biomaterials out there and attempts to test them *in vivo* have mainly proven successful. However, the objective of regenerating complex tissues has not yet been achieved in the clinic and will call for ongoing dedication and development in the industry.

KEYWORDS

- **bio-ceramics**
- **bioactive ceramics**
- **bioinert ceramics**
- **biomaterials**
- **biomimetic composites**
- **tissue engineering**
- **tissue growth**

REFERENCES

1. Tahmasebi, E., Alam, M., Yazdanian, M., Tebyanian, H., Yazdanian, A., Seifalian, A., & Mosaddad, S. A. (2020). Current biocompatible materials in oral regeneration: A comprehensive overview of composite materials. *Journal of Materials Research and Technology, 9*(5), 11731–11755. https://doi.org/10.1016/j.jmrt.2020.07.055.
2. Naseem, R., Tzivelekis, C., German, M. J., Gentile, P., Ferreira, A. M., & Dalgarno, K. (2021). Strategies for enhancing polyester-based materials for bone fixation applications. *Molecules, 26*(4), 992. https://doi.org/10.3390/molecules26040992.
3. Gritsch, L., Perrin, E., Chenal, J. M., Fredholm, Y., Maçon, A. L., Chevalier, J., & Boccaccini, A. R. (2021). Combining bioresorbable polyesters and bioactive glasses: Orthopedic applications of composite implants and bone tissue engineering scaffolds. *Applied Materials Today, 22*, 10092. https://doi.org/10.1016/j.apmt.2021.10092.
4. Sharma, A., Krishnan, M., Ganganahalli, G., Saraswathy, S., Biswas, P., Johnson, R., Abraham, K. M., & Iyer, S. R. (2021). In vitro evaluation of magnesium aluminate [$MgAl_2O_4$] spinel ceramic based polyphasic composite scaffold for craniofacial bone tissue engineering. *Ceramics International, 47*(10), 13678–13692. https://doi.org/10.1016/j.ceramint.2021.03.100.
5. Rahmani, R., Kamboj, N., Brojan, M., Antonov, M., & Prashanth, K. G. (2022). Hybrid metal-ceramic biomaterials fabricated through powder bed fusion and powder metallurgy for improved impact resistance of craniofacial implants. *Materialia, 22*, 101465. https://doi.org/10.1016/j.mtla.2022.101465.

6. Farshidfar, N., Amiri, M. A., Jafarpour, D., Hamedani, S., Niknezhad, S. V., & Tayebi, L. (2021). The feasibility of injectable PRF (I-PRF) for bone tissue engineering and its application in oral and maxillofacial reconstruction: From bench to chairside. *Materials Science and Engineering: C, 124*, 112557. https://doi.org/10.1016/j.msec.2021.112557.
7. Jones, J., Baino, F., & Boccaccini, A. R. (2019). 50 years of bioactive glasses: Celebratory special issue in "Biomedical Glasses." *Biomedical Glasses, 5*(1). https://doi.org/10.1515/bglass-2019-0002.
8. Hench, L. L., Splinter, R. J., Allen, W. C., & Greenlee, T. K. (1971). Bonding mechanisms at the interface of ceramic prosthetic materials. *Journal of Biomedical Materials Research, 5*(6), 117–141. https://doi.org/10.1002/jbm.820050603.
9. Brattström, V., & McWilliam, J. (1989). The influence of bone grafting age on dental abnormalities and alveolar bone height in patients with unilateral cleft lip and palate. *The European Journal of Orthodontics, 11*(4), 351–358. https://doi.org/10.1093/ejo/11.4.351.
10. Cha, H. S., Kim, J. W., Hwang, J. H., & Ahn, K. M. (2016). Frequency of bone graft in implant surgery. *Maxillofacial Plastic and Reconstructive Surgery, 38*(1), 1–4. https://doi.org/10.1186/s40940-016-0134-0.
11. Pilipchuk, S. P., Plonka, A. B., Monje, A., Taut, A. D., Lanis, A., Kang, B., & Giannobile, W. V. (2015). Tissue engineering for bone regeneration and osseointegration in the oral cavity. *Dental Materials, 31*(4), 317–338. https://doi.org/10.1016/j.dental.2015.01.020.
12. Cai, X., Ten Hoopen, S., Zhang, W., Yi, C., Yang, W., Yang, F., Jansen, J. A., Walboomers, X. F., & Yelick, P. C. (2017). Influence of highly porous electrospun PLGA/PCL/nHA fibrous scaffolds on the differentiation of tooth bud cells in vitro. *Journal of Biomedical Materials Research Part A, 105*(9), 2597–2607. https://doi.org/10.1002/jbm.a.36057.
13. Williams, D. F. (2008). On the mechanisms of biocompatibility. *Biomaterials, 29*(20), 2941–2953. https://doi.org/10.1016/j.biomaterials.2008.01.011.
14. Hench, L. L., & Wilson, J. (1984). Surface-active biomaterials. *Science, 226*(4675), 630–636. https://doi.org/10.1126/science.6477866.
15. Hench, L. (1998). Bio ceramics. *Journal of the American Ceramic Society, 81*(7), 1705–1728. https://doi.org/10.1111/j.1151-2916.1998.tb02794.x.
16. Neumann, A., & Kevenhoerster, K. (2009). Biomaterials for craniofacial reconstruction. *GMS Current Topics in Otorhinolaryngology, Head and Neck Surgery, 8*. https://doi.org/10.3205/cto000068.
17. Hench, L. (1980). Biomaterials. *Science, 208*(4446), 826–831. https://doi.org/10.1126/science.7403868.
18. Charnley, J. (1960). Anchorage of the femoral head prosthesis to the shaft of the femur. *The Journal of Bone and Joint Surgery. British Volume, 42*(1), 28–30. https://doi.org/10.1302/0301-620X.42B1.28.
19. Luhr, H. G. (1988). A micro-system for cranio-maxillofacial skeletal fixation: Preliminary report. *Journal of Cranio-Maxillofacial Surgery, 16*, 312–314. https://doi.org/10.1016/S1010-5182(88)80018-4.
20. Luhr, H. G. (1990). Indications for use of a microsystem for internal fixation in craniofacial surgery. *The Journal of Craniofacial Surgery, 1*(1), 35–52. https://doi.org/10.1097/00001665-199001000-00007.
21. Sidambe, A. T. (2014). Biocompatibility of advanced manufactured titanium implants—A review. *Materials, 7*(12), 8168–8188. https://doi.org/10.3390/ma7128168.

22. Adell, R., Lekholm, U., Rockler, B., & Brånemark, P. I. (1981). A 15-year study of osseointegrated implants in the treatment of the edentulous jaw. *International Journal of Oral Surgery, 10*(6), 387–416.
23. Hench, L. L. (2006). The story of Bio glass®. *Journal of Materials Science: Materials in Medicine, 17*(11), 967–978. https://doi.org/10.1007/s10856-006-0126-0.
24. Greenlee Jr, T. K., Beckham, C. A., Crebo, A. R., & Malmorg, J. C. (1972). Glass ceramic bone implants: A light microscopic study. *Journal of Biomedical Materials Research, 6*(3), 235–244. https://doi.org/10.1002/jbm.820060303.
25. Hench, L. L., & Paschall, H. A. (1973). Direct chemical bond of bioactive glass-ceramic materials to bone and muscle. *Journal of Biomedical Materials Research, 7*(3), 25–42. https://doi.org/10.1002/jbm.820070304.
26. Pina, S., Rebelo, R., Correlo, V. M., Oliveira, J. M., & Reis, R. L. (2018). Bio ceramics for osteochondral tissue engineering and regeneration. In *Osteochondral Tissue Engineering* (pp. 53–75). Wiley. https://doi.org/10.1002/9781119179893.ch3.
27. Kaur, M., & Singh, K. (2019). Review on titanium and titanium-based alloys as biomaterials for orthopedic applications. *Materials Science and Engineering: C, 102*, 844–862. https://doi.org/10.1016/j.msec.2019.01.066.
28. Hutmacher, D., Hürzeler, M. B., & Schliephake, H. (2000). A review of material properties of biodegradable and bioresorbable polymers for GTR and GBR. *Journal of Oral and Maxillofacial Implants, 11*(4), 667–678. https://doi.org/10.11607/jomi.11.4.667.
29. Upadhyay, A., Pillai, S., Khayambashi, P., Sabri, H., Lee, K. T., Tarar, M., Zhou, S., Harb, I., & Tran, S. D. (2020). Biomimetic aspects of oral and dentofacial regeneration. *Biomimetics, 5*(4), 1–45. https://doi.org/10.3390/biomimetics5040042.
30. Ward, B., Brown, S., & Krebsbach, P. H. (2010). Bioengineering strategies for regeneration of craniofacial bone: A review of emerging technologies. *Oral Diseases, 16*(8), 709–716. https://doi.org/10.1111/j.1601-0825.2010.01690.x.
31. Oppenheimer, A. J., Mesa, J., & Buchman, S. R. (2012). Current and emerging basic science concepts in bone biology: Implications in craniofacial surgery. *Journal of Craniofacial Surgery, 23*(1), 30–36. https://doi.org/10.1097/SCS.0b013e3182400120.
32. Pagni, G., Kaigler, D., Rasperini, G., Avila-Ortiz, G., Bartel, R., & Giannobile, W. V. (2012). Bone repair cells for craniofacial regeneration. *Advanced Drug Delivery Reviews, 64*(12), 1310–1319. https://doi.org/10.1016/j.addr.2012.04.010.
33. Ripamonti, U., Roden, L. C., Ferretti, C., & Klar, R. M. (2011). Biomimetic matrices self-initiating the induction of bone formation. *Journal of Craniofacial Surgery, 22*(5), 1859–1870. https://doi.org/10.1097/SCS.0b013e3182205f80.
34. Kawecki, F., Clafshenkel, W. P., Fortin, M., Auger, F. A., & Fradette, J. (2018). Biomimetic tissue-engineered bone substitutes for maxillofacial and craniofacial repair: The potential of cell sheet technologies. *Advanced Healthcare Materials, 7*(6). Wiley-VCH Verlag. https://doi.org/10.1002/adhm.201700692.
35. Kwan, M. D., & Longaker, M. T. (2008). Editorial note: Advances in science and technology: Impact on craniofacial surgery.
36. Kretlow, J. D., Young, S., Klouda, L., Wong, M., & Mikos, A. G. (2009). Injectable biomaterials for regenerating complex craniofacial tissues. *Advanced Materials, 21*(32–33), 3368–3393. https://doi.org/10.1002/adma.200900581.
37. Avila, G., Misch, K., Galindo-Moreno, P., & Wang, H. L. (2009). Implant surface treatment using biomimetic agents. *Implant Dentistry, 18*(1), 17–26. https://doi.org/10.1097/ID.0b013e318192fa10.

38. Marei, M. K., Nagy, N. B., Saad, M. S., Zaky, S. H., Elbackly, R. M., Eweida, A. M., & Alkhodary, M. A. (2013). Strategy for a biomimetic paradigm in dental and craniofacial tissue engineering. In *Biomimetics* (pp. 119–162). Wiley. https://doi.org/10.1002/9781118458565.ch5.
39. Miszuk, J. M., Hu, J., & Sun, H. (2020). Biomimetic nanofibrous 3D materials for craniofacial bone tissue engineering. *ACS Applied Bio Materials, 3*(10), 6538–6545. https://doi.org/10.1021/acsabm.0c00897.
40. Khadka, A., Li, J., Li, Y., Gao, Y., Zuo, Y., & Ma, Y. (2011). Evaluation of hybrid porous biomimetic nano-hydroxyapatite/polyamide 6 and bone marrow-derived stem cell construct in repair of calvaria critical size defect. *Journal of Craniofacial Surgery, 22*(5), 1852–1858. https://doi.org/10.1097/SCS.0b013e318230b4f1.
41. Mozzati, M., Gallesio, G., Staiti, G., Iezzi, G., Piattelli, A., & Mortellaro, C. (2017). Socket preservation using a biomimetic nanostructured matrix and atraumatic surgical extraction technique. *Journal of Craniofacial Surgery, 28*(4), 1042–1045. https://doi.org/10.1097/SCS.0000000000003471.
42. Li, Q., Reed, D. A., Min, L., Gopinathan, G., Li, S., Dangaria, S. J., Li, L., Geng, Y., Galang, M. T., Gajendrareddy, P., Zhou, Y., Luan, X., & Diekwisch, T. G. H. (2014). Lyophilized platelet-rich fibrin (PRF) promotes craniofacial bone regeneration through Runx2. *International Journal of Molecular Sciences, 15*(5), 8509–8525. https://doi.org/10.3390/ijms15058509.
43. Oliver, J. D., Madhoun, W., Graham, E. M., Hendrycks, R., Renouard, M., & Hu, M. S. (2020). Stem cells regenerating the craniofacial skeleton: Current state-of-the-art and future directions. *Journal of Clinical Medicine, 9*(10), 1–13. https://doi.org/10.3390/jcm9103216.
44. Levi, B., Glotzbach, J. P., Wong, V. W., Nelson, E. R., Hyun, J., Wan, D. C., Gurtner, G. C., & Longaker, M. T. (2012). Stem cells: Update and impact on craniofacial surgery. *Journal of Craniofacial Surgery, 23*(1), 319–322. https://doi.org/10.1097/SCS.0b013e31823c5e50.
45. Griffin, M., Kalaskar, D. M., Butler, P. E., & Seifalian, A. M. (2014). The use of adipose stem cells in cranial facial surgery. *Stem Cell Reviews and Reports, 10*(5), 671–685. https://doi.org/10.1007/s12015-014-9498-4.
46. Lee, D. K., Ki, M. R., Kim, E. H., Park, C. J., Ryu, J. J., Jang, H. S., Pack, S. P., Jo, Y. K., & Jun, S. H. (2021). Biosilicated collagen/β-tricalcium phosphate composites as a BMP-2-delivering bone-graft substitute for accelerated craniofacial bone regeneration. *Biomaterials Research, 25*(1). https://doi.org/10.1186/s40824-021-00231-5.
47. Francisco, I., Ribeiro, M. P., Marques, F., Travassos, R., Nunes, C., Pereira, F., Caramelo, F., Paula, A. B., & Vale, F. (2022). Application of three-dimensional digital technology in orthodontics: The state of the art. *Biomimetics, 7*(1). MDPI. https://doi.org/10.3390/biomimetics7010013.
48. Visscher, D. O., Farré-Guasch, E., Helder, M. N., Gibbs, S., Forouzanfar, T., van Zuijlen, P. P., & Wolff, J. (2016). Advances in bioprinting technologies for craniofacial reconstruction. *Trends in Biotechnology, 34*(9), 700–710. https://doi.org/10.1016/j.tibtech.2016.05.002.
49. Shah, G., & Costello, B. J. (2017). Soft tissue regeneration incorporating 3-dimensional biomimetic scaffolds. *Oral and Maxillofacial Surgery Clinics of North America, 29*(1), 9–18. https://doi.org/10.1016/j.coms.2016.09.003.

50. Raheem, A. A., Hameed, P., Whenish, R., Elsen, R. S., Aswin, G., Jaiswal, A. K., Prashanth, K. G., & Manivasagam, G. (2021). A review on development of bio-inspired implants using 3D printing. *Biomimetics, 6*(4). https://doi.org/10.3390/biomimetics6040075.
51. Nouri, A., RohaniShirvan, A., Li, Y., & Wen, C. (2021). Additive manufacturing of metallic and polymeric load-bearing biomaterials using laser powder bed fusion: A review. *Journal of Materials Science and Technology, 94*, 196–215. https://doi.org/10.1016/j.jmst.2021.03.042.
52. Best, S. M., Porter, A. E., Thian, E. S., & Huang, J. (2008). Bio ceramics: Past, present and for the future. *Journal of the European Ceramic Society, 28*(7), 1319–1327. https://doi.org/10.1016/j.jeurceramsoc.2007.11.015.
53. Singh, G. D., Heit, T., Preble, D., & Chandrashekhar, R. (2016). Changes in 3D nasal cavity volume after biomimetic oral appliance therapy in adults. *Cranio–Journal of Craniomandibular Practice, 34*(1), 6–12. https://doi.org/10.1080/08869634.2015.1062382.

CHAPTER 10

Physical and Biological Properties of Biocomposite Materials as Fixations or Sealers in Dentistry Applications

V. ANDAL,[1] R. LAKSHMIPATHY,[1] G. JAYANTHI,[1] and ARBIND PRASAD[2]

[1]*Department of Chemistry, KCG College of Technology, Chennai, Tamil Nadu, India*

[2]*Mechanical Engineering Department, Katihar Engineering College (Under Department of Science, Technology and Technical Education, Government of Bihar), Katihar, Bihar, India*

ABSTRACT

Bio-composite materials are a great choice for sealers in dental applications because of their outstanding biocompatibility, strength, aesthetics, tooth adherence, antibacterial properties, and superior physical and biological qualities. To stop apical periodontitis, sealants are utilized during root canal therapy. The characteristics that a sealant should have include strong sealing power, dimensional stability, slow setting time, insolubility, and biocompatibility. This chapter addresses recent developments in the development of bio-composite materials for use as sealants in dental applications, as well as their physical and biological properties. The chapter also focuses on the hybrid fillers for improving the physical and biological properties of composites.

10.1 INTRODUCTION

Numerous synthetic materials have been created in recent years with the purpose of rebuilding and maintaining a patient's oral function, health, and appearance [1, 2]. The materials that interact with biological systems

Bioabsorbable Polymers for Drug Carriers and Fixation Devices. Arbind Prasad and Sougata Jana (Eds.)

are known as biomaterials. They can be either natural or synthetic and are typically composed of several different parts. Composite materials are the combination of two or more biomaterials with different properties, which show enhanced bioactivity compared to the individual ones. Biocomposites are characterized as non-toxic composites that can effectively communicate with the human body *in vivo* and, ideally, contain one or more materials that promote the body's natural healing and implant absorption. As a result, for biocomposites, biological compatibility seems to be more crucial than any other kind [3–5].

Fissure sealants are extensively utilized in clinical settings in pediatric dentistry because they successfully prevent caries [6–8]. Due to their intricate architecture, pits and fissures are tough to brush clean and difficult to self-clean.

The two main sealant materials utilized nowadays are glass ionomer cement (GIC) and resin composite, with resin composite frequently employed in clinical settings due to its good mechanical strength and handleability [9]. In the meantime, therapeutically usable biocomposite-based sealant materials have recently been developed. GICs are resin-based sealants that efficiently attach to teeth and guard against root caries because of their antibacterial and anticariogenic qualities [10]. Glass ionomers solidify via an acid-base reaction, whereas composite resins solidify via a polymerization reaction that is typically triggered by a dental curing light [11]. Recent studies have concentrated on the potential for sealants to exhibit improved antibacterial activity. By lowering the possibility of bacterial colonization and biofilm formation at the tooth-sealant interface, the biocomposite-based sealants would benefit from enhancing the material's therapeutic effect.

Nanoparticles have been added to sealants to improve the mechanical, chemical, antibacterial, and remineralization properties of sealants. In this chapter, we are going to see the recent developments in sealants, such as (i) chitosan-based sealants and their biological properties; (ii) nanoparticles incorporated biocomposite sealants; and (iii) hybrid fillers in dental sealants. These days, plenty of materials are now in application, which have versatile applications in various biomedical fields. The major application of biobased nanomaterials is in orthopedics, implant fixation, and internal fixation devices. Dental restoration also has a wide scope in applications, including composite materials based on nanohydroxyapatite, antimicrobial materials such as nanosilver, and other multifunctional biobased materials [49–51].

This chapter aimed to review the development of biocomposite-based dental sealants and studied their physical and biological properties (Figure 10.1). In addition, the review focused on hybrid fillers for improving the physical and biological properties of composites.

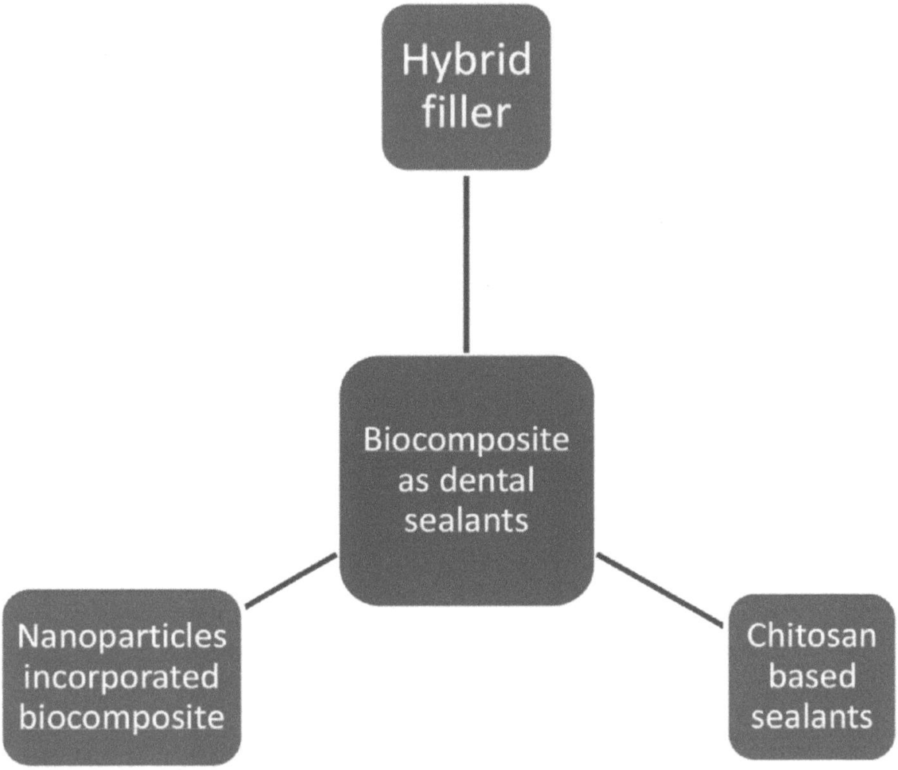

FIGURE 10.1 Schematic depiction of the summary of bio composite as dental sealants.

10.2 BIO-COMPOSITES AS A FIXATION AND SEALER IN DENTISTRY APPLICATIONS

In dentistry, various biomaterials are fabricated and processed for their intended application to last in the long term. Some of them have therapeutic properties. Based on the medication of the dental restoration, biobased materials are used for temporary dressings, cements, impressions, lining, and restorations. Some of the materials are listed in Table 10.1.

TABLE 10.1 Materials Used in Bio-Composite as Sealants

SL. No.	Materials	Merits	Demerits	References
1.	Stainless steel	Good physical and mechanical properties	Hypersensitivity reactions	[52]
2.	Zinc phosphate	Improves bone contact bio compatibility	Pulpal irritation, lack of antibacterial action, brittleness, lack of adhesion, and solubility in oral fluids	[53, 54]
3.	Nanohydroxyapatite	Osteo inductive capacity and improves bone-to-implant integration.	Limited usage in high stress area	[55, 56]
4.	Zirconium di oxide	Resistant to temperature change, better stain resistance, hypoallergenic, etc.	Opaque appearance, not natural	[57, 58]
5.	Calcium hydroxide	Intra canal medicament and prevents reinfection.	Less effective against *Enterococcus faecalis* and *Candida albicans*.	[59]
6.	Glass ionomer	Hydrophilic, release, and recharge fluoride.	Weakness and quick wear and tear.	[60]
7.	Titanium	Resistant to both corrosion and fatigue, strength, durability, lightweight, and biocompatibility.	Hypersensitivity	[61]
8.	Calcium silicate	Biocompatible, non-cyto-toxic, and non-genotoxic and hydrophilicity.	Improvement in physical properties required.	[62]
9.	Calcium hydroxide	Hard tissue formation and antimicrobial activity.	Not physically robust	[63]

10.3 CHITOSAN-BASED SEALANTS AND ITS BIOLOGICAL PROPERTIES

Bioactivity, biodegradability, and biocompatibility are characteristics of biological properties. When choosing any dental sealants, these are very important qualities that need to be taken into consideration. In order to prevent secondary caries, antibacterial additives to fissure sealants have been studied [12]. Due to their high moisture content, temperature fluctuations, and pH, the oral cavity presents substantial physical and chemical problems for resin-based sealants. The risk of recurrent caries increases with time due to the physical and mechanical dissociation of sealers. In order to create materials with therapeutic effects and better biological qualities, especially over the long term, it has been considered to add antibacterial agents to sealants [13, 14].

Chitosan is a natural antibacterial agent that is included in resin biocomposite. Chitosan is introduced in the form of chitosan, chitosan nanoparticles, and chitosan whiskers (Figure 10.2).

Chitosan has the chemical formula (1-4)-2-amino-2-deoxy-D-glucan. It comes from the deacetylation of chitin. The deprivation of an electron ion from the amino group causes the surface charge of chitosan to turn positive when the degree of deacetylation exceeds 50%. Chitosan molecules that are positively charged clash with negatively charged residues on the bacterial surface. It is possible to penetrate the irregular bacteria's wall and access the contents. The benefits of using chitosan include its inexpensive price, ability to prevent demineralization and the development of biofilms, as well as its ability to stimulate salivary flow without activating the immune system [15].

Bacteria, particularly *S. mutans* and *Lactobacillus* species, are the cause of dental caries because they produce acids. The cariogenic plaque contains a lot of *S. mutans*, which is anaerobic and generates organic acids at a pH of 5.5. The bacterial species *L. acidophilus* is another one that contributes to demineralization. *S. sanguis* is a different microbe that has been discovered in noncariogenic plaque; its presence in the plaque denotes that the plaque has little potential for causing caries [16].

Lai et al. created a fissure sealer containing chitosan/fluoride microparticles by modifying chitosan with NaF. They varied the concentration of chitosan and NaF and found that 2% chitosan/fluoride microparticles exhibited excellent biocompatibility and antibacterial properties against *S. mutans* [17].

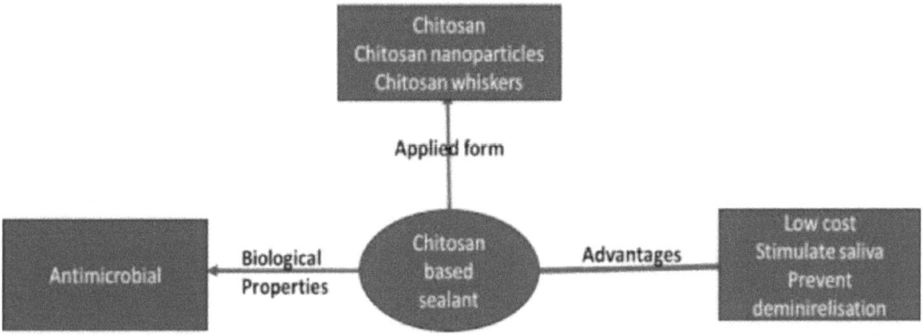

FIGURE 10.2 Schematic representation of chitosan based dental sealants.

Sara and his team investigated the sealant's optimum antibacterial effectiveness by incorporating the appropriate dosage of chitosan nanoparticles into it. By using a biofilm inhibition test and an eluted component test, they examined the antibacterial effectiveness. Incorporating 1 wt.% (weight percent) of chitosan into the fissure sealant was proven to be an efficient way to induce antibacterial activity, according to their analyses [18]. Ramar also studied the incorporation of chitosan nanoparticles in root canal sealants. Without affecting the flow of the root canal sealant in permanent teeth, they discovered that chitosan nanoparticles reduced the quantity of adherent bacteria in lateral canals. Therefore, to demonstrate its effectiveness, this material was chosen for use in primary teeth [19]. Suchit and his colleagues assessed the biological activity by adding nanoscale chitosan whiskers to the sealant. The incorporation of fibrous chitosan nano whiskers exhibited excellent antibacterial activity against *S. mutans* [20]. Similarly, Bottino et al. incorporated chitosan fibers in resin-based sealant to improve antibacterial properties.

Using chitosan, glycerophosphate pentahydrate (G-P), and povidone-iodine (PVP-I), Tao Jiang and his colleagues developed a chitosan hydrogel-based sealant. Chitosan's volume ratio was altered, and its antibacterial properties were investigated using the spread plate method. They determined through their analysis that the 16/4 volume ratio of chitosan hydrogel demonstrated remarkable sealing ability [21].

10.4 NANOPARTICLES INCORPORATED BIOCOMPOSITE SEALANTS

Microleakage and secondary caries are the two main clinical issues that pit and fissure sealants must address. To overcome this, Abdulaziz and his coworkers incorporated cobalt oxide nanoparticles in sealants and investigated their antibacterial potential against Streptococcus sobrinus. Compared to the normal sealants, it also showed enhanced antibiofilm potential [22]. Pozos-Guillén and his colleagues studied the effect of silver nanoparticles in pit and fissure sealants in the prevention of dental caries in children. In comparison to the traditional sealant, the silver nanoparticle-mixed sealant considerably reduced tooth demineralization and probably boosted remineralization [23]. In comparison to silver nanoparticles, zinc oxide nanoparticles (ZnO NPs) have better antibacterial capabilities because they produce reactive oxygen species

[24–26]. Hence, Swetha and her group members evaluated the antibacterial properties of ZnO and CaF_2 nanoparticles incorporated in pit and fissure sealants. Based on the results of the research, it can be concluded that standard sealants were outperformed by sealants containing 1 weight percent ZnO and CaF_2 NPs [27]. Similarly, Nejat and his team created ZnO nanoparticles and tested their root canal sealing effectiveness. Additionally, they made comparisons between the nanosized zinc oxide eugenol sealer and epoxy resin sealer (AH26) and the microsized zinc oxide eugenol sealer, concluding that the nanosized sealer had superior sealing performance [28]. The effectiveness of zinc(II) oxide nanoparticles in endodontic and orthodontic sealers has been demonstrated [29]. These particles have biocompatibility, low micro-density, and activity against *S. mutans, E. faecalis, S. mitis, Lactobacillus* spp., *P. gingivalis,* and *A. naeslundii.*

Incorporating hydroxyapatite nanoparticles into dental sealants has enabled Rafiee to study the remineralization ability and bond strength of the sealant. The shear bond strength of the sealants with higher concentrations of nanohydroxyapatite nanoparticles was greater than that of the standard sealants [30]. In resin-based dental sealants, Ibrahim has used nano amorphous calcium phosphate nanoparticles. They discovered that novel Ca and PO_4 dental sealants that are antibacterial and rechargeable have been developed to encourage remineralization and prevent cavities [31]. Hikmat J. Al-Judy investigated the effects of impact strength and surface roughness when boron nitride (BN) nanoparticles were added to the polymethyl methacrylate resin [32]. A protective composite against the advancement of enamel caries was reported to be made of reduced graphene oxide and silver nanoparticles. While reducing enamel surface roughness, lesion depth, and mineral loss, the nanoparticles also demonstrated antibacterial activity [33]. Compared to silver nanoparticles, copper oxide nanoparticles are less expensive. Copper oxide nanoparticles can be introduced into dental glue to stop early or carious white spot lesions, as they are antibacterial without affecting shear bond strength [34–36]. The antibacterial properties of other copper nanoparticles, such as copper iodide and copper fluoride nanoparticles, are also observed in *S. mutans*. They have a crystalline structure, high surface area, and good physical characteristics.

Figure 10.3 shows the nanoparticles as dental sealants and their chemical, mechanical, and biological properties.

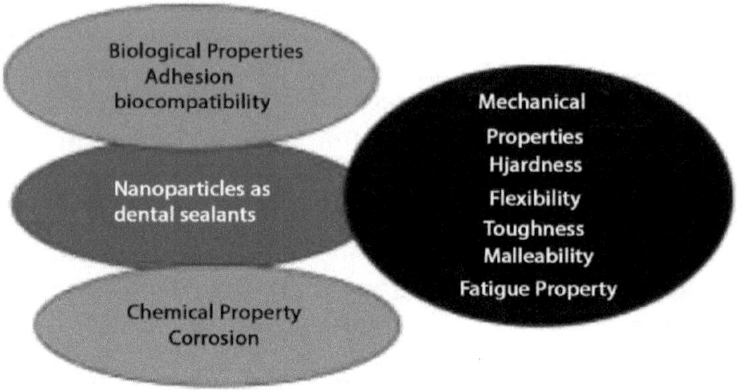

FIGURE 10.3 Nanoparticles as dental sealants.

Nanomaterials similar to carbon nanotubes are boron-nitride nanotubes (BNNTs). BNNTs have attracted a lot of interest in biomedical science due to their nanometric size, high surface-to-volume ratio, surface functionality, high elastic modulus, biocompatibility, hydrophobicity, chemical inertness, and sensitivity to precipitation in aqueous solutions. The effects of boron-nitride nanotubes (BNNTs) inserted at various concentrations on the characteristics of resin-based light-curing dental sealants were studied by Collares and his coworkers [37].

10.5 HYBRID FILLER IN DENTAL SEALANT

Surface sealants utilize fillers to stop the microleakage in resin composite. Most microleakage in composite resin happens as a result of poor adhesion, variations in thermal expansion coefficients, inadequate moisture control, etc. [38]. To enhance the mechanical and biological qualities, fillers are added to surface sealants [39]. The biomedical industry has highlighted the use of antimicrobial fillers, namely metals and oxides, as a potential method of combating diseases that are resistant to common medications [40]. The fillers' most important properties depend on size reduction, form enhancement (platelike, rod-like, and nanoparticle-like), functionalization, and bioactive capability [41–43]. The two types of hybrid sealants are giomer and compomer sealants [44] (Figure 10.4). Compomer is also known as a polyacid-modified composite resin. A polyacid-modified monomer, reactive silicate glass particles, a photo-initiator, and non-reactive inorganic filler particles are all present [45].

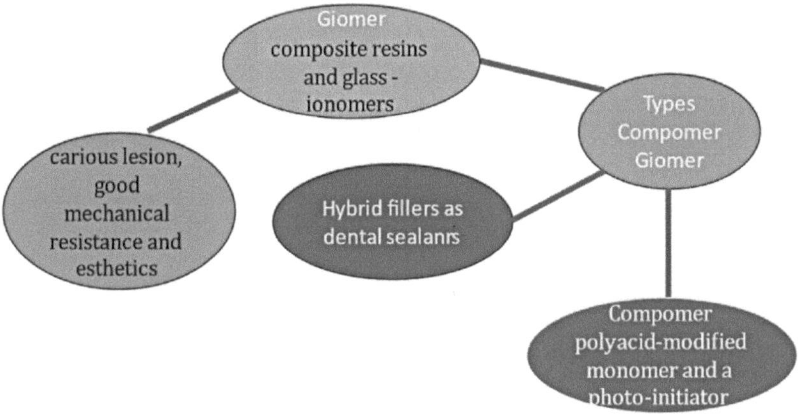

FIGURE 10.4 Hybrid fillers as dental sealants.

Giomer is made up of a matrix composed of resin-based monomers and pre-reacted glass ionomer (PRG) filler [46]. As a relatively new technology, hybrid sealants are not commonly used. Garcia and his group members synthesized hybrid Zn-based nanoparticles coated with ionic liquid (Simonkolleite (SKT) particles) as filler for sealants. They analyzed the physicochemical properties and antibacterial activity. It was found that the addition of fillers enhances antibacterial properties and prevents dental caries [47]. A possible hybrid filler for dental composites is S-rGO combined with surface-modified fumed SiO_2. The idea of using S-rGO/SiO_2 hybrid filler offers a number of opportunities to change the mechanical and physical characteristics of dental composites. New techniques for creating high-performance dental composites as sealants will emerge as a result of further adjustments and optimization of this hybrid filler [48].

10.6 CONCLUSION

In this chapter, we discuss about the dental sealant under the following heading:

- Chitosan based sealants and its biological properties;
- Nanoparticles incorporated bio composite sealants;
- Hybrid filler in dental sealant.

Dental sealants made of biocomposite materials work well to prevent dental cavities. They are used on deep pits and fissures of caries-prone teeth to stop the progression of the disease. Over time, sealant retention and effectiveness have increased thanks to developments in biocomposite materials and the creation of innovative procedures. There are several types of sealants, each with its own advantages. Sealants are incredibly effective at lowering dental cavities, as this review shows. Future studies on this topic should be expanded upon.

KEYWORDS

- **adhesive**
- **antibacterial properties**
- **biocompatibility**
- **bio-composites**
- **chitosan**
- **dental sealants**
- **dentistry**
- **sealant**

REFERENCES

1. Abdolahpour, Z., Saneipour, Z., & Azarhoosh, M. J. (2017). Application of biomaterials in dentistry. *Current Trends in Biomedical Engineering & Biosciences, 2*, 44–47. https://doi.org/10.19080/CTBEB.2016.01.555588.
2. Vert, M., Doi, Y., Hellwich, K. H., Hess, M., Hodge, P., Kubisa, P., Rinaudo, M., & Schué, F. (2012). Terminology for biorelated polymers and applications (IUPAC Recommendations 2012). *Pure and Applied Chemistry, 84*(2), 377–410. https://doi.org/10.1351/PAC-REC-10-12-04.
3. Böstman, O., & Pihlajamäki, H. (2000). Clinical biocompatibility of biodegradable orthopaedic implants for internal fixation: A review. *Biomaterials, 21*(26), 2615–2621. https://doi.org/10.1016/S0142-9612(00)00129-0.
4. John, M. J., & Thomas, S. (2008). Biofibers and bio composites. *Carbohydrate Polymers, 71*(3), 343–364. https://doi.org/10.1016/j.carbpol.2007.05.040
5. Rea, S. M., & Bonfield, W. (2004). Biocomposites for medical applications. *Journal of the Australian Ceramic Society, 40*(1), 43–57.
6. Kucukyilmaz, E., & Savas, S. (2015). Evaluation of different fissure sealant materials and flowable composites used as pit-and-fissure sealants: A 24-month clinical trial. *Pediatric Dentistry, 37*(6), 468–473.

7. Memarpour, M., Shafiei, F., Zarean, M., & Razmjoei, F. (2018). Sealing effectiveness of fissure sealant bonded with universal adhesive systems on saliva-contaminated and noncontaminated enamel. *Journal of Clinical and Experimental Dentistry, 10*(1), e1–e6. https://doi.org/10.4317/jced.54867.
8. Bodecker, C. F. (1964). Enamel fissure eradication. *New York State Dental Journal, 30*(3), 149–154.
9. Wilson, A. D., & McLean, J. W. (1988). *Glass-Ionomer Cement*. Quintessence Publishing.
10. Zalizniak, I., Palamara, J. E., Wong, R. H., Cochrane, N. J., Burrow, M. F., & Reynolds, E. C. (2013). Ion release and physical properties of CPP-ACP modified GIC in acid solutions. *Journal of Dentistry, 41*(5), 449–454. https://doi.org/10.1016/j.jdent.2012.12.002.
11. American Dental Association. (2008). ADA Professional Product Review: Academic Corner. Retrieved from: ADA website.
12. Rajabnia, R., Ghasempour, M., Gharekhani, S., & et al. (2016). Anti-Streptococcus mutans property of a chitosan-containing resin sealant. *Journal of the International Society of Preventive & Community Dentistry, 6*(1), 49–53. https://doi.org/10.4103/2231-0762.181307.
13. Garcia, I. M., Rodrigues, S. B., Leitune, V. C. B., & Collares, F. M. (2019). Antibacterial, chemical, and physical properties of sealants with polyhexamethylene guanidine hydrochloride. *Brazilian Oral Research, 33*, e019. https://doi.org/10.1590/1677-0501.20190019.
14. Poorzandpoush, K., Omrani, L. R., Jafarnia, S. H., Golkar, P., & Atai, M. (2017). Effect of addition of nano hydroxyapatite particles on wear of resin modified glass ionomer by tooth brushing simulation. *Journal of Clinical and Experimental Dentistry, 9*(3), e372–e376. https://doi.org/10.4317/jced.53946.
15. Ikono, R., Vibriani, A., Wibowo, I., & et al. (2019). Nanochitosan antimicrobial activity against Streptococcus mutans and Candida albicans dual-species biofilms. *BMC Research Notes, 12*(1), 383. https://doi.org/10.1186/s13104-019-4418-0.
16. Mosaddad, S. A., Tahmasebi, E., Yazdanian, A., & et al. (2019). Oral microbial biofilms: An update. *European Journal of Clinical Microbiology & Infectious Diseases, 38*(11), 2005–2019. https://doi.org/10.1007/s10096-019-03724-4.
17. Lai, C. C., Lin, C. P., & Wang, Y. L. (2022). Development of antibacterial composite resin containing chitosan/fluoride microparticles as pit and fissure sealant to prevent caries. *Journal of Oral Microbiology, 14*(1), 2008615. https://doi.org/10.1080/20002297.2021.2008615.
18. Zareian, H., Bahador, A., Pourhajibagher, M., Bashareh, Z., & Valizadeh, S. (2021). Evaluation of antibacterial effects of fissure sealants containing chitosan nanoparticles. *International Journal of Dentistry, 2021*. https://doi.org/10.1155/2021/8975948.
19. Ramar, K., & Vivek, N. (2022). Biocompatibility of chitosan nanoparticle in root canal sealant with Vero cell line. *International Journal of Clinical Pediatric Dentistry, 15*.
20. Mahapoka, E., Arirachakaran, P., Watthanaphanit, A., Rujiravanit, R., & Poolthong, S. (2012). Chitosan whiskers from shrimp shells incorporated into dimethacrylate-based dental resin sealant. *Dental Materials Journal, 31*(3), 273–279. https://doi.org/10.4012/dmj.2011-071.

21. Cao, X., Cai, X., Chen, R., Zhang, H., Jiang, T., & Wang, Y. (2019). A thermosensitive chitosan-based hydrogel for sealing and lubricating purposes in dental implant systems. *21*(19), 324–335.
22. Alkheraif, A. A., AlMufareh, N. A., AlQhtani, F. A., Asiri, W., Abuhadi, R. I., Hamoud, M., & Khan, A. A. (2022). Minocycline incorporated cobalt oxide nanoparticles in dental sealants: An in vitro study. *Microscopy Research and Technique, 85*(7), 2558–2566. https://doi.org/10.1002/jemt.24109.
23. Salas-López, E. K., Pierdant-Pérez, M., Hernández-Sierra, J. F., Ruíz, F., Mandeville, P., & Pozos-Guillén, A. J. (2017). Effect of silver nanoparticle-added pit and fissure sealant in the prevention of dental caries in children. *Journal of Clinical Pediatric Dentistry, 41*(1), 48–52. https://doi.org/10.17796/1053-4628-41.1.48.
24. Saqib, S., Nazeer, A., Ali, M., Zaman, W., Younas, M., Sunera, S., & Nisar, M. (2022). Catalytic potential of endophytes facilitates synthesis of bimetallic zinc oxide nanoparticles for agricultural application. *BioMetals, 35*(5), 967–985. https://doi.org/10.1007/s10534-022-00466-1.
25. Kasraei, S., Sami, L., Hendi, S., AliKhani, M. Y., Rezaei-Soufi, L., & Khamverdi, Z. (2014). Antibacterial properties of composite resins incorporating silver and zinc oxide nanoparticles on *Streptococcus mutans* and *Lactobacillus*. *Restorative Dentistry & Endodontics, 39*(2), 109–114. https://doi.org/10.5395/rde.2014.39.2.109.
26. Wu, W., Liu, T., He, H., Wu, X., Cao, X., Jin, J., Sun, Q. J., Roy, V. A. L., & Li, R. K. Y. (2018). Rheological and antibacterial performance of sodium alginate/zinc oxide composite coating for cellulosic paper. *Colloids and Surfaces B: Bio Interfaces, 167*, 538–543. https://doi.org/10.1016/j.colsurfb.2018.05.032.
27. Swetha, D. L., Vinay, C., Uloopi, K. S., RojaRamya, K. S., & Chandrasekhar, R. (2019). Antibacterial and mechanical properties of pit and fissure sealants containing zinc oxide and calcium fluoride nanoparticles. *Contemporary Clinical Dentistry, 10*(3), 477–482. https://doi.org/10.4103/ccd.ccd_805_18.
28. Javidi, M., Zarei, M., Naghavi, N., Mortazavi, M., & Nejat, A. H. (2014). Zinc oxide nanoparticles as sealer in endodontics and its sealing ability. *Contemporary Clinical Dentistry, 5*(1), 20–24. https://doi.org/10.4103/0976-237X.128656.
29. Kati, F. A. (2019). Effect of the incorporation of zinc oxide nanoparticles on the flexural strength of auto-polymerized acrylic resins. *Journal of Oral Research, 8*(1), 37–41. https://doi.org/10.1016/j.joor.2019.02.005.
30. Memarpour, M., Shafiei, F., Rafiee, A., Soltani, M., & Dashti, M. H. (2019). Effect of hydroxyapatite nanoparticles on enamel remineralization and estimation of fissure sealant bond strength to remineralized tooth surfaces: An in vitro study. *BMC Oral Health, 19*(1), 92. https://doi.org/10.1186/s12863-019-0787-x.
31. Ibrahim, M. S., AlQarni, F. D., Al-Dulaijan, Y. A., Weir, M. D., Oates, T. W., & et al. (2018). Tuning nano-amorphous calcium phosphate content in novel rechargeable antibacterial dental sealant. *Materials, 11*(9), 1544. https://doi.org/10.3390/ma11091544.
32. Hussein, H. M., & Al-Judy, H. J. (2023). Effect of incorporation of boron nitride nanoparticles on impact strength and surface roughness of heat cure poly methyl methacrylate resin: An in vitro study. *Dental Hypotheses, 14*(1), 19–21. https://doi.org/10.4103/denthyp.denthyp_71_22.
33. Wu, R., Zhao, Q., Lu, S., Fu, Y., Yu, D., & Zhao, W. (2018). Inhibitory effect of reduced graphene oxide-silver nanocomposite on progression of artificial enamel caries. *Journal of Applied Oral Science, 27*, e20180042. https://doi.org/10.1590/1678-7757-2018-0042.

34. Toodehzaeim, M. H., Zandi, H., Meshkani, H., & Hosseinzadeh Firouzabadi, A. (2018). The effect of CuO nanoparticles on antimicrobial effects and shear bond strength of orthodontic adhesives. *Journal of Dentistry, 19*(1), 1–5.
35. Gutiérrez, M. F., Malaquias, P., Matos, T. P., Szesz, A., Souza, S., Bermudez, J., Reis, A., Loguercio, A. D., & Farago, P. V. (2017). Mechanical and microbiological properties and drug release modeling of an etch-and-rinse adhesive containing copper nanoparticles. *Dental Materials, 33*(3), 309–320. https://doi.org/10.1016/j.dental.2016.12.011.
36. Sabatini, C., Mennito, A. S., Wolf, B. J., Pashley, D. H., & Renné, W. G. (2015). Incorporation of bactericidal poly-acrylic acid modified copper iodide particles into adhesive resins. *Journal of Dentistry, 43*(5), 546–555. https://doi.org/10.1016/j.jdent.2015.03.010.
37. Bohns, F. R., Degrazia, F. W., de Souza Balbinot, G., et al. (2019). Boron nitride nanotubes as filler for resin-based dental sealants. *Scientific Reports, 9*, 7710. https://doi.org/10.1038/s41598-019-44246-8.
38. Sadeghi, M., Davari, A., & Lynch, C. D. (2013). The effect of re-bonding using surface sealant or adhesive system on microleakage of class V resin composite restorations. *Dental Research Journal, 10*(5), 596–601. https://doi.org/10.4103/1735-3327.123657.
39. Lopes, M. B., Saquy, P. C., Moura, S. K., Wang, L., Graciano, F. M., Correr Sobrinho, L., & et al. (2012). Effect of different surface penetrating sealants on the roughness of a nanofiller composite resin. *Brazilian Dental Journal, 23*(6), 692–697. https://doi.org/10.1590/S0103-64402012000600007.
40. Makvandi, P., Wang, C., Zare, E. N., Borzacchiello, A., Niu, L., & Tay, F. R. (2020). Metal-based nanomaterials in biomedical applications: Antimicrobial activity and cytotoxicity aspects. *Advanced Functional Materials, 30*(22), 1–40. https://doi.org/10.1002/adfm.201910021.
41. Wang, Y., & Zhu, M. (2020). Functional fillers for dental resin composites. *Acta Biomaterialia, 122*, 1–13. https://doi.org/10.1016/j.actbio.2020.12.001.
42. Randolph, L. D., et al. (2016). Filler characteristics of modern dental resin composites and their influence on physico-mechanical properties. *Dental Materials, 32*(12), 1586–1599. https://doi.org/10.1016/j.dental.2016.09.001.
43. Habib, E., et al. (2016). Inorganic fillers for dental resin composites: Present and future. *ACS Biomaterials Science & Engineering, 2*(1), 1–11. https://doi.org/10.1021/acsbiomaterials.5b00270.
44. Ramamurthy, P., Rath, A., Sidhu, P., Fernandes, B., Nettem, S., & Muttalib, K. (2018). Sealants for preventing dental caries in primary teeth. *Cochrane Database of Systematic Reviews, 2018*(3), CD012981. https://doi.org/10.1002/14651858.CD012981.
45. Shen, C., Rawls, H. R., & Esquivel-Upshaw, J. F. (2022). *Phillips' Science of Dental Materials*. St. Louis, MO: Elsevier/Saunders.
46. Rusnac, M. E., Gasparik, C., Irimie, A. I., Grecu, A. G., Mesaroş, A. Ş., & Dudea, D. (2019). Giomers in dentistry–At the boundary between dental composites and glass-ionomers. *Medical & Pharmaceutical Reports, 92*, 123–129. https://doi.org/10.15386/mpr-1169.
47. Garcia, I. M., Souza, V. S., Souza, J. D., Visioli, F., Leitune, V. C. B., Scholten, J. D., & Collares, F. M. (2020). Zinc-based particle with ionic liquid as a hybrid filler for dental adhesive resin. *Journal of Dentistry, 102*, 103477. https://doi.org/10.1016/j.jdent.2020.103477.

48. Alrahlah, A., Khan, R., Al-Odayni, A. B., Saeed, W. S., Bautista, L. S., & Vohra, F. (2020). Evaluation of synergic potential of rGO/SiO_2 as hybrid filler for BisGMA/TEGDMA dental composites. *Polymers, 12*(12), 3025. https://doi.org/10.3390/polym12123025.
49. Prasad, A., Bhasney, S. M., & Prasannavenkadesan, V. (2023). Polylactic acid reinforced with nano-hydroxyapatite bioabsorbable cortical screws for bone fracture treatment. *Journal of Polymer Research, 30*, 177. https://doi.org/10.1007/s10965-023-03542-8.
50. Sarkar, K., Dutta, K., Chatterjee, A., Sarkar, J., Das, D., Prasad, A., Chattopadhyay, D., Acharya, K., Das, M., Verma, S. K., & De, S. (2023). Nanotherapeutic potential of antibacterial folic acid-functionalized nanoceria for wound-healing applications. *Nanomedicine, 18*(2). https://doi.org/10.2217/nnm-2022-0233.
51. Katiyar, V., Prasad, A., Sankar, M. R., & Bhasney, S. M. (2022). Process for the preparation of polymer composite-based cancellous screw and pins. Indian Patent No. 401811.
52. Kaswindiarti, S., Dinata, A. M., & Nurnaini, L. D. (2022). Dental fillings materials and dental management against hypersensitivity reaction of stainless-steel crown: A review. *Journal of Medicinal and Chemical Sciences, 5*, 153–161.
53. Kotha, A. K., Nicholson, J. W., & Booth, S. E. (2023). Biological evaluation of zinc phosphate cement for potential bone contact applications. *Biomedicines, 11*(2), 250. https://doi.org/10.3390/biomedicines11020250.
54. Parameswari, B. D., Rajakumar, M., Lambodaran, G., & Sundar, S. (2016). Comparative study on the tensile bond strength and marginal fit of complete veneer cast metal crowns using various luting agents: An in vitro study. *Journal of Pharmacy & Bio Allied Sciences, 8*(Suppl 1), S138. https://doi.org/10.4103/0975-7406.191944.
55. Pepla, E., Besharat, L. K., Palaia, G., Tenore, G., & Migliau, G. (2014). Nano-hydroxyapatite and its applications in preventive, restorative and regenerative dentistry: A review of literature. *Annali di Stomatologia, 5*(3), 108–114. https://www.ncbi.nlm.nih.gov/pmc/articles/PMC4252862/ (accessed on 8 August 2024).
56. Murugan, R., Yazid, F., Nasruddin, N. S., & Anuar, N. N. M. (2022). Effects of nanohydroxyapatite incorporation into glass ionomer cement (GIC). *Minerals, 12*(1), 9. https://doi.org/10.3390/min12010009.
57. Grech, J., & Antunes, E. (2019). Zirconia in dental prosthetics: A literature review. *Journal of Materials Research and Technology, 8*(5), 4956–4964. https://doi.org/10.1016/j.jmrt.2019.05.001.
58. Bapat, R. A., Yang, H. J., Chaubal, T. V., Dharmadhikary, S., Abdulla, A. M., Arora, S., Rawal, S., & Kesharwani, P. (2022). Review on synthesis, properties and multifarious therapeutic applications of nanostructured zirconia in dentistry. *RSC Advances, 12*, 12773–12793. https://doi.org/10.1039/D2RA01137D.
59. Revathi, N., & Sharath Chandra, S. M. (2014). Merits and demerits of calcium hydroxide as a therapeutic agent: A review. *International Journal of Dental Sciences and Research, 2*(6B), 1–4. https://doi.org/10.12691/ijdsr-2-6B-1.
60. Nicholson, J. W. (2016). The history and background to glass-ionomer dental cements. In *Glass-ionomers in Dentistry* (pp. 1–24). Springer.
61. Jayaraman, K., Elshereksi, N. W., Ghazali, M. J., Muchtar, A., Andanastuti, A., & Che, H. (2014). Perspectives for titanium-derived fillers usage on denture base composite construction: A review article. *Advances in Materials Science and Engineering, 2014*, 1–12. https://doi.org/10.1155/2014/734619.

62. Lim, M., Jung, C., Shin, D. H., Cho, Y. B., & Song, M. (2020). Calcium silicate-based root canal sealers: A literature review. *Restorative Dentistry & Endodontics, 45*(3), e35. https://doi.org/10.5395/rde.2020.45.e35.
63. Berman, L. H., Hargreaves, K., & Cohen, S. (2010). *Cohen's Pathways of The Pulp Expert Consult* (10th ed.). Maryland Heights, MO: Mosby Elsevier.

CHAPTER 11

New Frontiers of Hydrogels for Wound Healing Applications

SRIPARNA DE,[1] MADHURIMA BASAK,[1] DIPANJAN BHATTACHARJEE,[1] ARBIND PRASAD,[2] and BIDYANAND MAHTO[3]

[1]*Department of Allied Health Sciences, Brainware University, Kolkata, West Bengal, India*

[2]*Mechanical Engineering Department, Katihar Engineering College (Under Department of Science, Technology and Technical Education, Government of Bihar), Katihar, Bihar, India*

[3]*Government Engineering College, Vaishali (Under Department of Science, Technology, and Technical Education, Government of Bihar), Vaishali, Bihar, India*

ABSTRACT

Human skin furnishes an active rampart against several microbial perforations and infections. Owing to the characteristic features of direct exposure to the environment, the skin has also been considered one of the most vulnerable tissues. Tissues act as a safeguard and deliver an averting mechanism, which ultimately dismantles after surgeries, burns, skin diseases, etc. Unfortunately, this results in chronic wound development. Chronic wounds lead to colonization and infection caused by the genesis of a vascular eschar, facilitating the multiplication of microorganisms. Owing to the fascinating features such as compatibility with the native extracellular matrix and retention of moisture content after swelling, hydrogels are profoundly recognized for wound healing applications. However, certain flaws, including poor mechanical strength and multifunctionality, restrict their usage in the skin tissue regeneration process. To enhance the versatility of hydrogels, the

Bioabsorbable Polymers for Drug Carriers and Fixation Devices. Arbind Prasad and Sougata Jana (Eds.)

incorporation of biomaterials and nanostructures is an emerging avenue offering an induction template for tissue inflammation, proliferation, and remodeling, effective for wound healing. Advanced functions of hydrogel dressing, including antimicrobial properties, adhesion and hemostasis, anti-inflammatory, and anti-oxidation effects, self-healing, stimulus response, and conductivity, are cultivated in the proposed chapter. Furthermore, the application of hydrogel wound dressing for the treatment of different types of wounds, such as incisional and excisional wounds, is concise. Typically, other wounds, including infected wounds, burn wounds, and diabetic wounds, are also scrutinized. The chapter highlights traditional Chinese medicine (TCM)-based hydrogel material as a potential candidate in wound healing applications. The breakneck progression of antimicrobial hydrogels derived from the amalgamation of antimicrobial agents with hydrogel systems is also reviewed, and the relevant studies on technological advancements that offer a paradigm shift in the field of wound healing have also been summarized.

11.1 INTRODUCTION

The term "hydrogels" refers to cross-linked 3D networks that are created by water-rich environments filled with hydrophilic polymer chains, which have tunable physical and chemical attributes [1–3]. Hydrogels mimic the extracellular matrix (ECM) of biological soft tissues due to their biocompatibility, hydrophilic nature, and 3D network structure; as a result, they have established widespread applications in cell culture, tissue engineering, drug administration, soft actuators, etc. [4–7]. In 1894, the term "hydrogel" was originally used to describe a colloidal gel [8, 9]. DuPont scientists first described the production of poly(2-hydroxyethyl methacrylate) hydrogel in 1936. The need for creating a biomimetic, bio-plastic material that would have the properties of (i) a structure permitting the desired water content; (ii) inertness to normal biological processes; and (iii) permeability to metabolites was not recognized until the late 1950s. Due to these demands, Danno first described the creation of covalently crosslinked polyvinyl alcohol (PVA) hydrogel by gamma radiation in 1958. Since its beginnings, hydrogels have rapidly developed, making significant advancements [6, 12]. The focus of hydrogel research changed in the 1980s from straightforward synthesis to the creation of responsive hydrogels that could react to shifting environmental factors like pH and temperature. The improvement of hydrogel preparation resulted in the development of pH/thermo-responsive hydrogels that behave in various ways in response to different physiological stimuli. For the in-situ synthesis and regulated release of medicines, including medications, temperature-sensitive hydrogels are of special importance [13–15]. Ionic and hydrophobic interactions, respectively, are primarily responsible for the crosslinking of these pH- and temperature-responsive hydrogels. In the 1990s, different physical techniques were used to create responsive hydrogels and improve their mechanical, thermal, and degrading characteristics. Hoffman et al. reported the creation of dual-responsive hydrogels for amylase release in 1992. This was the first instance of a hydrogel responding to both pH and temperature as triggers. The hydrogel was created by combining thermally and pH-sensitive polymers with acrylic acid, divinyl silicone rubber, N-isopropyl acrylamide (NIPAM), and a small amount of crosslinker [16–18]. All living systems are responsive to stimuli (such as pH, temperature, physical strain, etc.), and self-assembly implies a case of self/non-self-recognition. Due to these advancements, hydrogels are now biomimetic in nature and useful for a range of biological applications. For the creation of the ordered structure of the hydrogel, the self-assembly of natural biomolecules such as polysaccharides, proteins, peptides, etc., was investigated.

Significant research advancements have recently been made in the biofabrication method for creating biocompatible nanocomposite hydrogels and mechanically stable, sticky hydrogels. Innovative biomimetic nanocomposite hydrogels with chemical, mechanical, and biological properties that match those of soft tissues are created when a nanomaterial and a biopolymer are combined. These materials are the most promising biomaterials for tissue engineering applications. The characteristics of ideal hydrogels for wound healing applications are shown in Figure 11.1. The stimulus response

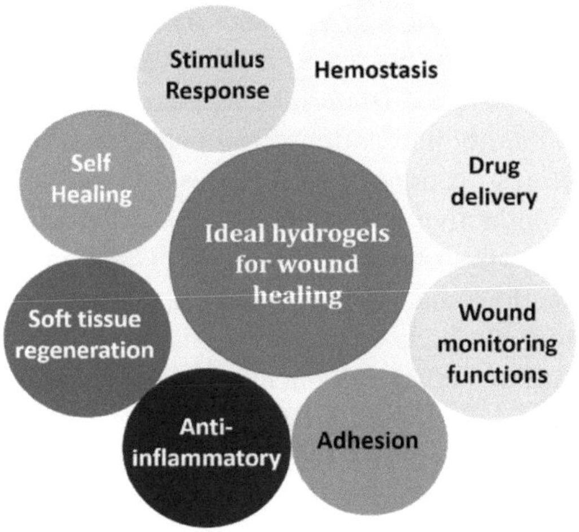

FIGURE 11.1 Ideal characteristics of hydrogels for wound healing applications.

activates the modeling of the wound for proper healing. Drug delivery in types of multifunctional materials is enhanced with hydrogels for efficient targeted curing of wounds [75, 76].

The biomimetic nanocomposite hydrogels are useful for surgical hemostasis, irregular bleeding wounds, and internal injuries due to their strong tissue adhesion and shear-thinning capabilities under wet conditions, electrical conductivity, and cell proliferation activity. The recent invention of stimuli-responsive bio-fabricated smart nanocomposite hydrogels has sparked a lot of attention in the field of trauma care management. The hemostatic and wound healing processes are improved when medicines, growth factors, cells, or other tiny molecules are released from smart hydrogels in the presence of external stimuli. This chapter focuses on a hydrogel material based on traditional Chinese medicine (TCM) that may be used in applications for wound healing. Additionally, it covers the rapid development of antimicrobial hydrogels produced by the fusion of antimicrobial agents with hydrogel systems, and provides a summary of the pertinent studies on technical advances that offer a paradigm change in the field of wound healing.

11.2 MULTIFACETED FEATURES OF HYDROGEL SYSTEM

Microbial hydrogel dressing is crucial for both chronic and acute wounds. The incorporation of conventional antibiotics within wound dressing systems exhibits some drawbacks. Therefore, current research relies on advanced antimicrobial hydrogel systems by amalgamating metallic nanoparticles (NPs), carbon-based nanomaterials, and nanofibers. The most abundant natural polymer, chitosan, possesses a positive charge that easily interacts with the negatively charged bacterial cell membrane. Another approach to tune the water solubility and antibacterial property is quaternized chitosan, which is a foremost candidate for chitosan-based dressings as injectable hydrogel. Conductive polymers such as polyaniline and polypyrrole can be grafted onto the chitosan backbone. This can be attributed to the synergistic interaction and electron transfer of polyaniline and bacterial cells, which ultimately leads to bacterial cell death [19–21]. A mechanistic insight into various nanomaterials such as zinc oxide (ZnO NPs) [22], silver NPs [23], and gold NPs [24] governs the antibacterial activities, wherein the penetration of nanoparticles within the bacterial membrane ultimately instigates the nucleic acid drainage of the outer peptidoglycan layer, thereby impeding protein synthesis. Recently, photothermal therapy (PTT), using a combination of near-infrared (NIR) light and light-absorbing materials, has been employed to cause heat damage and destroy locally prevalent harmful microorganisms. Due to its advantageous properties, including deep tissue penetration, low cytotoxicity, and minimal tissue damage, induced PTT in the NIR (700–1,100 nm) range has been reported to be effective for damaging bacterial cells. In order to enhance the multifunctional dressing with suitable results for adhesiveness and mechanical characteristics, several antibacterial techniques, such as PTT and PDT, can be integrated into a single scheme. The synergistic antibacterial effects based on the combination of photothermal nanoparticles and antibacterial medications have been researched as a viable method for wound healing to overcome tissue damage caused by PTT for antibacterial purposes.

Another pivotal feature of the hydrogel system is a protracted inflammatory response, wherein excessive reactive oxygen species (ROS) levels might hinder the healing of wounds since they are greater than the antioxidant capacity of the cells. In the case of diabetic chronic wounds, the overaccumulation of ROS can endanger oxidative stress through impaired angiogenesis and chronic inflammation. Among polyphenols, gallic acid and tannic acid are promising candidates that possess anti-collagenase activity and tissue adhesivity, respectively. GA-modified hydrogel systems impart enhanced neovascularization, highly ordered collagen, and hair follicle maturation. A porous, compact, interconnecting network structure could be fabricated using TA and silk fibroin. Increasing the concentration of TA could augment the adhesiveness of the hydrogels. Additionally, various antioxidant materials, e.g., mussel-inspired polydopamine (PDA) [25], curcumin [26], chitosan [27], hyaluronic acid [28], ceria nanocrystals, and ferulic acid [29, 30], are highly efficient as antioxidants with sustained bioactivity for wound healing applications. Rutin is another potent bioactive material that could be utilized as an efficient matrix for wound management [31].

Antibiotics are the most popular and efficient antibacterial agents. A promising platform for the local, controlled release of antimicrobial medicines is hydrogels laced with antibacterial medications [32]. The antibiotic was successfully encapsulated in hydrogels by dissolving the necessary amount of amoxicillin into the hydrogel precursor solution, and the hydrogels displayed effective antibacterial properties, creating amikacin-loaded hydrogels used in the treatment of wounds [33]. The hydrogels were created using a straightforward mixing technique, and the results revealed that the membranes had a noticeably higher zone of inhibition against *S. aureus* and *P. aeruginosa*.

11.3 TRADITIONAL CHINESE MEDICINE (TCM)-BASED HYDROGEL MATERIAL

Chronic wounds affect about 6 million people globally. Currently, surgical debridement and growth factor medications are the two main types of treatment for persistent wounds. The issue with surgical debridement is that it cannot effectively treat the chronic condition. The drawbacks of growth factor medications are their high cost and unwanted side effects, which can worsen patients' conditions. To give patients with wounds more options, research is still being conducted on the creation of innovative wound healing treatments. It has been known since ancient times that traditional Chinese medicines can be used to cure wounds. Ancient Chinese medical texts advise using a variety of botanical medications from traditional Chinese medicine to treat wounds. As time goes on, significant progress has been made in illuminating the probable processes of these botanical medications' wound healing abilities. Consequently, in this article, we will provide a summary of the plant medicines used in traditional Chinese medicine that have the ability to treat wounds. Several medications have undergone thorough research and have been shown to be clinically efficacious among all the plant medicines in traditional Chinese medicine that have been claimed to have wound-healing properties, including Centellae Herba, birch bark, calendula, aloe vera, and *Curcumae longae* rhizome [34].

A small herbal molecule, rhein, is extracted from the traditional Chinese medicine rhubarb. According to recent research, rhein has great anti-inflammatory qualities and may be used to treat rheumatoid arthritis, gout, and intestinal inflammation [35]. It has recently been shown that rhein's tiny molecules can self-assemble to create fibrous network hydrogels, which have been shown to have improved anti-inflammatory effectiveness. It is possible to J-type collect rhein molecules and then arrange them into left-handed helical nanofibers. Such a shape results in intense binding to the cellular receptor's active region [36]. Even while this is crucial for advancing the therapeutic effects of natural small molecules, it still confronts significant challenges due to its poor stability. Self-assembled rhein hydrogel dissociates particularly easily when used as a wound dressing due to the vibrations and outside forces that typically occur on the wound surface and other factors that typically impact the wound's surface [36]. As a result, the self-assembled rhein transforms back into a free substance and loses its therapeutic benefits. Creating a hydrogel system with an optimized structure may be a way to address this drawback of self-assembled rhein [37]. The integrated hydrogel will increase the stability of self-assembled rhein fibrils by working with a cross-linked network. For therapeutic effects on chronic inflammation, the integrity and stability of the rhein fibrils could be substantially maintained. This supramolecular hydrogel with enhanced therapeutic efficacy and oxidation responsiveness is anticipated to be used as a potential functional wound dressing in the treatment of chronic wounds in the future [37].

11.4 MULTIFUNCTIONAL HYDROGELS WITH NANO-STRUCTURAL COMPONENTS

Multifunctional hydrogels based on different nanostructures have attracted a lot of attention so far as a possible method to produce hydrogels with the right properties for wound healing [38]. Four general categories can be used to classify the nanoparticles used to create multifunctional hydrogels for wound healing: (i) based on nanofibers; (ii) based on metals; (iii) based on carbon; and (iv) based on minerals (Figure 11.2). This section introduces new advancements in multipurpose hydrogels with nanostructures for wound healing.

11.4.1 NANOFIBER-BASED COMPOSITES FOR USE IN WOUND HEALING

For tissue regeneration and wound healing, dressings based on both nanofibers and hydrogels have recently been studied. In the next subsections, we concentrate on recent advancements in the creation of nano-reinforced composite hydrogels with suitable characteristics for use in wound healing. As potential structures for wound healing applications, we initially focus on various methods to fabricate nanofiber-hydrogel-based scaffolds, primarily concentrating on bilayers, nanofiber reinforcement dressings, and self-assembled scaffolds while taking into account the difficulties of individual electrospun nanofibers and hydrogels. Three methods can be used to create nanofiber-based multifunctional hydrogels: integrating nanofibrous structures into hydrogels, incorporating nanofibers into hydrogels, and creating hydrogels that self-assemble using peptides. The hydrogels have been given functionality using each of the methods mentioned above. The manufacturing of nanofiber-hydrogel composites has been studied using a variety of techniques [38]. Electrospun nanofibers have received a lot of attention among different nanostructures for their use in wound healing.

11.4.2 METAL-BASED COMPOSITES FOR USE IN WOUND HEALING

In the field of wound healing, metal-based nanomaterials have generated a lot of interest. Due to their unique antibacterial actions, previous investigations have shown that metallic NPs display lower bacterial resistance than traditional antibiotics. ZnO NPs, a class of metal-based nanomaterials, have drawn a lot of interest because of their exceptional qualities, which include minimal cytotoxicity, antibacterial activity, the ability to stimulate fibroblast growth, angiogenesis, keratinocyte migration, and re-epithelialization. Therefore, the use of ZnO-based nanocomposite hydrogels for wound healing applications is of tremendous interest [39].

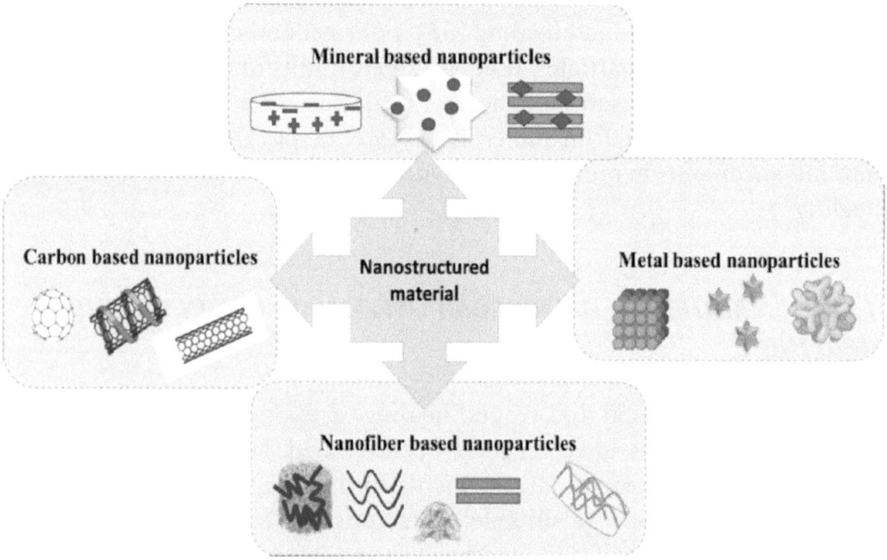

FIGURE 11.2 Various nanostructured materials used for wound healing applications.

11.4.3 CARBON-BASED COMPOSITES FOR USE IN WOUND HEALING

Carbon-based nanomaterials with promising electrochemical, optical, and catalytic capabilities, like graphene, carbon nanotubes (CNT), and carbon dots, are widely used in the field of wound healing. Graphene oxide (GO) and two-dimensional (2D) graphene sheets are thought to be effective nanomaterials for tissue engineering. GO is a strong contender for the loading of pharmaceuticals and biological molecules due to its active functional groups, including carboxyl, hydroxyl, and epoxy. Without employing any organic crosslinkers, GO nanosheets can be used as 2D materials to create a dual network nanocomposite hydrogel. Reduced GO (rGO) nanosheets have been made using a variety of techniques, but one that has shown promise is green chemistry [39].

Carbon-based multifunctional nanostructures have also attracted a lot of attention as a result of recent advances in the design of novel nanomaterials to speed up wound healing. In order to benefit from the synergistic effects of the photothermal and photodynamic antibacterial activity for wound healing, hybrid nanosheets of graphitic carbon nitride (g-C_3N_4)-Zn^{2+}@GO (SCN-Zn^{2+}@GO) were created. Bacterial activity may be decreased by the production of hyperthermia at 808 nm light irradiation caused by the presence of GO. On the other hand, the hybrid nanosheets' photocatalytic activity at 660 nm can kill the bacteria by causing damage to their membranes, denaturing their proteins, and disrupting their metabolic processes [40]. Wound dressings incorporating electroactive materials such as metal NPs and carbon nanomaterials can be a promising approach for accelerating wound healing, especially in light of the significant drawbacks of conductive polymers (e.g., polyaniline, polypyrrole, and polythiophene) such as poor solubility and non-degradability that limit their biomedical applications [41].

11.4.4 MINERAL-BASED COMPOSITES FOR USE IN WOUND HEALING

In the fields of bioactive molecule delivery and regenerative medicine, 2D nanomaterials like nanoclays, which have a sheet- or disc-like shape and special structural and surface properties, have been exploited as potential biomaterials [42]. Additionally, these clays can successfully interact with the polymer interface, disperse uniformly throughout the polymeric matrix, and crosslink molecules to affect the mechanical characteristics of hydrocarbons [43].

For biomedical applications, 2D nanomaterials with properties like dual-charged surfaces, absence of heavy metals, high cationic exchange, and low cytotoxicity are commonly employed. The essential building blocks of laponite nanosheets, which are naturally found in the human body, are minerals. Additionally, under physiological settings, these laponite nanosheets are biocompatible and biodegradable [44–45]. Laponite has been found to enhance the physiological stability, injectability, and *in vivo* hemostatic efficacy of hydrogels [46]. The swellability of laponite and montmorillonite (MMT) clays, the charged stimulation of initiating blood coagulation, and their disk-like structure all influence their hemostatic function [37, 48]. Laponite is a suitable nanostructure for use as an auxiliary material in the self-supported method of direct 3D printing hydrogel composite scaffolds. Due to their advantageous characteristics, such as their crystal structure, they can combine with a range of hydrogel inks because of their positive and negative charges. Laponite's capacity to reconstruct its "house of cards" structure maintains the ability to support itself, enabling direct 3D printing of scaffolds in the air. Laponite's enhanced mechanical characteristics can also help maintain the shape of printed scaffolds following deposition [49]. Laponite is utilized as a delivery system for growth factors that are released gradually, such as VEGF, or vascular endothelial growth factor. Due to the significant interaction between the growth factor and laponite, there may be no VEGF release. Laponite-containing injectable hydrogels have been studied for angiogenesis. Without releasing VEGF, it was shown that the VEGF-laponite gels accelerated tubulogenesis. Long-term VEGF maintenance at the site of implantation resulted in increased efficacy [50].

11.5 VERSATILITY OF HYDROGELS IN WOUND HEALING APPLICATIONS

11.5.1 CONDUCTIVE HYDROGEL

Conductive hydrogels are unique hydrogels that have high conductivity. Conductive hydrogels have been created using a range of conductive materials, including graphite, carbon nanotubes (CNTs), free ions, liquid metals, and conducting polymers (CPs). Due to their excellent electrical properties and flexible mechanical characteristics, CPs have been identified as one of the most promising materials for the creation of conductive hydrogels. It has also been shown that conducting polymer-based hydrogels (CPHs) are a suitable design platform for stretchy and wearable strain sensors. Hydrogel-based conductive materials have drawn more and more interest due to their exceptional flexibility, adaptability, and superior biocompatibility. First, various conductive hydrogels are discussed, including pure single-network hydrogels based on conductive polymers, single-network hydrogels with additional conductive additives (such as nanoparticles, nanowires, and nanosheets), double-network hydrogels based on conductive polymers, and double-network hydrogels with additional conductive additives [51]. The second section introduces in-depth conductive hydrogels with a range of capabilities, such as shape memory, self-healing, super toughness, self-growing, stickiness, anti-swelling, and antibacterial properties. Third, examples of hydrogel applications in flexible devices are provided. These include strain sensors, supercapacitors, touch screens, triboelectric nanogenerators, bioelectronic devices, and robots. The present difficulties that hydrogels are encountering are then briefly discussed [52].

11.5.2 HYDROGEL DRESSINGS

Three-dimensional networks of hydrophilic polymers make up hydrogel dressings. In the area of the wound, they offer a moist environment that encourages tissue regeneration through granulation and re-epithelialization [53, 54]. The treatment of chronic wounds has been made simple by the use of hydrogel dressings. The characteristics of hydrogel-based dressings can be easily altered in comparison to other chronic wound therapy methods. Hydrogel dressings can be loaded with cells, antibacterial, antiviral, and antifungal drugs, growth factors, and biomolecules to hasten wound contraction and healing due to their flexible and customizable qualities. Based on the size, severity, and location of a certain wound, hydrogel dressings can be created for that particular lesion. These dressings can also be put on deep or uneven wounds with ease since they can create cytocompatibility *in situ* chemical cross-linking [55–57]. Furthermore, the applications of functional hydrogel for chronic wound healing will be discussed in the next sections.

11.5.3 FUNCTIONAL HYDROGELS FOR CHRONIC WOUND HEALING

The potential for multifunctional properties in hydrogels is very high. Hydrogels for chronic wound healing can integrate a variety of functional characteristics, such as biocompatibility, biodegradability, adhesiveness, and vascularization potential, as well as antibacterial, anti-inflammatory, and pro-angiogenic capabilities (Figure 11.3). A hydrogel must be biocompatible to maintain tissue homeostasis by providing an appropriate matrix throughout chronic wound healing without causing damage to the surrounding tissue. Other crucial factors include the hydrogels' biodegradability and rate of decomposition since they provide a temporary template for fibroblast proliferation, re-epithelialization, neovascularization, and chronic wound remodeling. Bioadhesivity is crucial for the long-term durability of hydrogel dressings around the wound site because it enhances the homeostatic action, keeps the wound moist, and absorbs exudates from the healing tissues. Antimicrobial hydrogels can be helpful in preventing infections since the extended healing of chronic wounds might raise the chance of infection, which can negatively impair the healing process. The primary cause of the prolonged healing of chronic wounds is the inflammatory phase. By easing the transition from the inflammatory to the proliferative stage, anti-inflammatory hydrogels can speed up the healing of wounds. Another factor contributing to prolonged chronic wound healing is the restricted transport of nutrients and oxygen to the wound region. Pro-angiogenic hydrogels can encourage angiogenesis, which will help to speed up the healing of chronic wounds by supplying the necessary nutrients and oxygen to the wound bed. The incorporation of various medications or therapeutic substances into hydrogels can enhance their functionality even more. In general, hydrogel-based wound dressings provide hopeful answers for a variety of issues related to the management of chronic wounds [58, 59]. The capabilities of these hydrogels are further covered in the section after, with examples from recent literature for chronic wound healing.

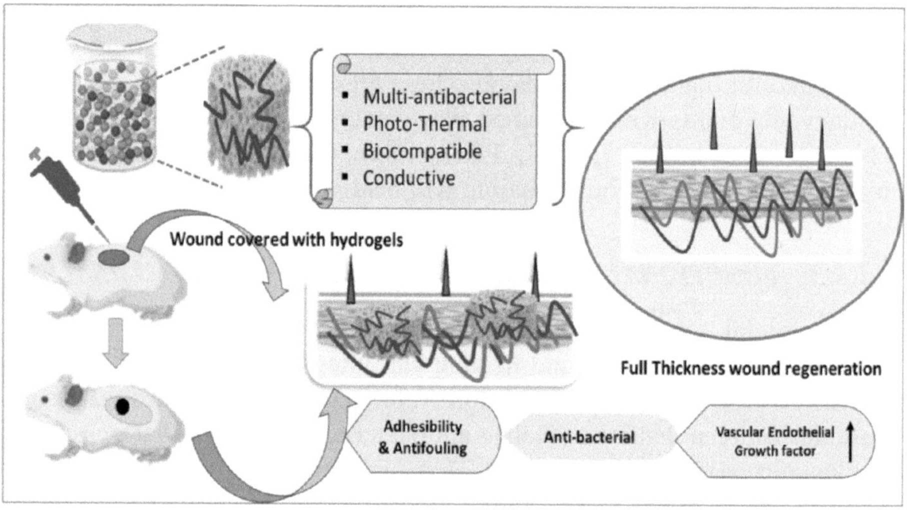

FIGURE 11.3 Multifunctional hydrogel for wound healing applications.

11.5.4 BIODEGRADABLE HYDROGELS FOR CHRONIC WOUND HEALING

The ability of a material to break down after coming into contact with a biological environment is known as biodegradability. When healing and regenerating chronic wounds, particularly those that are deeper [60], such as third-degree burns [61] and diabetic foot ulcers [62], the pace of hydrogel biodegradation is crucial. The pace of degradation should, ideally, be equal to the rate of production and remodeling of new tissues. Various tactics can be used to modify the rate of biodegradability, such as altering the degree of crosslinking between polymer chains, mixing or combining various types of polymers at different ratios, or adding chemical functional groups that are protease sensitive [63]. Biodegradable hydrogels are frequently made using protein-based polymers originating from the extracellular matrix (ECM), like collagen and gelatin [64]. Because of their inherent cell recognition molecules, these biomaterials are advantageous for cell attachment and regulated enzymatic biodegradation during cell proliferation and tissue remodeling. By physically crosslinking in response to temperature change, gelatin and collagen can both create hydrogels. At physiological temperatures, however, gelatin is unable to preserve the entire hydrogel structure. Gelatin-based hydrogels are frequently stabilized using cytocompatible chemical crosslinking techniques. Methacrylate groups (GelMA) are frequently added to gelatin to facilitate the fast and *in situ* photo-crosslinking of hydrogels [65, 66]. While the rapid disintegration of gelatin-based hydrogels can be negative, changing the gelatin concentration and the degree of crosslinking between polymer chains can assist in tuning the degradation behavior during the healing process [67].

Studies on the treatment of chronic wounds frequently use biodegradable materials with polysaccharide bases, such as chitosan, alginate, dextran, and hyaluronic acid. These substances can accelerate granulation, migration, and neo-angiogenesis while exhibiting a slower rate of biodegradation than protein-based polymers formed from the ECM [68]. Proteins and polysaccharides were combined to generate hydrogels that had acceptable degradation behavior during the healing process [68]. For instance, combining methacrylate chitosan (ChMA) with gelatin (Gel), depending on the degree of photo-crosslinking and gelatin concentration, reduced the chitosan's degrading behavior. A hybrid hydrogel was created in a different work by photo-crosslinking GelMA and hyaluronic acid (HA). In comparison to pristine GelMA hydrogels, the hydrogel's resistance to collagenase biodegradation was improved by the creation of stronger covalent connections between GelMA and HA.

11.5.5 BIOADHESIVE HYDROGELS FOR CHRONIC WOUND HEALING

Bioadhesive hydrogels can help a hydrogel dressing adhere to a moist wound bed and offer long-term stability. The hydrogel's presence in the wound comforts the patient because of its elasticity and stretchability.

Bioadhesive hydrogels are more biologically friendly and easier to remove from the wound than traditional wound dressings like gauze and films. By modifying the hydrogel dressings with polyphenol-derived moieties such as catechol, dopamine, gallic acid, or tannic acid [63], it is possible to give them the bioadhesive feature. To fulfill the requirements of the specific wound type, the degree of adhesiveness can be modified by varying the chemical alterations that polyphenol-derived moieties undergo. For shallow and small chronic wounds, highly adhesive hydrogel dressings were found to be advantageous, but less adhesion was favored for deep and large chronic wounds. For instance, Sun et al. modified chitosan (CS-GA) with gallic acid (GA) using varying amounts of grafting (CS-GA1, CS-GA2, CS-GA3) [70]. The finished CS-GA product was highly stretchy, sticky, and biocompatible. The grafted GA concentrations were shown to improve the bioadhesion capacity. A concentration-dependent ROS scavenging activity (antioxidant), as well as antibacterial activity, were also made possible by the GA alteration. In an *in vivo* full-thickness skin defect model, the use of CS-GA hydrogels led to better healing than gauze, gelatin sponge, and pure CS. The increased adhesivity and antioxidant activity of the hydrogel dressings were credited for the more effective wound closure with CS-GA dressings compared to the pristine CS dressings in this study.

11.5.6 BIO-INSPIRED HYDROGEL PATCH FOR WOUND HEALING

The bio-inspired hydrogel patch is a cutting-edge method for wound healing that takes its cues from nature to quicken the healing process (Figure 11.4). This patch is made of a specialized hydrogel polymer that has characteristics similar to those of human skin and contains bioactive ingredients to speed up healing. The most unique features and significant applications of adhesives are hemostasis and closure. Tissue organisms reconcile spontaneously after injury [71]. Meanwhile, the natural hemostasis process is not adequate to heal massive uncontrolled hemorrhage. After hemostasis, adhesives need to seal the wound site, which ultimately impedes external adverse physicochemical factors and the risk of infection. Adhesives are anticipated to produce tissue adhesion during wound healing, acting as an extracellular matrix. Chen et al. created a type of adhesive for wound repair that had hemostatic, antimicrobial, and angiogenesis properties after being inspired by the healing process [72]. Sundaram adopted a hybrid strategy of hydrogels and inorganic ions to integrate potassium aluminum sulfate and calcium chloride, wherein potassium aluminum sulfate plays the role of a vasoconstrictor and calcium chloride acts as a coagulation activator [73].

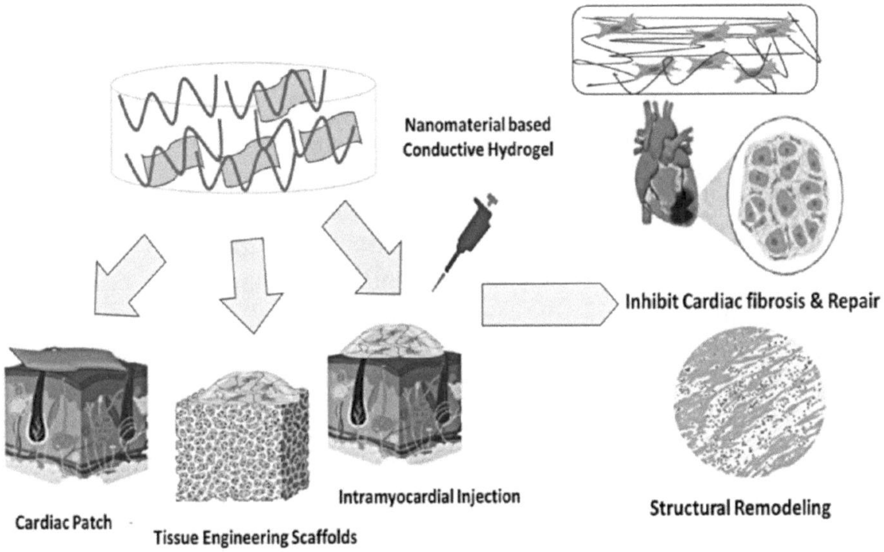

FIGURE 11.4 Bioinspired hydrogel patch for wound closure applications.

The hydrogel patch is designed to provide moisture, encourage oxygenation, and facilitate the interchange of nutrients and waste products in order to create the ideal environment for wound healing. It can better integrate with the wound site and promote cell migration and tissue regeneration because its structure and chemistry closely mimic the extracellular matrix of human skin. The presence of bioactive ingredients like growth factors, antimicrobials, and anti-inflammatory compounds is one of the fundamental characteristics of the bio-inspired hydrogel patch. These ingredients are carefully incorporated into the hydrogel matrix, and their regulated release aids in modulating the healing process and reducing the risk of infection and inflammation. A variety of wounds, including burns, chronic wounds, and surgical incisions, can be treated using the patch. It may adhere firmly to the wound surface due to its flexibility and conformability, creating a barrier that protects against external contaminants while still allowing the exchange of gases and fluids. This feature also enables the patch to be removed painlessly during dressing changes, reducing patient discomfort [74]. Although this still requires a broad interdisciplinary approach to conceptual research aptitude in the material design sector, with the fabrication of various multifaceted, stimuli-responsive, and potent hydrogel systems to advance the avant-garde bio-inspired adhesive hydrogel towards sustainable and high-indexing directions.

11.6 PERSPECTIVE CHALLENGES

The challenges associated with bio-based materials are processing, mechanical strength, and rate of degradation. It was observed that the mechanical strength required for wound dressing, implant devices, skin treatment, and wound healing applications [11, 47, 69]. Hydrogels utilized in drug delivery are generally shaped outside the body and impregnated with drugs before insertion of the hydrogel-drug complex in the body. An extensive variety of cross-linking methodologies can be utilized, including UV photopolymerization and various chemical cross-linking strategies. Such cross-linking strategies are beneficial provided that harmful reagents can be completely eliminated prior to hydrogel implantation, which might be challenging to accomplish without also leaching loaded drugs out of the hydrogel. The main weakness of such methodologies is that the preformed material must be embedded, since bulk hydrogels have a defined dimensionality and often high viscosity, which generally prevents their extrusion through a needle. The latter issue can sometimes be avoided by forming the preformed gel into micro or nanoparticles. The researchers are exploring all these domains to adapt the ideal characteristics of the hydrogel for their wound healing applications.

11.7 SUMMARY

This chapter deals with the new frontiers of hydrogel applications in wound healing. Critical headway has been made in working on the properties of hydrogels utilized for drug delivery and expanding the scope of medications and kinetics that can be accomplished using a hydrogel-based delivery vehicle. However, several challenges remain to improve the clinical relevance of hydrogels for drug delivery and the rate of delivery to its targeted sites. Progress on any of these challenges would greatly expand the potential of hydrogel-based drug delivery to convey the upcoming generation of designed drugs at the optimal rate and location in the body effectively. There are numerous broad and specialty applications not covered in this review where there is ample room for improvement. There is a need for continuous advancement in the delivery of not only hydrophobic particles but also others such as proteins, antibodies, or nucleic acids, which can readily be deactivated or unfolded by interactions with the hydrogel delivery vehicle. Conductive hydrogels, along with other materials such as metal-based composites, carbon-based composites, and functional composites, would be able to extend the application of wound dressing in more effective ways.

KEYWORDS

- **antimicrobial hydrogels**
- **chronic wound**
- **diabetic wound**
- **hydrogel**
- **inflammation**
- **mechanical strength**
- **remodeling**

REFERENCES

1. Robson, M. C. (1997). Wound infection: A failure of wound healing caused by an imbalance of bacteria. *Surgical Clinics of North America, 77*(3), 637–650. https://doi.org/10.1016/S0039-6109(97)80020-0.
2. Jones, S. G., Edwards, R., & Thomas, D. W. (2004). Inflammation and wound healing: The role of bacteria in immune-regulation of wound healing. *The International Journal of Lower Extremity Wounds, 3*(4), 201–208. https://doi.org/10.1177/1534734604269748.
3. Fan, Z., Liu, B., Wang, J., Zhang, S., Lin, Q., Gong, P., Ma, L., & Yang, S. (2014). A novel wound dressing based on Ag/graphene polymer hydrogel: Effectively kill bacteria and accelerate wound healing. *Advanced Functional Materials, 24*(31), 4673–4682. https://doi.org/10.1002/adfm.201401219.
4. Norahan, M. H., Pedroza-Gonzalez, S. C., Sanchez-Salazar, M. G., Alvarez, M. M., & Trujillo de Santiago, G. (2023). Structural and biological engineering of 3D hydrogels for wound healing. *Bioactive Materials, 24*, 197–235. https://doi.org/10.1016/j.biomat.2023.01.029.
5. Krizek, T. K., Robson, M. C., & Kho, E. (1967). Bacterial growth and skin graft survival. *Surgical Forum, 18*, 518–519.
6. Lindsay, S., Oates, A., & Bourdillon, K. (2017). The detrimental impact of extracellular bacterial proteases on wound healing. *International Wound Journal, 14*(1), 56–62. https://doi.org/10.1111/iwj.12650.

7. Lee, K. Y., & Mooney, D. J. (2001). Hydrogels for tissue engineering. *Chemical Reviews, 101*(7), 1869–1880. https://doi.org/10.1021/cr0001068.
8. Stadelmann, W. K., Digenis, A. G., & Tobin, G. R. (1998). Impediments to wound healing. *Excerpta Medica, 176*(Suppl 2A), 39S–47S. https://doi.org/10.1016/S0070-217X(98)80008-1.
9. Stephens, P., Wall, I. B., Wilson, M. J., et al. (2003). Anaerobic cocci populating the deep tissues of chronic wounds impair cellular wound healing responses in vitro. *British Journal of Dermatology, 148*(3), 456–466. https://doi.org/10.1046/j.1365-2133.2003.05154.x.
10. Prasad, A., Devendar, B., Ravi Sankar, M., & Robi, P. S. (2015). Micro-scratch based tribological characterization of hydroxyapatite (HAp) fabricated through fish scales. *Materials Today: Proceedings, 2*(4–5), 1216–1224. https://doi.org/10.1016/j.matpr.2015.07.091.
11. Prasad, A. (2021a). Bioabsorbable polymeric materials for biofilms and other biomedical applications: Recent and future trends. *Materials Today: Proceedings, 44*, 2447–2453. https://doi.org/10.1016/j.matpr.2020.12.489.
12. Shi, L., Ramsay, S., Ermis, R., & Carson, D. (2011). pH in the bacteria contaminated wound and its impact on Clostridium histolyticum collagenase activity: Implications for the use of collagenase wound debridement agents. *Journal of Wound, Ostomy, and Continence Nursing, 38*(5), 514–521. https://doi.org/10.1097/WON.0b013e31822d9a4f.
13. Samarghandian, S., Farkhondeh, T., & Samini, F. (2017). Honey and health: A review of recent clinical research. *Pharmacognosy Research, 9*(3), 121–127. https://doi.org/10.4103/0974-8490.204647.
14. Negut, I., Grumezescu, A. M., & Grumezescu, V. (2018). Treatment strategies for infected wounds. *Molecules, 23*(9), 2392. https://doi.org/10.3390/molecules23092392.
15. Kurek-Gorecka, A., Gorecki, M., Rzepecka-Stojko, A., Balwierz, R., & Stojko, J. (2020). Bee products in dermatology and skin care. *Molecules, 25*(3), 556. https://doi.org/10.3390/molecules25030556.
16. Requier, F., Garnery, L., Kohl, P. L., Njovu, H. K., Pirk, C. W. W., Crewe, R. M., & Steffan-Dewenter, I. (2019). The conservation of native honey bees is crucial. *Trends in Ecology & Evolution, 34*(6), 520–532. https://doi.org/10.1016/j.tree.2019.04.008.
17. Agresti, R., Triulzi, T., Sasso, M., Ghirelli, C., Aiello, P., Rybinska, I., Campiglio, M., Sfondrini, E., Tagliabue, E., & Bianchi, F. (2019). Wound healing fluid reflects the inflammatory nature and aggressiveness of breast tumors. *Cells, 8*(2), 181. https://doi.org/10.3390/cells8020181.
18. Ansari, M. J., Rajendran, R. R., Mohanto, S., Agarwal, U., Panda, K., Dhotre, K., Manne, R., Deepak, A., Zafar, A., & Pramanik, S. (2022). Poly(N-isopropylacrylamide)-based hydrogels for biomedical applications: A review of the state-of-the-art. *Gels, 8*(7), 454. https://doi.org/10.3390/gels8070454.
19. Zhao, X., Li, P., Guo, B., & Ma, P. X. (2015). Antibacterial and conductive injectable hydrogels based on quaternized chitosan-graft-polyaniline/oxidized dextran for tissue engineering. *Acta Biomaterialia, 26*, 236–248. https://doi.org/10.1016/j.actbio.2015.07.010.
20. Qu, J., Zhao, X., Ma, P. X., & Guo, B. (2018). Injectable antibacterial conductive hydrogels with dual response to an electric field and pH for localized "smart" drug release. *Acta Biomaterialia, 72*, 55–69. https://doi.org/10.1016/j.actbio.2018.03.005.
21. Dong, R., Zhao, X., Guo, B., & Ma, P. X. (2016). Self-healing conductive injectable hydrogels with antibacterial activity as cell delivery carriers for cardiac cell therapy.

ACS Applied Materials & Interfaces, 8(27), 17138–17150. https://doi.org/10.1021/acsami.6b04796.

22. Khorasani, M. T., Joorabloo, A., Moghaddam, A., Shamsi, H., & MansooriMoghadam, Z. (2018). Incorporation of ZnO nanoparticles into heparinized polyvinyl alcohol/chitosan hydrogels for wound dressing application. *International Journal of Biological Macromolecules, 114*, 1203–1215. https://doi.org/10.1016/j.ijbiomac.2018.03.159.
23. GhavamiNejad, A., Park, C. H., & Kim, C. S. (2016). In situ synthesis of antimicrobial silver nanoparticles within antifouling zwitterionic hydrogels by catecholic redox chemistry for wound healing application. *Biomacromolecules, 17*(3), 1213–1223. https://doi.org/10.1021/acs.biomac.5b01366.
24. Arafa, M. G., El-Kased, R. F., & Elmazar, M. (2018). Thermoresponsive gels containing gold nanoparticles as smart antibacterial and wound healing agents. *Scientific Reports, 8*(1), 1–16. https://doi.org/10.1038/s41598-018-32220-5.
25. Tang, P., Han, L., Li, P., Jia, Z., Wang, K., Zhang, H., et al. (2019). Mussel-inspired electroactive and antioxidative scaffolds with incorporation of polydopamine-reduced graphene oxide for enhancing skin wound healing. *ACS Applied Materials & Interfaces, 11*(8), 7703–7714. https://doi.org/10.1021/acsami.8b21554.
26. Huynh, N. T., Pham, N. O., Nguyen, C. T., Vu, M. T., & Tran, N. Q. (2019). Injectable nanocurcumin dispersed gelatin–pluronic nanocomposite hydrogel platform for burn wound treatment. *Bulletin of Materials Science, 42*(2), 71. https://doi.org/10.1007/s12034-019-1777-5.
27. Pham, L., Truong, M. D., Nguyen, T. H., Le, L., Nam, N. D., Bach, L. G., et al. (2019). A dual synergistic effect of curcumin and gelatin on thermal-responsive hydrogel based on chitosan-P123 in wound healing application. *Biomedicine & Pharmacotherapy, 117*, 109183. https://doi.org/10.1016/j.biopha.2019.109183.
28. Zhang, S., Hou, J., Yuan, Q., Xin, P., Cheng, H., Gu, Z., et al. (2019). Arginine derivatives assist dopamine-hyaluronic acid hybrid hydrogels to have enhanced antioxidant activity for wound healing. *Chemical Engineering Journal, 371*, 123775. https://doi.org/10.1016/j.cej.2019.123775.
29. Wei, Q., Duan, J., Ma, G., Zhang, W., Wang, Q., Hu, Z., et al. (2019). Enzymatic crosslinking to fabricate antioxidant peptide-based supramolecular hydrogel for improving cutaneous wound healing. *Journal of Materials Chemistry B, 7*(13), 2220–2225. https://doi.org/10.1039/C9TB00207B.
30. Sarkar, K., Dutta, K., Chatterjee, A., Sarkar, J., Das, D., Prasad, A., Chattopadhyay, D., Acharya, K., Das, M., Verma, S. K., & De, S. (2023). Nanotherapeutic potential of antibacterial folic acid-functionalized nanoceria for wound healing applications. *Nanomedicine, 18*(2), 167–181. https://doi.org/10.2217/nnm-2022-0233.
31. Almeida, J., Benvegnú, D., Boufleur, N., Reckziegel, P., Barcelos, R., Coradini, K., et al. (2012). Hydrogels containing rutin intended for cutaneous administration: Efficacy in wound healing in rats. *Drug Development and Industrial Pharmacy, 38*(7), 792–799. https://doi.org/10.3109/03639045.2011.609184.
32. Song, J., Yuan, C., Jiao, T., Xing, R., Yang, M., Adams, D. J., & Yan, X. (2020). Multifunctional antimicrobial biometallohydrogels based on amino acid-coordinated self-assembly. *Small, 16*(8), e1907309. https://doi.org/10.1002/smll.201907309.
33. Abbasi, A. R., Sohail, M., Minhas, M. U., Khaliq, T., Kousar, M., Khan, S., Hussain, Z., & Munir, A. (2020). Bioinspired sodium alginate-based thermosensitive hydrogel

membranes for accelerated wound healing. *International Journal of Biological Macromolecules, 155*, 751–765. https://doi.org/10.1016/j.ijbiomac.2020.03.248.

34. Zhuang, S., Zhong, J., Zhou, Q., Zhong, Y., Liu, P., & Liu, Z. (2019). Rhein protects against barrier disruption and inhibits inflammation in intestinal epithelial cells. *International Immunopharmacology, 71*, 321–327. https://doi.org/10.1016/j.intimp.2019.03.030.
35. Zheng, J., Fan, R., Wu, H., Yao, H., Yan, Y., Liu, J., Ran, L., Sun, Z., Yi, L., Dang, L., Gan, P., Zheng, P., Yang, T., Zhang, Y., Tang, T., & Wang, Y. (2019). Directed self-assembly of herbal small molecules into sustained release hydrogels for treating neural inflammation. *Nature Communications, 10*(1), 1604. https://doi.org/10.1038/s41467-019-09601-3.
36. Zhao, W., Li, Y., Zhang, X., Zhang, R., Hu, Y., Boyer, C., & Xu, F. J. (2020). Photo-responsive supramolecular hyaluronic acid hydrogels for accelerated wound healing. *Journal of Controlled Release, 323*, 24–35. https://doi.org/10.1016/j.jconrel.2020.04.014
37. Zhao, W., Zhang, X., Zhang, R., Li, Y., Zhang, K., Li, Y., & Xu, F. J. (2020). Self-assembled herbal medicine encapsulated by an oxidation-sensitive supramolecular hydrogel for chronic wound treatment. *ACS Applied Materials & Interfaces, 12*(51), 56898–56907. https://doi.org/10.1021/acsami.0c15916.
38. Asadi, N., Pazoki-Toroudi, H., Rahmani Del Bakhshayesh, A., Akbarzadeh, A., Davaran, S., & Annabi, N. (2021). Multifunctional hydrogels for wound healing: Special focus on bio macromolecular based hydrogels. *International Journal of Biological Macromolecules, 170*, 728–750. https://doi.org/10.1016/j.ijbiomac.2020.12.202.
39. Gnanasekar, S., Palanisamy, P., Jha, P. K., Murugaraj, J., Kandasamy, M., Mohammed Khan, A., & Sivaperumal, S. (2018). Natural honeycomb flavone chrysin (5,7-dihydroxyflavone)-reduced graphene oxide nanosheets fabrication for improved bactericidal and skin regeneration. *ACS Sustainable Chemistry & Engineering, 6*(1), 349–363. https://doi.org/10.1021/acssuschemeng.7b02603.
40. Li, Y., Liu, X., Tan, L., Cui, Z., Yang, X., Zheng, Y., Yeung, K. W. K., Chu, P. K., & Wu, S. (2018). Rapid sterilization and accelerated wound healing using Zn^{2+} and graphene oxide modified g-C_3N_4 under dual light irradiation. *Advanced Functional Materials, 28*(30), 1800299. https://doi.org/10.1002/adfm.201800299.
41. Qu, J., Zhao, X., Liang, Y., Xu, Y., Ma, P. X., & Guo, B. (2019). Degradable conductive injectable hydrogels as novel antibacterial, anti-oxidant wound dressings for wound healing. *Chemical Engineering Journal, 362*, 548–560. https://doi.org/10.1016/j.cej.2019.01.028.
42. Prasad, A., Sankar, M. R., & Katiyar, V. (2017). State of art on solvent casting particulate leaching method for orthopedic scaffolds fabrication. *Materials Today: Proceedings, 4*(2), 898–907. https://doi.org/10.1016/j.matpr.2017.01.101.
43. Pacelli, S., Paolicelli, P., Moretti, G., Petralito, S., Di Giacomo, S., Vitalone, A., & Casadei, M. A. (2016). Gum methacrylate and laponite as an innovative nanocomposite hydrogel for biomedical applications. *European Polymer Journal, 77*, 114–123. https://doi.org/10.1016/j.eurpolymj.2016.02.007.
44. Lokhande, G., Carrow, J. K., Thakur, T., Xavier, J. R., Parani, M., Bayless, K. J., & Gaharwar, A. K. (2018). Nanoengineered injectable hydrogels for wound healing application. *Acta Biomaterialia, 70*, 35–47. https://doi.org/10.1016/j.actbio.2018.01.045.
45. Dawson, J. I., & Oreffo, R. O. C. (2013). Clay: New opportunities for tissue regeneration and biomaterial design. *Advanced Materials, 25*(30), 4069–4086. https://doi.org/10.1002/adma.201301034.

46. Prasad, A., Bhasney, S., Katiyar, V., & Sankar, M. R. (2017). Biowastes processed hydroxyapatite filled poly (lactic acid) bio-composite for open reduction internal fixation of small bones. *Materials Today: Proceedings, 4*(9), 10153–10157. https://doi.org/10.1016/j.matpr.2017.01.101.
47. Prasad, A., Chakraborty, G., & Kumar, A. (2022). Bio-based environmentally benign polymeric resorbable materials for orthopedic fixation applications. In *Advanced Materials for Biomedical Applications* (pp. 251–266). CRC Press.
48. Rajabi, N., Kharaziha, M., Emadi, R., Zarrabi, A., Mokhtari, H., & Salehi, S. (2020). An adhesive and injectable nanocomposite hydrogel of thiolated gelatin/gelatin methacrylate/Laponite® as a potential surgical sealant. *Journal of Colloid and Interface Science, 564*, 155–169. https://doi.org/10.1016/j.jcis.2019.12.048.
49. Sarkar, K., Dutta, K., Chatterjee, A., Sarkar, J., Das, D., Prasad, A., Chattopadhyay, D., Acharya, K., Das, M., Verma, S. K., & De, S. (2023). Nanotherapeutic potential of antibacterial folic acid-functionalized nanoceria for wound-healing applications. *Nanomedicine, 18*(2). https://doi.org/10.2217/nnm-2022-0233.
50. Clarkin, C. E., Mani, R., Khan, N. A., Dawson, J. I., & Evans, N. D. (2019). Injectable nanoclay gels for angiogenesis. *Acta Biomaterialia, 100*, 378–387. https://doi.org/10.1016/j.actbio.2019.09.023.
51. He, H., Li, H., Pu, A., Li, W., Ban, K., & Xu, L. (2023). Hybrid assembly of polymeric nanofiber network for robust and electronically conductive hydrogels. *Nature Communications, 14*(1), 759. https://doi.org/10.1038/s41467-023-37195-6.
52. Lu, H., & Zhang, N. (2023). Electroconductive hydrogels for biomedical applications. *Wiley Nanomedicine and Nanotechnology, 15*(1). https://doi.org/10.1002/wnan.1568.
53. Aswathy, S., Narendrakumar, U., & Manjubala, I. (2020). Commercial hydrogels for biomedical applications. *Heliyon, 6*(12), e03719. https://doi.org/10.1016/j.heliyon.2020.e03719.
54. Gupta, B., Agarwal, R., & Alam, M. (2011). Biomedical hydrogels. In *Hydrogels for Wound Healing Applications* (pp. 184–227). Woodhead Publishing.
55. Chandel, A. K. S., Nutan, B., & Jewrajka, S. K. (2018). Self-assembly of partially alkylated dextran-graft-poly [(2-dimethylamino) ethyl methacrylate] copolymer facilitating hydrophobic/hydrophilic drug delivery and improving network hydrogel properties. *Biomacromolecules, 19*(3), 1142–1153. https://doi.org/10.1021/acs.biomac.8b00015.
56. Chandel, A. K. S., Kannan, D., Nutan, B., Singh, S., & Jewrajka, S. K. (2017). Dually crosslinked injectable hydrogels of poly (ethylene glycol) and poly [(2-dimethylamino) ethyl methacrylate]-b-poly (N-isopropyl acrylamide) as a wound healing promoter. *Journal of Materials Chemistry B, 5*(31), 4955–4965. https://doi.org/10.1039/C7TB00848A.
57. Nichol, J. W., Koshy, S. T., Bae, H., Hwang, C. M., Yamanlar, S., & Khademhosseini, A. (2010). Cell-laden micro engineered gelatin methacrylate hydrogels. *Biomaterials, 31*(21), 5536–5544. https://doi.org/10.1016/j.biomaterials.2010.03.064.
58. Yue, K., Trujillo-de Santiago, G., Alvarez, M. M., Tamayol, A., Annabi, N., & Khademhosseini, A. (2015). Synthesis, properties, and biomedical applications of gelatin methacryloyl (GelMA) hydrogels. *Biomaterials, 73*, 254–271. https://doi.org/10.1016/j.biomaterials.2015.08.045.

59. Xiong, Y., Zhang, X., Ma, X., Wang, W., Yan, F., Zhao, X., Chu, X., Xu, W., & Sun, C. (2021). A review of the properties and applications of bio adhesive hydrogels. *Polymer Chemistry, 12*(20), 3721–3739. https://doi.org/10.1039/D1PY00282A.
60. Arif, M. M., Khan, S. M., Gull, N., Tabish, T. A., Zia, S., Khan, R. U., Awais, S. M., & Butt, M. A. (2021). Polymer-based biomaterials for chronic wound management: Promises and challenges. *International Journal of Pharmaceutics, 598*, 120270. https://doi.org/10.1016/j.ijpharm.2021.120270.
61. He, J. J., McCarthy, C., & Camci-Unal, G. (2021). Development of hydrogel-based sprayable wound dressings for second-and third-degree burns. *Advanced NanoBiomed Research, 1*(1), 2100004. https://doi.org/10.1002/anbr.202100004.
62. Prasad, A. (2022). Biomaterial-based nanofibers scaffolds in tissue engineering application. In *Functional Biomaterials* (pp. 245–264). Springer.
63. Firlar, I., Erdal, M., & Çelikel, C. (2022). Functional hydrogels for treatment of chronic wounds. *Gels, 8*(2), 127. https://doi.org/10.3390/gels8020127.
64. Kang, J. I., & Park, K. M. (2021). Advances in gelatin-based hydrogels for wound management. *Journal of Materials Chemistry B, 9*(6), 1503–1520. https://doi.org/10.1039/D0TB02582H.
65. Ågren, M. (Ed.). (2016). *Wound Healing Biomaterials* (Vol. 2). Woodhead Publishing.
66. Prasad, A. (2021b). State of art review on bioabsorbable polymeric scaffolds for bone tissue engineering. *Materials Today: Proceedings, 44*, 1391–1400.
67. Hancock, M. J., Piraino, F., Camci-Unal, G., Rasponi, M., & Khademhosseini, A. (2011). Anisotropic material synthesis by capillary flow in a fluid stripe. *Biomaterials, 32*(26), 6493–6504. https://doi.org/10.1016/j.biomaterials.2011.05.057.
68. Essawy, A. A., Hefni, H., & El-Nggar, A. (2019). Biocompatible and biodegradable chitosan composites in wound healing application. In *Sustainable Polymer Composites and Nanocomposites* (pp. 143–183). Springer.
69. Prasad, A., Bhasney, S. M., Prasannavenkadesan, V., & Kumar, A. (2023). Polylactic acid reinforced with nano-hydroxyapatite bioabsorbable cortical screws for bone fracture treatment. *Journal of Polymer Research, 30*(3), 177. https://doi.org/10.1007/s10965-023-02819-1.
70. Sun, C., Zeng, X., Zheng, S., Wang, Y., Li, Z., Zhang, H., Nie, L., Zhang, Y., Zhao, Y., & Yang, X. (2022). Bio-adhesive catechol-modified chitosan wound healing hydrogel dressings through glow discharge plasma technique. *Chemical Engineering Journal, 427*, 130843. https://doi.org/10.1016/j.cej.2021.130843.
71. Li, W., Zheng, Y., Pang, W., & Lai, P. (2023). Bio-inspired adhesive hydrogel for wound healing. *Biomedical Technology, 1*(1), 65–72.
72. Chen, K., Wu, Z., Liu, Y., Yuan, Y., & Liu, C. (2022). Injectable double-crosslinked adhesive hydrogels with high mechanical resilience and effective energy dissipation for joint wound treatment. *Advanced Functional Materials, 32*(31), 2109687. https://doi.org/10.1002/adfm.202109687.
73. Sundaram, M. N., Mony, U., Varma, P. K., & Rangasamy, J. (2021). Vasoconstrictor and coagulation activator entrapped chitosan based composite hydrogel for rapid bleeding control. *Carbohydrate Polymers, 258*, 117634. https://doi.org/10.1016/j.carbpol.2021.117634.
74. Zhu, J., Zhou, H., Gerhard, E. M., Zhang, S., Rodríguez, F. I. P., Pan, T., Yang, H., Lin, Y., Yang, J., & Cheng, H. (2023). Smart bio adhesives for wound healing and closure. *Bioactive Materials, 19*, 360–375.

75. Bhoi, S., Prasad, A., Kumar, A., Sarkar, R. B., Mahto, B., Meena, C. S., & Pandey, C. (2022). Experimental study to evaluate the wear performance of UHMWPE and XLPE material for orthopedics application. *Bioengineering, 9*(11), 676. https://doi.org/10.3390/bioengineering9110676.
76. Gupta, A., Agarwal, R., & Alam, M. (2017). Multifunctional nanohydroxyapatite-promoted toughened high-molecular-weight stereo complex poly (lactic acid)-based bio nanocomposite for both 3D-printed orthopedic implants and high-temperature engineering applications. *ACS Omega, 2*(7), 4039–4052. https://doi.org/10.1021/acsomega.7b00640.

CHAPTER 12

3D Printing of Bioabsorbable Polymeric Composites in Biomedical Applications

SUDIPTO DATTA,[1] YUSUF OLATUNJI WAIDI,[1] and RANJIT BARUA[2]

[1]*Indian Institute of Science, C.V. Raman Avenue, Bangalore, Karnataka, India*

[2]*Indian Institute of Engineering Science and Technology, Howrah, West Bengal, India*

ABSTRACT

Bioresorbable material has been promising for various biomedical applications in the last few years. This is due to its inherent minimal cytotoxicity, patient compliance, and the avoidance of the need for revisiting surgery. The 3D printing technique has also received ample attention in biomedical applications due to the possibility of manufacturing or fabricating patient-specific constructs. By coupling both bioresorbable materials and additive manufacturing methods, many limitations of traditional methods can be overcome. In this chapter, we have summarized various aspects of 3D printing of different bioresorbable composites, which include 3D printing techniques and applications, various bioresorbable polymeric materials for several biomedical 3D applications, conclusions, and perspectives.

12.1 INTRODUCTION

Incorporating additive manufacturing (AM) systems into the biomedical field has resulted in significant medical technological advancements. Lost tissues may now be treated and restored using scaffolds made of

Bioabsorbable Polymers for Drug Carriers and Fixation Devices. Arbind Prasad and Sougata Jana (Eds.)

biocompatible materials, allowing cells to develop into fresh and healthy tissues [1]. 3D printing, when combined with modern imaging capabilities, assists in producing sophisticated scaffold designs that imitate the human body structure [2]. Its ability to create microarchitecture dimension scaffolds improves cell response growth, while the capacity to change porosity allows for flexibility over cell adhesion and migration [3]. With regenerative medicine, tissue engineering, and 3D printing, we now have the tools to repair or regenerate tissues and perhaps organs using cell-laden scaffolds much closer to typical human body functions [4]. 3D-printed components utilized in various sections of the human body present diverse problems and opportunities. 3D printing of biomaterials must meet six material requirements, namely: (i) printability; (ii) biodegradability; (iii) biocompatibility; (iv) the absence of hazardous by-products; (v) desired mechanical qualities; and (vi) replicating the architecture of natural tissue [2]. Even though a material's printability perspective influences whether it is a viable option for 3D bioprinting in the first instance, all of the above factors are equally relevant. Each intended use has unique requirements influencing the material selection and printing technology. Biomaterials are classified as resorbable or non-resorbable based on whether they degrade or do not degrade. Biodegradable polymers are preferred in the biomedical field, particularly in tissue engineering, to prevent extra surgery for retrieving implants, scaffolds, or other materials implanted within the human body. Because biodegradable materials degrade over time, cells continually invade the matrix, producing structural proteins like collagen and elastin, which progressively substitute degradable components. Vert et al. [5, 6] categorized polymeric biodegradable materials into three classes based on their characteristics and biological uses:

1. Biodegradable polymers are polymeric substances that degrade *in vivo* to create degradation macromolecular products but are not entirely eliminated. Polyurethane is a typical example. (This description eliminates deterioration caused by the environment, fungi, or bacteria).
2. Bioresorbable polymers are polymeric substances that degrade in bulk and are entirely absorbed in the body. In this case, all the polymeric substances are removed either by the excretion of breakdown byproducts or through further metabolization. Bioresorption denotes the complete removal of any foreign substance, including the breakdown of byproducts with no residual left behind. Poly(D,L-lactide) is a typical example.

3. Bioerodibles are polymers that degrade on their surfaces indefinitely until the substance is removed. Bioerosion also represents the complete removal of any foreign substance, including the by-products from the surface degradation, with no residual left. Examples of erodible polymers are crosslinked polyester hydrogels, poly(a-hydroxy acids), polyanhydrides, and poly(orthoesters).
4. Polymeric bioabsorbable substances are those polymers that dissolve gradually in human fluids without causing the polymer chain to cleave or making the molecular weight diminish. Polyethylene glycol is a famous example [7–9]. If the dissolved macromolecules are discharged from the body, a bioabsorbable polymer may also be referred to as bioresorbable [10–12]. Despite the various benefits of polymers, their clinical usages require further improvement, given their poor mechanical features for load-bearing functions. Polymers have been mixed with other substances to gain improved characteristics to overcome this limitation [13, 14]. These combinations are composed of two or more phases called fillers and matrices with various chemical or physical features spanning between nanometer and macron-sized ranges [13–16]. For a given application, multiple kinds of filler dispersion substances embedded inside the matrix would provide a variety of biological and mechanical characteristics [13, 14]. For example, a bone scaffold that entails a ceramic/polymer composite is structured to use the mechanical, biological, and physical capabilities of bioactive ceramics and polymers combined. Few of those examples involve PLA/hydroxyapatite (HA) constructs having significantly higher cell proliferation than PLA constructs [14, 17–19], improved mechanical characteristics of polylactic-co-glycolic acid (PLGA)/HA employed for bone load-bearing replacement [20–23], and the composite of PEEK/HA exhibiting better osseointegration and bone-implant contact [24–26].

12.2 APPLICATION OF 3D PRINTING TECHNOLOGY

With additive manufacturing technology, it is now thinkable to fabricate 3D constructs with complicated forms and regulated interior porous structures. These were formerly unattainable via traditional production [27, 28]. AM technologies like powder-based selective laser sintering (SLS), resin-based stereolithography (SLA), and nozzle-based fused deposition modeling

(FDM) are employed to make scaffolds and implants [28, 29]. CAD (Computer-aided design) tools like Fusion 360, Autodesk, Creo, CATIA, and SolidWorks are first used to create a 3D model or by scanning made accessible by imaging [28–30]. The 3D structure is made from 2D images by slicing using 3D printer-friendly software for slicing [28–30]. 2D graphics instruct the printers on creating each layer of 3D objects [29, 30]. Polymers, metals, and ceramics may all be processed by SLS. This approach is noted for its excellent accuracy and precision since the laser source and the input raw material determine it. In a layer-wise style, the particles are fused in a proper dimension by laser to build a 3D component [27, 28, 31]. SLA is another conventional approach recognized for its speed and precision, in which ultraviolet (UV) radiation cures raw materials, often liquid photopolymers [29, 31, 32]. Fused filament fabrication (FFF), on the other hand, is a type of extrusion-based 3D printing in which a thermoplastic polymer filament is fed through a nozzle that has been heated. This tracks the intended structure of the item substance deposited, which hardens upon cooling to produce a 3D component layer by layer [28, 30, 31]. In contrast, the Binder Jetting (BJ) technique employs powder-based and liquid bonding agents to make components directly. A print head creates three-dimensional structures by selectively jetting a liquid agent and gluing powder components together [33–35]. Despite their promise, these manufacturing technologies have obstacles and constraints, including poor surface finishing, low speed, inadequate precision, end-of-component dimensions, the construction of suspended surfaces, mechanical anisotropic characteristics, exorbitant prices, poor production effectiveness, and restricted material utilization [36–40]. Only specific polymers reinforced with short fibers or particles, and thermoplastic polymers may be employed in Fused Deposition Modeling (FDM) printing, restricting the range of raw materials available [36, 37, 40]. Stereolithography (SLA) printing, on the other hand, requires specific materials since the method relies on photopolymerization, and the substance is often a hybrid combination of acrylate or epoxy [36, 40]. One disadvantage of Selective Laser Sintering (SLS) printing techniques is that it is impossible to create closed objects since the unprocessed particles are confined within the dimension [36, 40–42]. In the case of BJ, another post-processing phase termed densification is necessary to cure the initially weak piece [37, 40]. Table 12.1 presents the biomaterials and the additive manufacturing (AM) approaches used. The underlying production faults in these manufacturing procedures are an additional issue of the existing AM approach. These inaccuracies cause a shape difference between the planned and AM components fabricated, which is a significant contributor to developed samples with attributes that deviate from predicted values. The issue is exacerbated in applications requiring complicated geometries with specialized internal properties, such as porous bone scaffolds. A dimensional discrepancy can lead to pore occlusion and walls that are narrower than intended, both of which can limit the ingrowth of bone and negatively influence mechanical characteristics [41, 42]. Theoretical investigations employing finite element analysis (FEA) aid in examining the deviation in as-designed and as-fabricated components, demonstrating the limits of AM techniques that must be resolved [41–43]. Micromechanical modeling and FEA analysis as input for AM technologies have been presented as an efficient way to change the material's characteristics to desired values [43].

TABLE 12.1 Various Kinds of Biomaterials and Their Additive Manufacturing Techniques

Biomaterial	AM Technology
Alginate	Extrusion, SLA
Collagen	Extrusion, SLA
Chitosan	Extrusion, SLA
Hyaluronic acid	Extrusion, SLA
Silk-fibroin	Extrusion, SLA
Fibrin	SLA
Gelatin	Extrusion, SLA
PHA	SLS, ME-AM, SE-AM
Cellulose	Extrusion

12.3 BIORESORBABLE POLYMER COMPOSITE FOR 3D PRINTING

12.3.1 BIORESORBABLE POLYMERS COMPOSITE

Bioresorbable polymers have been employed to create bioresorbable suture threads used in surgery to substitute non-absorbable sutures. Recently, bioresorbable polymeric materials have gained interest in a variety of applications, including artery stents [44], bone repair screws [45], assisted tissue engineering [46], and drug delivery [10]. Bioresorbable polymeric materials can be broken down through the bonds of chemical hydrolysis that link the units of monomers or degradation via enzymatic catalysis, which occurs over time *in vivo*. Lengthy polymer macromolecules are decomposed to become oligomers or monomers expelled from the body or processed further via metabolic processes. To induce the development of new tissues, three major techniques have been used: (i) autogenous cells immediately inserted directly inside the affected region; (ii) scaffolds for culturing tissues for eventual damaged tissue implantation substitutes; or (iii) chemical compounds that are implantable to trigger tissue repair [8, 47].

Bioresorbable polymeric composites must have the following inherent features for tissue engineering: composition and chemical structure; hydrophobicity or hydrophilicity; amorphous/crystalline ratio; and the starting molecular weight. The breakdown rate of bioresorbable polymeric materials is also influenced by physical, structural, and environmental factors like pH and enzyme activity [48, 49]. Many bioresorbable materials are manufactured from biomaterials, including collagen, chitosan, poly(orthoesters), poly(anhydrides), aliphatic poly(amino acids), poly(amides), poly(phosphazenes), and poly(esters). All of the polymeric materials are appealing because of their wide availability, simplicity of production for tissue regeneration, and their rigid/elastic and chemical characteristics given their application. As a result of their reduced toxic effect and superior biocompatibility, aliphatic poly(esters) are still the biomedical area's most investigated biodegradable polymeric materials. These are some examples: poly(glycolic acid) (PGA), poly(lactic-co-glycolic acid) (PLGA) [50, 51].

12.3.2 3D-PRINTED BIORESORBABLE NATURAL POLYMER-BASED COMPOSITES

Several tissue engineering (TE) fields, such as cartilage, skin, bone, ligaments, and blood vessels, have been developed using natural polymers. The key benefits of natural polymers include their good biodegradability, exceptional biocompatibility, and the fact that several of them occur naturally in the extracellular matrix (ECM). These polymers are biologically sourced and thus appropriate for cell attachment, differentiation, and proliferation. The principal drawbacks of these polymers include weak mechanical characteristics and constrained processability, which may impede their broad usage in therapeutic developments [52]. Natural polymers are categorized into three types according to their origin: (a) polyhydroxyalkanoate (PHA); (b) polysaccharide-based polymers; and (c) protein-based polymers [53–55]. Each of them has its pros and cons. For example, polysaccharide-based natural polymers (e.g., hyaluronic acid, alginate, starch, chitosan, dextran) offer nontoxicity, high hemocompatibility, better cell interaction, and reduced cost when compared to other biopolymers like collagen, supporting their usage as materials for scaffolding in TE systems. Protein-based natural polymers, including gelatin, fibrin, elastin, and collagen, have received much consideration as favorable materials for cell transport in TE. Numerous commercially available TE scaffolds have been developed using collagen derived from animals. PHAs are quite an intriguing family of biodegradable polymeric materials for TE applications that are created through bacterial fermentation using sugars or carbon as energy sources. Various PHAs like poly(4-hydroxybutyrate), poly(3-hydroxybutyrate), poly(3-hydroxybutyrate-co-3-hydroxyvalerate), poly(3-hydroxyoctanoate), and poly(3-hydroxybutyrate-co-3-hydroxyhexanoate) are explored to devise resorbable implantable gadgets like sutures, wound dressings, adhesion barriers, and tissue engineering scaffolds. The inherent bioactivity of collagen and chitosan has been demonstrated, and products based on these polymeric materials have been employed in tissue regeneration applications [56, 57]. Chitosan, a well-known natural biopolymer, is the subject of several reports due to its biodegradability, antibacterial activity, wound healing-stimulating characteristics, biocompatibility, large-scale availability, bio-adhesive character, and low cost [58]. Recently, Sadeghianmaryan et al. combined 3D printing and impregnating methods to fabricate nano-hydroxyapatite (nHA) embedded chitosan/alginate scaffolds. This resulted in a hybrid but new structure of scaffolds for possible cartilage engineering. First and foremost, they introduced nHA into chitosan ink, 3D fabricated it to make scaffolds, and then investigated printability by comparing the printed platforms to their designs. After that, alginate containing nHA was impregnated into the chitosan 3D-printed scaffolds to produce a hybrid scaffold framework. The constructs were mechanically and physiologically characterized, with an emphasis on determining the effect of alginate and nHA for possible cartilage engineering. The introduction of nHA enhanced the scaffold's elastic moduli in compression testing. At the same time, the live/dead assay demonstrated how nHA substantially increased the adhesion and survival of ATCD5 cells seeded on the constructs. Additionally, their findings revealed that scaffolds impregnated with nHA in alginate ink enhanced cell adhesion and survival. Furthermore, the antimicrobial effect of hybrid constructs was investigated. The results suggest that scaffolds made from chitosan natural polymer had a promising antibacterial capacity, which was further boosted with nHA-embedded chitosan constructs [59]. Yang et al. in their study, employed FDM printing to create a drug delivery device with high biocompatibility, regulated and effective drug release, and individualized delivery. Hot-melt extrusion was used to develop drug-loaded strands for the FDM technique (HME). The delivery carrier and drug model employed were polycaprolactone and ibuprofen, respectively. Importantly, chitosan was solubilized to generate efficient and regulated release routes. Several features, such as printability, physical and chemical characteristics, changed through the FDM and HME steps of filament making, and the vehicle's drug release characteristics, mechanism, and biocompatibility were all examined. The findings indicate that as the drug and chitosan concentration increases, the tensile strength of the filament reduces. The release of drug efficiency might attain >% and continue for 120 hours, owing mostly to the diffusion-erosion process [60]. Patel et al. on the other hand, 3D-printed biodegradable scaffolds consisting of chitosan/silk fibroin (CS/SF/CNPs) reinforced with cellulose nanoparticles and then analyzed them using several spectroscopic methods. Remarkably, CS/SF/CNPs hydrogels have better recovery and rheological strength than pure hydrogels. After incubation for three days, a considerable shift from M1 macrophage polarization was discovered in the treated scaffold group containing CS/SF/CNPs compared to the control group, demonstrating its capacity for immune modulation. The osteo-immunomodulatory implications of the manufactured constructs on human bone marrow-derived mesenchymal stem cells (hBMSCs) were investigated using a macrophage-derived conditioned medium (M-CM). The calvaria defect rat model showed increased bone regeneration, implying that manufactured scaffolds are potential regimens for bone repair [61]. Figure 12.1 shows the biomedical applications of additive manufacturing technology.

12.3.3 3D-PRINTED BIORESORBABLE SYNTHETIC-BASED POLYMER COMPOSITES

When aiming to develop scaffolds for biomedical applications, synthetic bioresorbable polymers offer several benefits over natural polymers: (a) they are easy to process; (b) they may be manufactured at a low cost using a reproducible approach on a large scale; (c) their kinetics of degradation and mechanical characteristics may be readily modified for appropriate utilization; and (d) they pose no danger of immunogenicity. Their primary disadvantages include being less biocompatible than natural polymers, often lacking active cell sites, and their byproducts usually are not natural metabolites. They may create issues if stored in the body [62, 63]. Poly(a-hydroxy acids) aliphatic polyesters are one of the principal families of synthetic

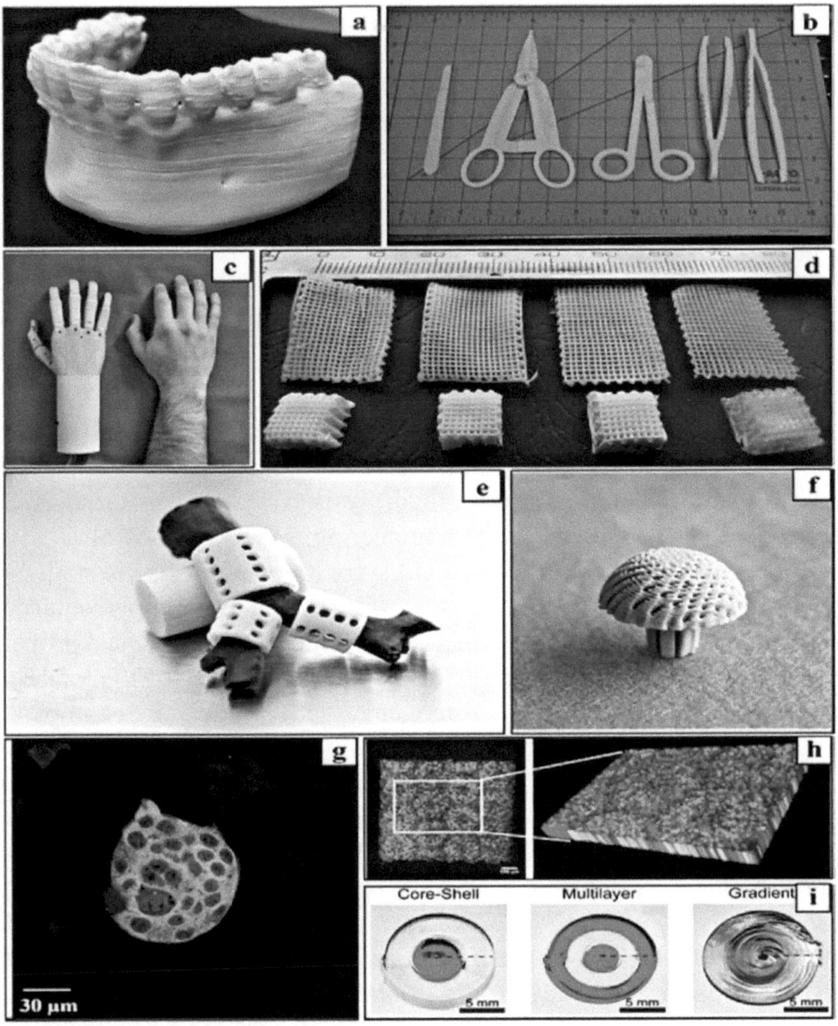

FIGURE 12.1 Various applications of additive manufacturing in biomedical engineering. (a) FDM-fabricated poly(D,L-lactide) (PDLLA) model of the mandible. (b) SLS-printed modified set of surgical nylon. (c) SLS-printed prototype of a hand made with nylon fiber-reinforced composite. (d) Computer-aided wet-spinning (CAWS) printed surgical implants using porous poly(methyl methacrylate) (PMMA). (e) SLS-printed surgical biodegradable PCL implants. (f) FDM-printed bone scaffold using PCL/hydroxyapatite (HAp). (g) Micrograph of confocal laser scanning microscopy (CLSM) 3D tissue modeling human pancreatic cancer cell spheroids. (h) CLSM micrograph of an integrated organ-on-a-chip by gelatin methacryloyl (GelMA), supporting cells (red), and hepatic cells (green) patterns. (i) Drug loading system configuration.

Source: Reproduced with permission from Ref. [96]. Copyright © 2020 Elsevier Ltd.

bioresorbable polymeric materials. The most commonly utilized bioresorbable polymers are stereoisomers of poly(lactic acid) (PLA), poly(D-lactic acid), poly(a-hydroxy acids) like PGA, and copolymers of poly(lactic-co-glycolic acid) and poly(L-lactic acid) (PLLA) [64, 65].

12.3.3.1 POLY(LACTIC-COGLYCOLIC) ACID (PLGA) BIORESORBABLE 3D PRINTED COMPOSITES

The advancement of organ repair and cell growth has led to the use of the copolymer PLGA for medical purposes, such as human body implants, materials for tissue engineering, and cell scaffold fabrication [66, 67]. This type of copolymer has good biocompatibility and mechanical properties. Many PLGA copolymers degrade inside the human body, producing CO_2 and H_2O through non-enzymatic hydrolysis [68]. This material is being extensively used for bone tissue engineering. Various series of HA/PLGA scaffolds with different contents of HA were reported by Jiawei et al. A 60% weight percentage of HA mimics the natural bone mineral percentage. The characterization of the biomaterial was conducted for mechanical properties, *in vitro* degradability, structure, and composition. The HA/PLGA fabricated scaffolds were assessed for osteogenic activity and cytocompatibility through *in vivo* rabbit femoral defect healing experiments and *in vitro* cell culture. From the results, it is reported that a 45% weight percentage of the composite scaffold of HA/PLGA showed the maximum material strength (compressive), which is more than 40 MPa, approximately six times greater than the clean scaffolds of PLGA. Mixing microspheres of HA into the PLGA matrix significantly improved the osteogenic proliferation, cell differentiation, and adhesion of the bone marrow stem cells (BMSCs) that were seeded and cultured on the scaffold's outer surface. From another report, it is shown that the composite of HA/PLGA with 45 wt% HA exhibited excellent osteogenic performance and structural maintenance *in vivo* [69]. Pierre et al. designed a new system of drug delivery using biodegradable polymer and TPGS for constructing nanoparticles loaded with methotrexate for a 3D printable hydrogel of alginate-gelatin ink, forming a tablet that is a solid 3D printed structure for oral drug delivery. Using a 25G needle, the highest accuracy is obtained for the 3D printed tablets, achieving greater than 95%. To simulate the gastrointestinal environment, the drug release profile *in vitro* was examined at pH levels ranging from 1.2 to 7.4. A prolonged and controlled release profile of methotrexate was observed for up to 24 hours.

From the gastrointestinal location, the study of the silicon modeling showed that inhibition of P-gp ATPase simplified and improved the absorption of MTX [70]. Elsewhere, Chen et al. developed a bioactive glass containing a mesoporous lithium-containing structure (Li-MBG) and studied the *in vitro* characteristics in controlling the osteogenic differentiation, relocation, and proliferation of bone marrow stem cells (BMSCs) in a high-glucose micro-environment, as well as the functional operations. Furthermore, composite scaffolds of Li-MBG/PLGA were fabricated by bioprinting, and their effects were examined *in vivo* for the healing of complex skull defects in mice. It was found that Li-MBG reversed the maximum glucose-induced suppression of osteogenic differentiation, migration, and proliferation of bone marrow stem cells by enabling signaling pathways such as β-catenin/Tcf7/Ccn4 and upregulating Itga3. They concluded that the composite scaffold of Li-MBG/PLGA can successfully heal skull defects in diabetic mice by recruiting stem cells and demonstrating a significant effect on osteogenesis [71].

12.3.3.2 POLY(LACTIC ACID) 3D PRINTED BIORESORBABLE COMPOSITES

In various orthopedic and dental applications, the polymer poly(lactic acid) (PLA), which is a bioabsorbable polymer, is being used [72, 73]. However, some opposing effects of this biomaterial in clinical settings have also been reported when it is used individually [74]. To overcome these inflammatory and allergic reactions in the human body, it is incorporated with other biomaterials like hydroxyapatite (HA) or tricalcium phosphate (TCP) [75–77]. Composites of PLA, such as PLA/TCP, are being widely used in tissue engineering applications. An artificial scaffold fabricated by coating decellularized extracellular matrix (bdECM) and bone demineralized on the present polycaprolactone/tricalcium phosphate (PCL/TCP) 3D printed construct to improve osteoinductivity and osteoconductivity was reported by Lee et al. From their earlier studies, injecting adipose-derived stem cells (ADSCs) in combined form showed promising results. They continued their study by investigating the scaffold's effect on ossification during the reconstruction of the mandible in beagle dogs. They created two different groups: group A (ADSC injection; n = 5 + PCL/TCP/bdECM) and group B (PCL/TCP/bdECM; n = 5). After intermediation, the data were studied at four as well as eight weeks. From CT data, they concluded that group A has greater diffuse osteoblast tissue compared to group B. Proof of immune rejection or infection was noticed by histological examination. In the pores of the scaffold, the Goldner trichrome (G/T) staining showed excess ossification. Using polymerase chain reaction (PCR), the expressions of genes like Runx2, Osteocalcin, and ColI were identified. The gene expressions are more prominent in group A. By using the western blotting technique, group A displayed better gene expressions of the genes that encode Runx2, Osteocalcin, and ColI proteins. They concluded that the intrusion group A, where the beagle dogs received extra ADSC injection as well as the bioprinted bdECM coated PCL/TCP, presented rectified mandibular ossification around and in the scaffold pores [78]. For the treatment of GBR, Salamanca et al. compared and tested the efficacy and properties of many ratios of PLA and β-TCP that were used to develop the 3D printed material filament to find the most suitable material combination. Various combinations of PLA to β-TCP ratios were examined, including ratios of PLA/β-TCP 80%/20% (PLA-20), 85%/15% (PLA-15), 90%/10% (PLA-10), and 95%/5% (PLA-5). The qPCR and *in vitro* testing were also done for the material characterization. After incorporating β-TCP into PLA, elongation and tensile strengths decreased, cell promotion and proliferation improved, and retention of hardness was present. They reported that 3D printed filaments developed at a ratio of 10% β-TCP and 90% PLA were effective for the case of GBR compared to the PLA filament [79]. For bone reconstruction, the commonly used bioactive material is Hydroxyapatite (HA), which improves the mechanical and osseointegration properties of PLA polymers [80–82]. The technology of Fused Deposition Modeling (FDM) was used for the fabrication of the material composite of nano-hydroxyapatite (n-HA) and polylactic acid (PLA), as described by Wang et al. They optimized the material composite by performing mechanical property tests, biocompatibility tests for *in vitro* bone marrow mesenchymal stem cells, and material characterization. Ultimately, the rabbit model was used to assess the PLA/n-HA scaffolds' osteogenic ability *in vivo*. The data showed that the composite of PLA/n-HA is easily printable, and the struts of the printed structure presented varying mechanical strengths obtained by the percentage of the composition of n-HA. Compared to the pure scaffold of PLA, the osteogenic induction property and biocompatibility are much better. For the repair of extreme and complex defects of bone, the composite scaffold of n-HA and PLA yielded promising results [83]. The combination of PLLA (L-polylactic acid) and nano-HA (nHA) optimized composite, along with Fused Deposition Modeling (FDM) technology for preparing the PLLA/nHA constructs for bone repair, is reported by

Zhang et al. It is also shown that the composite ink of PLLA/nHA not only improved the smoothness and accuracy of the printing but also met the requirements for customized bone healing applications. nHA high-loaded scaffolds have appropriate compressive strength, which is greater than that of cancellous bone and pure HA ceramic scaffolds. In addition to the *in vitro* study, the *in vivo* study also showed appropriate osteogenic properties [30]. By using Fused Deposition Modeling (FDM), Wu et al. investigated the possibilities of resembling natural bone with respect to biodegradability and mechanical properties, where the composite filament of hydroxyapatite (HA), poly(lactic acid) (PLA), and degradable polymers were used. Three compositions of PLA/HA were used, having weight percentages of 5%, 10%, and 15% HA. Using these materials, a model of human trabecular bone was printed. The morphogenic and mechanical properties of the 3D printed model were evaluated using screw pull-out, compression, and micro-computed tomography tests. By using a scaling factor of 2–4, the architecture of the trabecular bone can be produced with PLA and FDM. By mixing particles of HA, the concerning morphology and printing accuracy were reduced, but the mechanical properties were enhanced. The scaled-up models showed slightly improved mechanical strength compared to the generally used synthetic bone models using polymeric foam like Sawbones [84]. For osteosynthesis studies, PLA/CF and PLA are being used with carbon fibers (CF). The CFs have high chemical and thermal stability, low density, and excellent tensile strength, along with other characteristics [85, 86]. Using a self-designed 3D printer, Zhao et al. developed a composite scaffold incorporating continuous carbon fiber (CF) reinforced with HA (CF/HA). The HA inks tailored the viscoelastic properties, and the optimized nozzle structure ensured the extraction of the compound of multifilament and monofilament CF with rods of HA. Using the computer-aided design (CAD) program, the composite scaffold is fabricated, and the sintering is performed through an appropriate process, resulting in a classified macro/microporous structure containing 50% β-TCP and HA. The presence of continuous CF simultaneously improves both the toughness and strength of the scaffold. For 5CF/HA and 1CF/HA, the compressive forces were 16.3 ± 2.6 MPa and 11.4 ± 1.7 MPa, respectively, compared to the pure HA scaffolds, which were much higher. The fracture toughness of 1CF/HA was double that of the pure HA scaffold, which is approximately close to that of cortical bone. It also has bone regeneration capacity and apatite formation ability, as demonstrated by *in vivo* and *in vitro* studies [87].

12.3.3.3 POLY(LACTIC ACID) 3D PRINTED BIORESORBABLE COMPOSITES

Poly(lactic acid) PCL is an aliphatic polyester that is biodegradable and is being used as a biological construct for many applications in tissue engineering [88]. Apart from some advantages of PCL, such as chemical inertness, excellent thermal stability, and biocompatibility, the disadvantages of PCL must also be taken into account, as it is hydrophobic. Because of this, it shows poor cell-material interaction and proliferation *in vivo*. To overcome these problems, blending PCL with other polymers and surface modification is needed [89–92]. Park et al. fabricated a composite scaffold of PCL/b-TCP by 3D bioprinting for bone tissue engineering applications. They investigated the increasing effect of the content of b-TCP from 0 wt.% to 30 wt.% on the scaffold of PCL/b-TCP, as well as its capability for osteogenic differentiation. From the data, it was observed that with the increasing content of b-TCP, the mechanical strength improved. For bone tissue engineering applications, 30 wt.% of b-TCP in the platform of PCL/b-TCP is highly suitable. By using this technology, the fabrication of a composite scaffold of (PCL)/SrHA was reported by Liu et al. SEM images of the 3D printed constructs revealed that SrHA is uniformly distributed within the interior of the scaffold strut. From the *in vitro* release studies, it was observed that Ca and Sr ions were released in a sustained manner from the scaffolds of PCL/SrHA. For determining the performance of the composite scaffolds used in bone tissue engineering, the osteogenic differentiation and cell proliferation in mesenchymal stem cells (BMSCs) from rat bone marrow, which were developed on the platform, were assessed. From the experimental data, it was found that combining SrHA with PCL 3D printed scaffolds considerably enhanced cell proliferation. A higher level of BMSCs differentiation was shown by the PCL/SrHA scaffolds compared to the PCL/HA scaffolds and PCL scaffolds, as indicated by osteo-related gene expression and ALP activity. Additionally, a study reported that adding SrHA to the PCL 3D printed constructs promoted bone regeneration [93]. Using the 3D printing electrohydrodynamic jet (EHD-jet) method, Vijayavenkataraman et al. fabricated scaffolds of PCL/rGO. The material and mechanical characterization were also performed on the PCL/rGO and PCL bioprinted scaffolds. For neural differentiation, softer scaffolds were prepared by adding rGO. *In vitro* studies on neural differentiation were conducted using PC12 cells. The PCL/rGO scaffolds showed higher cell proliferation compared to the pure PCL construct. The results of immunocytochemistry and reverse transcription polymerase chain reaction indicated that the neural differentiation of PC12 cells was supported by the PCL/rGO scaffolds [94]. Using an extrusion-based bioprinter that is mechanically operated, Kim et al. fabricated scaffolds of PCL/nHA. At various wt.% concentrations of nHA (0, 10, 20, and 30), the quantitative analysis of the scaffold-like cell mineralization and proliferation, mechanical strength, chemical composition, and scaffold morphology was conducted. From the data, the optimization criteria such as osteoconductivity, cellular interactions, printability, and mechanical properties for the composite scaffolds of PCL/nHA 3D-printed were investigated [95]. Figure 12.2 represents various AM techniques that are commonly employed for biodegradable polymer processing.

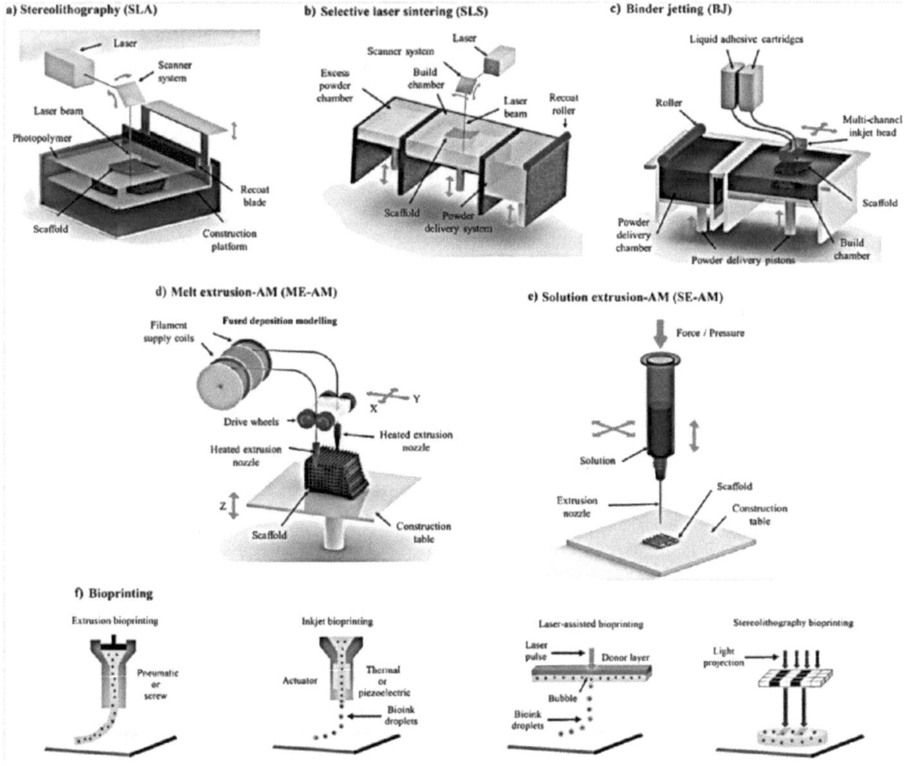

FIGURE 12.2 Commonly used AM techniques. (a) Stereolithography; (b) selective laser sintering; (c) binder jetting; (d) melt extrusion-AM; (e) solution extrusion-AM; and (f) extrusion bioprinting.

Source: Reproduced with permission from Ref. [96]. Copyright © 2020 Elsevier Ltd.

12.4 CONCLUSION

Currently, biodegradable polymers are being investigated in various tissue engineering applications. This method is in its infancy stage; few of these materials are used clinically. These bioabsorbable biomaterials are used for internal fixations, which exclude the need for surgical intervention a second time for material removal after healing has occurred. These material composites are gaining a lot of attention in the tissue engineering domain because they provide suitable mechanical properties for the healing process of tissues and allow cells to grow and attach. The rate of degradation of these materials must be within a sustainable range for the specific location where the material is intended to serve in the human body. For applications like this, poly(lactic acid) fulfills all these conditions because of its chiral structure and its ability to undergo copolymerization reactions with other polymers for the formation of composites. Nanocomposite materials have one problem: the biological material is absorbed in the human body, but the nanoparticles migrate to adjacent tissues. Additionally, a multidisciplinary approach is needed to broadly examine these nanocomposite materials before they can be extensively available for grafting in patients. Furthermore, these nanocomposite materials need to be manufactured on a large scale. Academic institutes and biotechnology companies have started using this technology for tissue engineering applications, by which body parts and organs are being developed. The major advantage of this technology is that it enables the manufacturing of objects with complicated internal structures and geometries that can be developed according to the requirements of a particular patient by using 3D medical scanned data. This technology is widely used in biomedical applications for these reasons, particularly in the field of tissue engineering. Synthetic as well as natural polymers are developed for tissue engineering applications using this technology, and new materials are also being investigated. Particles and fibers are added to these polymers for the fabrication of materials with better chemical and physical properties, biocompatibility, and bioactivity. For much wider 3D printing applications, the printing of organs and tissues must be studied further; also, more materials need to be developed that can be used as materials for 3D printing, and finally, the cost of 3D printing technology should be reduced. Moreover, the study of cell growth, differentiation, and attachment inside the 3D-printed material must be conducted. For the development of biocompatible products, the essential criteria are biomimicry, safe by-products, biodegradability, desirable mechanical properties, biocompatibility, and material printability. The printability factor of the material can be optimized by regulating the parameters of the 3D printer, such as infill, bed temperature, printing speed, etc. In the case of FDM-DIW, a thick paste for the ink can be obtained by adding thixotropic agents like additives and fillers in nanoscale and microscale sizes. Moreover, the use of non-toxic polymeric material for 3D printing allows for the reduction of volatile organic compounds (VOCs) and toxic particles. The filaments and biopolymer inks are environmentally friendly because they are biodegradable, benign, and usually require low temperatures during printing. The selection of the additive manufacturing (AM) method is necessary for optimizing energy consumption and environmental impacts. The printing process can be fully utilized by using optimized operational parameters such as extruder movement, UV exposure time, wavelength, post-curing temperature, bed, and printing speed. Minute process monitoring at all stages of printing is necessary for the biocompatibility of 3D-printed materials. The aspects of stimuli-responsive polymer systems and 4D printing applied in biomedical applications should be considered for future work. All these opportunities involve the use of polymeric 3D-printed materials that demonstrate diagnostic (theranostic) and therapeutic functionality, as well as sensory, actuation, and shape memory capabilities.

KEYWORDS

- **3D printing**
- **biomedical applications**
- **bioresorbable**
- **composite**
- **polymer**

REFERENCES

1. Wu, Z., Su, X., Xu, Y., Kong, B., Sun, W., & Mi, S. (2016). Bioprinting three-dimensional cell-laden tissue constructs with controllable degradation. *Scientific Reports, 6*, 24474. https://doi.org/10.1038/srep24474.
2. Guvendiren, M., Molde, J., Soares, R. M. D., & Kohn, J. (2016). Designing biomaterials for 3D printing. *ACS Biomaterials Science & Engineering, 2*(7), 1679–1693. https://doi.org/10.1021/acsbiomaterials.6b00124.
3. Barrère, F., Mahmood, T. A., de Groot, K., & van Blitterswijk, C. A. (2008). Advanced biomaterials for skeletal tissue regeneration: Instructive and smart functions. *Materials*

Science and Engineering: R: Reports, 59(1), 38–71. https://doi.org/10.1016/j.mser.2007.09.002.

4. Mason, C., & Dunnill, P. (2008). A brief definition of regenerative medicine. *Regenerative Medicine, 3*(1), 1–5. https://doi.org/10.2217/17460751.3.1.1.
5. Vert, M. (1989). Bioresorbable polymers for temporary therapeutic applications. *Die Angewandte Makromolekulare Chemie, 166*(1), 155–168. https://doi.org/10.1002/apmc.1989.050166011.
6. Vert, M., Li, S. M., Spenlehauer, G., & Guerin, P. (1992). Bioresorbability and biocompatibility of aliphatic polyesters. *Journal of Materials Science: Materials in Medicine, 3*(5), 432–446. https://doi.org/10.1007/BF00122754.
7. Uhrich, K. E., & Abdelhamid, H. (2016). Biodegradable and bio erodible polymers for medical applications. In *Biosynthetic Polymers for Medical Applications* (pp. 63–83). Elsevier.
8. Hajebi, S., Mohammadi Nasr, S., Rabiee, N., Bagherzadeh, M., Ahmadi, S., Rabiee, M., Tahriri, M., Tayebi, L., & Hamblin, M. R. (2021). Bioresorbable composite polymeric materials for tissue engineering applications. *International Journal of Polymeric Materials and Polymeric Biomaterials, 70*(12), 926–940. https://doi.org/10.1080/00914037.2020.1827490.
9. Akinapelli, A., Chen, J. P., Roy, K., Donnelly, J., Dawkins, K., Huibregtse, B., & Hou, D. (2017). Current state of bioabsorbable polymer-coated drug-eluting stents. *Current Cardiology Reviews, 13*(2), 139–154. https://doi.org/10.2174/1573403X13666170215160 14.
10. Dhaliwal, K., & Dosanjh, P. (2018). Biodegradable polymers and their role in drug delivery systems. *Biomedical Journal of Scientific & Technical Research, 11*(5), 8315–8320. https://doi.org/10.26717/BJSTR.2018.11.002191.
11. Sheridan, M., Shea, L. D., Peters, M. C., & Mooney, D. J. (2000). Bioabsorbable polymer scaffolds for tissue engineering capable of sustained growth factor delivery. *Journal of Controlled Release, 64*(1–3), 91–102. https://doi.org/10.1016/S0168-3659(99)00239-1.
12. Alexy, R. D., & Levi, D. S. (2013). Materials and manufacturing technologies available for production of a pediatric bioabsorbable stent. *BioMed Research International, 2013*, 137985. https://doi.org/10.1155/2013/137985.
13. Navarro, M., Michiardi, A., Castano, O., & Planell, J. A. (2008). Biomaterials in orthopedics. *Journal of the Royal Society Interface, 5*(27), 1137–1158. https://doi.org/10.1098/rsif.2008.0204.
14. Liu, H., & Webster, T. J. (2007). Bioinspired nanocomposites for orthopedic applications. In *Nanotechnology for the Regeneration of Hard and Soft Tissues* (pp. 1–51).
15. Steinberg, E. L., Rath, E., Shlaifer, A., Chechik, O., Maman, E., & Salai, M. (2013). Carbon fiber reinforced PEEK Optima—A composite material biomechanical properties and wear/debris characteristics of CF-PEEK composites for orthopedic trauma implants. *Journal of the Mechanical Behavior of Biomedical Materials, 17*, 221–228. https://doi.org/10.1016/j.jmbbm.2012.12.010.
16. Gide, K. M., Islam, S., & Bagheri, Z. S. (2022). Polymer-based materials built with additive manufacturing methods for orthopedic applications: A review. *Journal of Composites Science, 6*(7), 262. https://doi.org/10.3390/jcs6070262.
17. Chen, X., Gao, C., Jiang, J., Wu, Y., Zhu, P., & Chen, G. (2019). 3D printed porous PLA/nHA composite scaffolds with enhanced osteogenesis and osteoconductivity

in vivo for bone regeneration. *Biomedical Materials, 14*(6), 065003. https://doi.org/10.1088/1748-605X/ab4bfb.

18. Tanodekaew, S., Channasanon, S., Kaewkong, P., & Uppanan, A. (2013). PLA-HA scaffolds: Preparation and bioactivity. *Procedia Engineering, 59*, 144–149. https://doi.org/10.1016/j.proeng.2013.07.022.
19. Jeong, S. I., Ko, E. K., Yum, J., Jung, C. H., Lee, Y. M., & Shin, H. (2008). Nanofibrous poly (lactic acid)/hydroxyapatite composite scaffolds for guided tissue regeneration. *Macromolecular Bioscience, 8*(4), 328–338. https://doi.org/10.1002/mabi.200700251.
20. Liu, H., & Webster, T. J. (2010). Mechanical properties of dispersed ceramic nanoparticles in polymer composites for orthopedic applications. *International Journal of Nanomedicine, 5*, 299–309. https://doi.org/10.2147/IJN.S7413.
21. Jose, M. V., Thomas, V., Johnson, K. T., Dean, D. R., & Nyairo, E. (2009). Aligned PLGA/HA nanofibrous nanocomposite scaffolds for bone tissue engineering. *Acta Biomaterialia, 5*(1), 305–315. https://doi.org/10.1016/j.actbio.2008.07.014.
22. Kang, Y., Scully, A., Young, D. A., Kim, S., Tsao, H., Sen, M., & Yang, Y. (2011). Enhanced mechanical performance and biological evaluation of a PLGA coated β-TCP composite scaffold for load-bearing applications. *European Polymer Journal, 47*(9), 1569–1577. https://doi.org/10.1016/j.eurpolymj.2011.06.002.
23. Ebrahimian-Hosseinabadi, M., Ashrafizadeh, F., Etemadifar, M., & Venkatraman, S. S. (2011). Evaluating and modeling the mechanical properties of the prepared PLGA/nano-BCP composite scaffolds for bone tissue engineering. *Journal of Materials Science & Technology, 27*(12), 1105–1112. https://doi.org/10.1016/S1005-0302(11)60154-8.
24. Vaezi, M., Black, C., Gibbs, D. M., Oreffo, R. O., Brady, M., Moshrefi-Torbati, S., & Yang, S. (2016). Characterization of new PEEK/HA composites with 3D HA network fabricated by extrusion free forming. *Molecules, 21*(5), 687. https://doi.org/10.3390/molecules21050687.
25. Vaezi, M., & Yang, S. (2015). A novel bioactive PEEK/HA composite with controlled 3D interconnected HA network. *International Journal of Bioprinting, 1*(1), 23–34. https://doi.org/10.18063/ijb.v1i1.23.
26. Uddin, M., Dhanasekaran, P. S., & Asmatulu, R. (2019). Mechanical properties of highly porous PEEK bio nanocomposites incorporated with carbon and hydroxyapatite nanoparticles for scaffold applications. *Progress in Biomaterials, 8*(3), 211–221. https://doi.org/10.1007/s40204-019-0107-2.
27. Niinomi, M., Narushima, T., & Nakai, M. (2015). Advances in metallic biomaterials: Tissues, materials and biological reactions. Springer. https://doi.org/10.1007/978-3-319-06977-5.
28. Bagaria, V., Bhansali, R., & Pawar, P. (2018). 3D printing—Creating a blueprint for the future of orthopedics: Current concept review and the road ahead! *Journal of Clinical Orthopaedics and Trauma, 9*(3), 207–212. https://doi.org/10.1016/j.jcot.2017.07.001.
29. D'Alessio, J., & Christensen, A. (2019). 3D printing for commercial orthopedic applications: Advances and challenges. In *3D Printing in Orthopedic Surgery* (pp. 65–83).
30. Zhang, B., Wang, L., Song, P., Pei, X., Sun, H., Wu, L., Zhou, C., Wang, K., Fan, Y., & Zhang, X. (2021). 3D printed bone tissue regenerative PLA/HA scaffolds with comprehensive performance optimizations. *Materials & Design, 201*, 109490. https://doi.org/10.1016/j.matdes.2021.109490.

31. Tappa, K., & Jammalamadaka, U. (2018). Novel biomaterials used in medical 3D printing techniques. *Journal of Functional Biomaterials, 9*(1), 17. https://doi.org/10.3390/jfb9010017.
32. Fan, D., Li, Y., Wang, X., Zhu, T., Wang, Q., Cai, H., Li, W., Tian, Y., & Liu, Z. (2020). Progressive 3D printing technology and its application in medical materials. *Frontiers in Pharmacology, 11*, 122. https://doi.org/10.3389/fphar.2020.00012.
33. Du, W., Ren, X., Pei, Z., & Ma, C. (2020). Ceramic binder jetting additive manufacturing: A literature review on density. *Journal of Manufacturing Science and Engineering, 142*(4), 040801. https://doi.org/10.1115/1.4047422.
34. Zhou, Z., Lennon, A., Buchanan, F., McCarthy, H. O., & Dunne, N. (2020). Binder jetting additive manufacturing of hydroxyapatite powders: Effects of adhesives on geometrical accuracy and green compressive strength. *Additive Manufacturing, 36*, 101645. https://doi.org/10.1016/j.addma.2020.101645.
35. Szymczyk-Ziółkowska, P., Łabowska, M. B., Detyna, J., Michalak, I., & Gruber, P. (2020). A review of fabrication polymer scaffolds for biomedical applications using additive manufacturing techniques. *Biocybernetics and Biomedical Engineering, 40*(3), 624–638. https://doi.org/10.1016/j.bbe.2020.05.006.
36. Abdulhameed, O., Al-Ahmari, A., Ameen, W., & Mian, S. H. (2019). Additive manufacturing: Challenges, trends, and applications. *Advances in Mechanical Engineering, 11*(8), 1687814018822880. https://doi.org/10.1177/1687814018822880.
37. Kumar, M. B., & Sathiya, P. (2021). Methods and materials for additive manufacturing: A critical review on advancements and challenges. *Thin-Walled Structures, 159*, 107228. https://doi.org/10.1016/j.tws.2021.107228.
38. Jared, B. H., Aguilo, M. A., Beghini, L. L., Boyce, B. L., Clark, B. W., Cook, A., Kaehr, B. J., & Robbins, J. (2017). Additive manufacturing: Toward holistic design. *Scripta Materialia, 135*, 141–147. https://doi.org/10.1016/j.scriptamat.2016.08.015.
39. Guessasma, S., Zhang, W., Zhu, J., Belhabib, S., & Nouri, H. (2015). Challenges of additive manufacturing technologies from an optimization perspective. *International Journal for Simulation and Multidisciplinary Design Optimization, 6*(1), A9. https://doi.org/10.1051/smdo/2015001.
40. Somireddy, C. (2021). Fabrication of composite structures via 3D printing. In *Fused Deposition Modeling Based 3D Printing* (pp. 255–276). Springer. https://doi.org/10.1007/978-3-030-49263-4_13.
41. Melancon, D., Bagheri, Z. S., Johnston, R., Liu, L., Tanzer, M., & Pasini, D. (2017). Mechanical characterization of structurally porous biomaterials built via additive manufacturing: Experiments, predictive models, and design maps for load-bearing bone replacement implants. *Acta Biomaterialia, 63*, 350–368. https://doi.org/10.1016/j.actbio.2017.08.031.
42. Bagheri, Z. S., Melancon, D., Liu, L., Johnston, R. B., & Pasini, D. (2017). Compensation strategy to reduce geometry and mechanics mismatches in porous biomaterials built with selective laser melting. *Journal of the Mechanical Behavior of Biomedical Materials, 70*, 17–27. https://doi.org/10.1016/j.jmbbm.2017.01.022.
43. Piat, R., Sinchuk, Y., Vasoya, M., & Sigmund, O. (2011). Minimal compliance design for metal–ceramic composites with lamellar microstructures. *Acta Materialia, 59*(14), 4835–4846. https://doi.org/10.1016/j.actamat.2011.04.041.
44. Eberhart, R. C., Su, S. H., Nguyen, K. T., Zilberman, M., Tang, L., Nelson, K. D., & Frenkel, P. (2003). Bioresorbable polymeric stents: Current status and future promise.

Journal of Biomaterials Science, Polymer Edition, 14(3), 299–312. https://doi.org/10.1163/156856203321408583.
45. Chazono, M., Tanaka, T., Komaki, H., & Fujii, K. (2004). Bone formation and bio resorption after implantation of injectable β-tricalcium phosphate granules–hyaluronate complex in rabbit bone defects. *Journal of Biomedical Materials Research Part A, 70*(3), 542–549. https://doi.org/10.1002/jbm.a.30053.
46. Ignjatović, N., Wu, V., Ajduković, Z., Mihajilov-Krstev, T., Uskoković, V., & Uskoković, D. (2016). Chitosan-PLGA polymer blends as coatings for hydroxyapatite nanoparticles and their effect on antimicrobial properties, osteoconductivity, and regeneration of osseous tissues. *Materials Science and Engineering: C, 60*, 357–364. https://doi.org/10.1016/j.msec.2015.11.033.
47. Santos Jr, A. R. (2010). Bioresorbable polymers for tissue engineering. In *Tissue Engineering* (pp. 235–246).
48. Shikinami, Y., Okazaki, K., Saito, M., Okuno, M., Hasegawa, S., Tamura, J., Fujibayashi, S., & Nakamura, T. (2006). Bioactive and bioresorbable cellular cubic-composite scaffolds for use in bone reconstruction. *Journal of the Royal Society Interface, 3*(9), 805–821. https://doi.org/10.1098/rsif.2006.0152.
49. Wuisman, P., & Smit, T. (2006). Bioresorbable polymers: Heading for a new generation of spinal cages. *European Spine Journal, 15*(1), 133–148. https://doi.org/10.1007/s00586-005-0957-3.
50. Ulery, B. D., Nair, L. S., & Laurencin, C. T. (2011). Biomedical applications of biodegradable polymers. *Journal of Polymer Science Part B: Polymer Physics, 49*(12), 832–864. https://doi.org/10.1002/polb.22358.
51. Wu, A. (2008). Ceramic/metal bonding. In Y. Zhou (Ed.), *Microjoining and Nanojoining* (pp. 277–306). Woodhead Publishing.
52. Wang, J., Wang, L., Zhou, Z., Lai, H., Xu, P., Liao, L., & Wei, J. (2016). Biodegradable polymer membranes applied in guided bone/tissue regeneration: A review. *Polymers, 8*(4), 115. https://doi.org/10.3390/polym8040115.
53. Gupta, P., & Nayak, K. K. (2015). Characteristics of protein-based biopolymer and its application. *Polymer Engineering & Science, 55*(2), 485–498. https://doi.org/10.1002/pen.23978.
54. Nasef, M. M., & Hegazy, E. S. A. (2004). Preparation and applications of ion exchange membranes by radiation-induced graft copolymerization of polar monomers onto non-polar films. *Progress in Polymer Science, 29*(6), 499–561. https://doi.org/10.1016/j.progpolymsci.2004.04.003.
55. Lenz, R. W., & Marchessault, R. H. (2005). Bacterial polyesters: Biosynthesis, biodegradable plastics and biotechnology. *Biomacromolecules, 6*(1), 1–8. https://doi.org/10.1021/bm0498603.
56. Paul, W., & Sharma, C. (2008). Natural bioresorbable polymers. In *Degradation Rate of Bioresorbable Materials* (pp. 67–94). Elsevier. https://doi.org/10.1016/B978-0-08-045137-7.50010-2.
57. Sampath, U. G. T., Ching, Y. C., Chuah, C. H., Sabariah, J. J., & Lin, P. C. (2016). Fabrication of porous materials from natural/synthetic biopolymers and their composites. *Materials, 9*(12), 991. https://doi.org/10.3390/ma9120991.
58. Suh, J., & Matthew, H. W. (2000). Application of chitosan-based polysaccharide biomaterials in cartilage tissue engineering: A review. *Biomaterials, 21*(25), 2589–2598. https://doi.org/10.1016/S0142-9612(00)00162-7.

59. Sadeghianmaryan, A., Naghieh, S., Yazdanpanah, Z., Alizadeh Sardroud, H., Sharma, N. K., Wilson, L. D., & Chen, X. (2022). Fabrication of chitosan/alginate/hydroxyapatite hybrid scaffolds using 3D printing and impregnating techniques for potential cartilage regeneration. *International Journal of Biological Macromolecules, 204*, 62–75. https://doi.org/10.1016/j.ijbiomac.2022.01.060.
60. Yang, Y., Wu, H., Fu, Q., Xie, X., Song, Y., Xu, M., & Li, J. (2022). 3D-printed polycaprolactone-chitosan based drug delivery implants for personalized administration. *Materials & Design, 214*, 110394. https://doi.org/10.1016/j.matdes.2022.110394.
61. Patel, D. K., Dutta, S. D., Hexiu, J., Ganguly, K., & Lim, K. T. (2022). 3D-printable chitosan/silk fibroin/cellulose nanoparticle scaffolds for bone regeneration via M2 macrophage polarization. *Carbohydrate Polymers, 281*, 119077. https://doi.org/10.1016/j.carbpol.2021.119077.
62. Guan, J., Sacks, M. S., Beckman, E. J., & Wagner, W. R. (2004). Biodegradable poly (ether ester urethane) urea elastomers based on poly (ether ester) triblock copolymers and putrescine: Synthesis, characterization, and cytocompatibility. *Biomaterials, 25*(1), 85–96. https://doi.org/10.1016/S0142-9612(03)00525-0.
63. Jenkins, M., & Stamboulis, A. (2012). *Durability and Reliability of Medical Polymers*. Elsevier.
64. Albertsson, A. C., & Varma, I. K. (2002). Aliphatic polyesters: Synthesis, properties, and applications. In *Degradable Aliphatic Polyesters* (pp. 1–40).
65. Homaeigohar, S., & Boccaccini, A. R. (2022). Nature-derived and synthetic additives to poly(ε-caprolactone) nanofibrous systems for biomedicine: An updated overview. *Frontiers in Chemistry, 9*, 809676. https://doi.org/10.3389/fchem.2021.809676.
66. Xiao, L., Wang, B., Yang, G., & Gauthier, M. (2012). Poly (lactic acid)-based biomaterials: Synthesis, modification, and applications. *Biomedical Science, Engineering and Technology, 11*, 247–282.
67. Cheng, Y., Deng, S., Chen, P., & Ruan, R. (2009). Polylactic acid (PLA) synthesis and modifications: A review. *Frontiers of Chemistry in China, 4*(3), 259–264. https://doi.org/10.1007/s11458-009-0019-7.
68. Makadia, H. K., & Siegel, S. J. (2011). Poly lactic-co-glycolic acid (PLGA) as biodegradable controlled drug delivery carrier. *Polymers, 3*(3), 1377–1397. https://doi.org/10.3390/polym3031377.
69. Wei, J., Yan, Y., Gao, J., Li, Y., Wang, R., Wang, J., Zou, Q., Zuo, Y., Zhu, M., & Li, J. (2022). 3D-printed hydroxyapatite microspheres reinforced PLGA scaffolds for bone regeneration. *Biomaterials Advances, 133*, 112618. https://doi.org/10.1016/j.biadv.2022.112618.
70. Kondiah, P. P., Rants'o, T. A., Makhathini, S. S., Mdanda, S., & Choonara, Y. E. (2022). An oral 3D printed PLGA-Tocopherol PEG succinate nanocomposite hydrogel for high-dose methotrexate delivery in maintenance chemotherapy. *Biomedicines, 10*(6), 1470. https://doi.org/10.3390/biomedicines10061470.
71. Chen, Y., Chen, L., Wang, Y., Lin, K., & Liu, J. (2022). Lithium-containing bioactive glasses enhanced 3D-printed PLGA scaffolds for bone regeneration in diabetes. *Composites Part B: Engineering, 230*, 109550. https://doi.org/10.1016/j.compositesb.2022.109550.
72. Persson, M., Lorite, G. S., Kokkonen, H. E., Cho, S. W., Lehenkari, P. P., Skrifvars, M., & Tuukkanen, J. (2014). Effect of bioactive extruded PLA/HA composite films on focal adhesion formation of preosteoblastic cells. *Colloids and Surfaces B: Bio Interfaces, 121*, 409–416. https://doi.org/10.1016/j.colsurfb.2014.05.037.

73. Weis, S., Lee, T. T., del Campo, A., & García, A. J. (2013). Dynamic cell-adhesive microenvironments and their effect on myogenic differentiation. *Acta Biomaterialia, 9*(8), 8059–8066. https://doi.org/10.1016/j.actbio.2013.03.002.
74. Hong, Z., Zhang, P., He, C., Qiu, X., Liu, A., Chen, L., Chen, X., & Jing, X. (2005). Nano-composite of poly(L-lactide) and surface grafted hydroxyapatite: Mechanical properties and biocompatibility. *Biomaterials, 26*(29), 6296–6304. https://doi.org/10.1016/j.biomaterials.2005.01.015.
75. Mathieu, L., Montjovent, M. O., Bourban, P. E., Pioletti, D. P., Månson, J. A., & Pioletti, D. P. (2005). Bioresorbable composites prepared by supercritical fluid foaming. *Journal of Biomedical Materials Research Part A, 75*(1), 89–97. https://doi.org/10.1002/jbm.a.30246.
76. Lee, M. R., Lee, G. W., Kim, J. E., Yun, W. B., Choi, J. Y., Park, J. J., Kim, H. R., Song, B. R., Park, J. W., & Kang, M. J. (2019). Biocompatibility of a PLA-based composite containing hydroxyapatite derived from waste bones of dolphin *Neophocaena asiaeorientalis*. *Journal of the Australian Ceramic Society, 55*(2), 269–279. https://doi.org/10.1080/0002811X.2019.1631161.
77. Rakmae, W., Ruksakulpiwat, Y., Sutapun, W., & Suppakarn, S. (2011). Physical properties and cytotoxicity of surface-modified bovine bone-based hydroxyapatite/poly (lactic acid) composites. *Journal of Composite Materials, 45*(12), 1259–1269. https://doi.org/10.1177/0021998310380782.
78. Lee, J. S., Park, T. H., Ryu, J. Y., Kim, D. K., Oh, E. J., Kim, H. M., Shim, J. H., Yun, W. S., Huh, J. B., & Moon, S. H. (2021). Osteogenesis of 3D-printed PCL/TCP/bdECM scaffold using adipose-derived stem cells aggregates; an experimental study in the canine mandible. *International Journal of Molecular Sciences, 22*(10), 5409. https://doi.org/10.3390/ijms22105409.
79. Salamanca, E., Tsao, T. C., Hseuh, H. W., Wu, Y. F., Choy, C. S., Lin, C. K., Pan, Y. H., Teng, N. C., Huang, M. C., & Lin, S. M. (2021). Fabrication of Polylactic Acid/β-Tricalcium Phosphate FDM 3D printing fiber to enhance osteoblastic-like cell performance. *Frontiers in Materials*, 171. https://doi.org/10.3389/fmat.2021.804217.
80. Sánchez-Arévalo, F., Muñoz-Ramírez, M., Álvarez-Camacho, M., Rivera-Torres, F., Maciel-Cerda, A., Montiel-Campos, R., & Vera-Graziano, R. (2017). Macro-and micromechanical behaviors of poly (lactic acid)–hydroxyapatite electrospun composite scaffolds. *Journal of Materials Science, 52*(6), 3353–3367. https://doi.org/10.1007/s10853-016-0797-x.
81. McManus, A. J., Doremus, R. H., Siegel, R. W., & Bizios, R. (2005). Evaluation of cytocompatibility and bending modulus of nanoceramic/polymer composites. *Journal of Biomedical Materials Research Part A: An Official Journal of The Society for Biomaterials, The Japanese Society for Biomaterials, and The Australian Society for Biomaterials and the Korean Society for Biomaterials, 72*(1), 98–106. https://doi.org/10.1002/jbm.a.30180.
82. Akindoyo, J. O., Beg, M. D., Ghazali, M., Heim, H. P., & Feldmann, M. (2017). Effects of surface modification on dispersion, mechanical, thermal and dynamic mechanical properties of injection molded PLA-hydroxyapatite composites. *Composites Part A: Applied Science and Manufacturing, 103*, 96–105. https://doi.org/10.1016/j.compositesa.2017.09.007.
83. Wang, W., Zhang, B., Li, M., Li, J., Zhang, C., Han, Y., Wang, L., Wang, K., Zhou, C., Liu, Y., Fan, Y., & Zhang, X. (2021). 3D printing of PLA/n-HA composite scaffolds

with customized mechanical properties and biological functions for bone tissue engineering. *Composites Part B: Engineering, 224*, 109192. https://doi.org/10.1016/j.compositesb.2021.109192.
84. Wu, D., Spanou, A., Diez-Escudero, A., & Persson, C. (2020). 3D-printed PLA/HA composite structures as synthetic trabecular bone: A feasibility study using fused deposition modeling. *Journal of the Mechanical Behavior of Biomedical Materials, 103*, 103608. https://doi.org/10.1016/j.jmbbm.2020.103608.
85. Xiaosong, H. (2009). Fabrication and properties of carbon fibers. *Materials, 2*(4), 2369–2403. https://doi.org/10.3390/ma2042369.
86. Wan, Y., Wang, Y., Xu, X., & Li, Q. (2001). In vitro degradation behavior of carbon fiber-reinforced PLA composites and influence of interfacial adhesion strength. *Journal of Applied Polymer Science, 82*(1), 150–158. https://doi.org/10.1002/app.1833.
87. Zhao, X., Liu, A., Zhou, L., Yang, Z., Wei, S., Zhao, Z., Fan, Q., & Ma, L. (2022). 3D printing of bioactive macro/microporous continuous carbon fiber reinforced hydroxyapatite composite scaffolds with synchronously enhanced strength and toughness. *Journal of the European Ceramic Society, 42*(13), 4396–4409. https://doi.org/10.1016/j.jeurceramsoc.2022.06.021.
88. Oh, S. H., Park, I. K., Kim, J. M., & Lee, J. H. (2007). In vitro and in vivo characteristics of PCL scaffolds with pore size gradient fabricated by a centrifugation method. *Biomaterials, 28*(10), 1664–1671. https://doi.org/10.1016/j.biomaterials.2006.12.006.
89. Sousa, I., Mendes, A., & Bártolo, P. J. (2013). PCL scaffolds with collagen bio activator for applications in tissue engineering. *Procedia Engineering, 59*, 279–284. https://doi.org/10.1016/j.proeng.2013.01.027.
90. Dell'Erba, R., Groeninckx, G., Maglio, M., Malinconico, M., & Migliozzi, A. (2001). Immiscible polymer blends of semicrystalline biocompatible components: Thermal properties and phase morphology analysis of PLLA/PCL blends. *Polymer, 42*(16), 7831–7840. https://doi.org/10.1016/S0032-3861(01)00207-7.
91. Coombes, A., Rizzi, S., Williamson, M., Barralet, J., Downes, S., & Wallace, W. (2004). Precipitation casting of polycaprolactone for applications in tissue engineering and drug delivery. *Biomaterials, 25*(2), 315–325. https://doi.org/10.1016/S0142-9612(03)00548-0.
92. Averous, L., & Moro, L. (2000). *Polymer (Guildf), 41*(11), 4157–4170. https://doi.org/10.1016/S0032-3861(00)00636-9.
93. Liu, D., Nie, W., Li, D., Wang, W., Zheng, L., Zhang, J., Zhang, J., Peng, C., Mo, X., & He, C. (2019). 3D printed PCL/SrHA scaffold for enhanced bone regeneration. *Chemical Engineering Journal, 362*, 269–279. https://doi.org/10.1016/j.cej.2019.01.131.
94. Vijayavenkataraman, S., Thaharah, S., Zhang, S., Lu, W. F., & Fuh, J. Y. H. (2019). 3D-printed PCL/rGO conductive scaffolds for peripheral nerve injury repair. *Artificial Organs, 43*(6), 515–523. https://doi.org/10.1111/aor.13632.
95. Kim, M. H., Yun, C., Chalisserry, E. P., Lee, Y. W., Kang, H. W., Park, S. H., Jung, W. K., Oh, J., & Nam, S. Y. (2018). Quantitative analysis of the role of nanohydroxyapatite (nHA) on 3D-printed PCL/nHA composite scaffolds. *Materials Letters, 220*, 112–115. https://doi.org/10.1016/j.matlet.2018.03.138.
96. Puppi, D., & Chiellini, E. (2020). Biodegradable polymers for biomedical additive manufacturing. *Applied Materials Today, 20*, 100700. https://doi.org/10.1016/j.apmt.2020.100700.

CHAPTER 13

Clinical Translational Studies and Challenges of Bioabsorbable Polymeric Composites

YUSUF OLATUNJI WAIDI,[1] NIPUN JAIN,[1] RANJIT BARUA,[2] and SUDIPTO DATTA[1]

[1]Department of Materials Engineering, Indian Institute of Science, C.V. Raman Avenue, Bangalore, Karnataka, India

[2]Indian Institute of Engineering Science and Technology, Howrah, West Bengal, India

ABSTRACT

Bioabsorbable polymers have hydrolyzable bonds that undergo chemical degradation either by enzyme-catalyzed active hydrolysis or by reactive hydrolysis. Synthetic bioabsorbable polymers degrade by chemical hydrolysis. The degradation pace is regulated by changing the crystalline structure or molecular mass. Examples of these polymers are polyethylene glycol, polyanhydrides, poly(orthoesters), cross-linked polyester hydrogels, poly(α-hydroxy acids), poly(lactic-co-glycolic) acid, polylactide, and polyurethane. The book chapter will cover composites of bioabsorbable polymeric composite materials utilized for various tissue engineering-based research. Finally, the chapter will discuss the challenges of these polymeric composites and the anticipated future.

13.1 INTRODUCTION

Significant tissue degeneration or damage remains one of the most common and severe challenges in biomedical settings. The current therapeutic

Bioabsorbable Polymers for Drug Carriers and Fixation Devices. Arbind Prasad and Sougata Jana (Eds.)

techniques used to repair or replace damaged tissues include allografts, autografts, xenografts, or implantation of biomedical devices. These currently established methods have been criticized for shortcomings, such as infection susceptibility, donor availability, probable implant rejection, and poor integration [1, 2]. Nowadays, regenerative medicine encompasses a variety of technologies for the engineering of tissue replacement or new tissue, such as cell cloning, non-cellular structure manufacturing, and biological constructions involving live cells. The latter method has been demonstrated to be an effective technique for engineering purposes, better known as tissue engineering (TE). TE is an interdisciplinary area that combines engineering concepts and applications with biological sciences to mimic the original patient tissue through structure-function relationships that link the laboratory-engineered tissue substitute. In addition, tissue engineering (TE) encompasses a mix of chemical and physical elements involving tissue stability preservation, enhancing compromised tissue functionalities, or restoring the biological processes of damaged or missing tissue [3–5]. TE aims to create various tissues in the body that can be easily incorporated, endured, and prosper within the transplanted person's body. Hence, it serves as a lasting remedy for restoring injured tissues, avoiding ongoing maintenance, and lowering treatment costs [6]. Many diverse tissues, including cartilage, bone, skin, and blood vessels, have been repaired via tissue engineering. The engineered tissues require the necessary structural traits and mechanical qualities to operate optimally. For example, for cells to live and multiply in regenerated tissue, the engineered scaffold should mimic the natural 3D environment *in vivo* by altering external variables (*ex vivo*). The targeted tissue cells are also cultured and seeded on the platforms to accomplish these goals.

Furthermore, the fabricated scaffolds are intended to emulate the existing extracellular matrix by employing a porous framework that promotes cell adherence and mobility. The use of biodegradable implant scaffolds, which may be absorbed *in vivo* after performing their desired function, is another viable approach [7–10]. The primary sources of biomaterials are broadly classified into natural or synthetic (or composite between the two) utilized within the human body. Biomaterials like sutures, bone plates, yarns, joints, intraocular lenses, cardiac valves, and several others are now commonly employed to restore or alter injured organs' operation due to advancements in synthetic processes. These implants aid in repairing, improving performance, correcting and eliminating structural problems, and improving the recipient's quality of life. Biomaterials employed *in vivo* are now classified as polymers, metals, ceramics, and composites. Above all, biomaterials must be biocompatible; that is, the interaction of the typical bodily environment with external materials should not result in hazardous by-products or an excessive inflammatory or fibrotic response. Recently, researchers have been looking for materials that can be eliminated or absorbed in the body after serving their purpose [11–14]. Approximately 90% of the materials studied as implanted scaffolds are polymeric. These polymers' comparatively simple production procedure and reduced Young's modulus promote cell adhesion and migration. Polymers have a better capacity for tension transmission to the bone surface, improving bone regeneration and lifespan [73]. Polymeric compounds are grouped into two types based on source: natural and artificial. Collagen, alginate, and chitosan are the most effective biomaterials produced from natural polymers. Non-biodegradable synthetic polymers are distinguished from biodegradable synthetic polymers. Biodegradable polymers are preferred in tissue engineering (TE) to minimize extra surgical procedures for implant or scaffold removal. Since biodegradable polymers are continuously degrading *in vivo*, elastin and collagen, examples of structural proteins, are produced by the penetrated cells, thus replacing the degraded material. Biodegradable polymers are broadly classified into four categories by Vert et al. [74, 75] based on their characteristics and biological applications:

1. Biodegradable polymers can be described as polymeric biomaterials that create macromolecule by-products that are not eliminated upon degradation. Polyurethane is one example. (It should be noted that environmental materials such as bacterial and fungal deterioration are excluded from this definition).
2. Bioresorbable polymers can be described as polymeric biomaterials that degrade fully *in vivo*. Polymers are excreted as breakdown by-products or after further metabolization. Biosorption is the complete removal of the first foreign substance derived and the breakdown of products (molecules with low molecular weight), resulting in no leftover substance. Poly-D, L-lactide is an example.
3. Bio-erodible polymers are polymeric biomaterials that degrade on their surfaces indefinitely until the substance is completely removed. Bioerosion also indicates the complete removal of the surface degradation by-products and first foreign material, resulting in no leftover substance. Crosslinked polyester hydrogels, poly(a-hydroxy acids), polyanhydrides, and poly(orthoesters) are erodible polymers.
4. Bioabsorbable polymers can be described as polymeric biomaterials that dissolve sluggishly in the human body (*in vivo*) without causing

polymer chain cleavage or a loss in molecular mass. Polyethylene glycol is one example [16–18]. If the dissolved product is expelled from the body, bioabsorbable polymeric biomaterials can also be called bioresorbable [19–21]. Several bone tissue engineering scaffolds are made from polymer-based materials (composite). Composite materials are made up of more than one substance which, when combined, mitigate the shortcomings of one piece when employed alone. Therefore, composite is vital since every human hard tissue, aside from enamel (tooth), may be considered composite nanostructures. Notably, the cell and tissue growth should be equivalent to the pace of the implanted composite material resorption. In addition, the composite must have better mechanical characteristics than each polymer alone, offering flexibility and structural integrity superior to brittle materials like ceramics [22, 23]. In the subsequent sections of this chapter, we present a thorough overview of bioresorbable composite polymeric biomaterials for TE, such as biodegradation systems and design methodologies. Furthermore, we also summarize the latest research on various bioresorbable polymeric substances employed and their usage in TE.

13.2 APPLICATION OF BIORESORBABLE POLYMERS

Bioabsorbable polymers are utilized in surgical operations and continuously replace non-resorbable sutures. Nowadays, bioresorbable polymers are used in an array of functions such as guided cell regeneration [25], targeted medicine delivery [19], bone repair screws, and vascular stents [24]. Bioresorbable polymers can be broken down either by the action of enzymes that takes place gradually or by straightforward hydrolysis, in which the monomers are released after catalyzing the chemical bonds. Long chains of polymers are cut down into monomeric units, which are eliminated or metabolized in certain specific pathways. The three primary methods employed to promote the development of healthy tissues include the application of implants to trigger the regenerative processes, using tissues cultured on matrices as implants, or the direct delivery of cells onto the area of injury [26, 27]. The right hydrophilicity/hydrophobicity, percent crystallinity, starting molecular weight, and chemical structure and composition should all be present in bioresorbable polymer composites to promote tissue regeneration. The breakdown rate is also influenced by physical parameters, structural constituents, and environmental factors, like pH and enzyme variability [28, 29].

Biomaterials, including chitosan, collagen, polyester, polyanhydride, polyorthoesters, polyamides, polyamino acids, and polyphosphazenes, are used to make the majority of bioresorbable structures. These compounds are desirable for regenerative medicine applications due to their availability, simplicity of synthesis, chemical composition, and elastic/rigid characteristics based on usage. Due to its decreased toxicity and improved biocompatibility, the aliphatic poly(esters) family is the biodegradable polymer that has been the subject of the most research in tissue engineering practice. These even comprise the copolymers of polylactic and glycolic acid [30, 31].

13.3 FEATURES OF BIORESORBABLE POLYMERS DEGRADATION

In the degradation process, polymer chains are hydrolyzed into oligomers and, ultimately, monomers. Degradation may take either at the polymer's surface or throughout the bulk of the material. The degradation process is started when water enters the polymer matrix. There are two approaches to eroding polymers: (a) bulk degradation, which causes the water to seep through the substrate more quickly than hydrolysis; and (b) surface erosion, where hydrolysis is more rapid than water absorption [32, 33]. Figure 13.1 shows the bioresorbable polymer degradation process.

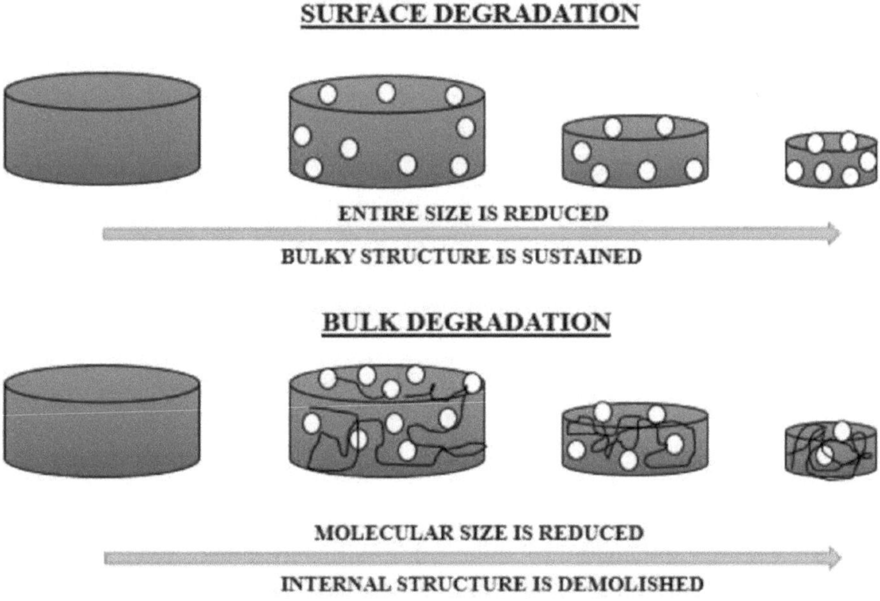

FIGURE 13.1 Bioresorbable polymer degradation.

The time needed for resorption or breakdown will increase with the increase in molecular weight (MW) of the substrate. Bioresorbable polymers have hydrolyzable linkages that can be broken down chemically through enzyme- or chemical-catalyzed hydrolysis reactions [34]. Compared to the crystalline parts of polymers, amorphous regions are more prone to experience passive hydrolysis. Through certain metabolic pathways, the broken-down products (mostly water and carbon dioxide) are expelled from the body by the action of certain organs like the kidneys. Degradation should also occur by generating the least harmful compounds possible [35].

13.3.1 NATURAL POLYMERS-BASED BIORESORBABLE COMPOSITES

Utilizing polymers derived from natural sources is common for major tissue engineering purposes, such as skin, cartilage, blood capillaries, ligaments, tendons, and bones. Isolated mainly from the ECM tissue, they offer superior cell compatibility and high degradation, making them preferable for cell attachment, growth, and differentiation. The principal drawbacks of these polymers are poor mechanical characteristics and restricted processing that prevent their extensive application in therapeutics [36]. Depending on their origin, these can be categorized as (a) polysaccharides; (b) proteins; and (c) polyesters [37–39]. Polysaccharide polymeric compounds such as chitosan, starch, alginate, etc., provide certain specific benefits over conventional polymers, such as low toxicity, good biocompatibility, excellent cell connections, and reduced cost, which justifies their usage as a scaffolding component for tissue engineering. Collagen, gelatin, fibrin, and elastin are protein-based polymers that have received much attention as prospective cell delivery agents. Several scaffolds currently on the market were developed using animal collagen and are being employed regularly for tissue engineering since it has been demonstrated to possess inherent biological activity [11, 40–42]. PHA (polyhydroxyalkanoates), another intriguing class, is created by bacterial fermentation of carbohydrates. Poly(3-hydroxybutyrate), poly(3-hydroxy octanoate), and related compounds were recently utilized for creating scaffolds, adhesion barriers, sutures, and other degradable device implants. Chitosan is lately becoming the focus of many studies across polysaccharides since it exhibits inherent antimicrobial properties, biodegradability, compatibility, wound healing capabilities, cell adhesive nature, wide accessibility, and is inexpensive [8]. Shavandi and co-workers created a chitosan (derived from squid pens), hydroxyapatite, and tricalcium phosphate-based composite structure to investigate its physiological characteristics for bone tissue regeneration [43]. The group also demonstrated that while the extent of deterioration accelerated in specimens with high concentrations of HA/TCP, the samples also displayed improved mechanical characteristics. The natural polymer-based scaffold architecture has been crucial for promoting blood vessel formation and cellular growth. A good range of pore sizes for bone regeneration is documented in the literature, ranging from 30 to 1,000 nm.

13.3.2 SYNTHETIC POLYMERS-BASED BIORESORBABLE COMPOSITES

With regard to the creation of support frameworks for tissue engineering purposes, artificial degradable polymers possess several benefits over organic polymers, such as:

- High repeatability at a macroscale level economically;
- Ease of production and modification;
- Minimum immunogenic and inflammation risk; and
- Product degradation and mechanical characteristics that could be customized based on requirements. However, they also have certain drawbacks, such as being less biocompatible than natural polymers, inadequate cell binding sites, and the degraded products produced are typically not natural metabolites, which could be problematic if they build up inside an organism [44, 45]. The main categories of artificial biodegradable polymers are primarily from the aliphatic category of polyhydroxy acids like PLA, PLLA, PDLA, and PLGA. These are frequently employed as bioabsorbable compounds for various uses in regenerative medicine [46, 47].

13.3.3 POLY(LACTIC-CO-GLYCOLIC) ACID-BASED BIORESORBABLE POLYMERS

PLGA combines polyglycolic and polylactic acid (Figure 13.2). In the past few years, they have been utilized in tissue regeneration, scaffolds for cell attachment and growth, and surgical implants inside the human body to encourage cell development and heal organs [48, 49]. A few favorable characteristics of this copolymer are structural strength and biocompatibility. Additionally, the PLGA copolymer can be broken down through hydrolysis without any enzyme action, and the breakdown leftovers are expelled as water and CO_2 [50]. PLGA can create skin-based grafts because it has compliant mechanical attributes and a controllable breakdown rate [51]. Zuber et al. [52] researched thin film creation as cellular grafts in skin regeneration. These new culture substrates were examined and explored with primary human skin cell growth, attachment, migration, and differentiation abilities alongside TCP polystyrene, which is widely used as an ideal substrate to cultivate cells. It was later shown that the fundamental activity of skin fibroblasts and keratinocytes in cell growth was unaffected by PLGA-based films. This blended polymer possesses suitable biomechanical properties, biocompatibility, and biodegradability, thus becoming an intriguing option for orthopedic services like bone reconstruction and fixation. Due to their outstanding hardness and strength, these resilient polymer composites, such as PLGA, have gained popularity in bone tissue engineering and scaffolding activities over the past few years [52, 53]. CieGlik et al. [66] assessed PLGA+HA and PLGA+carbon fiber (CF) based composite blends for restoring bone tissue. The *in vivo* data revealed that these composites are biocompatible and show non-toxicity toward growing cells. As discussed above, chitosan is a naturally occurring polymer with numerous advantages and provides certain physical qualities for utilization as a component in bone regeneration. However, it can initiate and cause reactions that form blood clots. Conversely, PLGA is an artificial polymeric compound suitable for tissue engineering and continuous drug delivery. Still, the by-products released from degradation might impede healing and promote inflammation at the unwanted site. Utilizing PLGA and chitosan-based blended composite materials could be one way to increase biological compatibility.

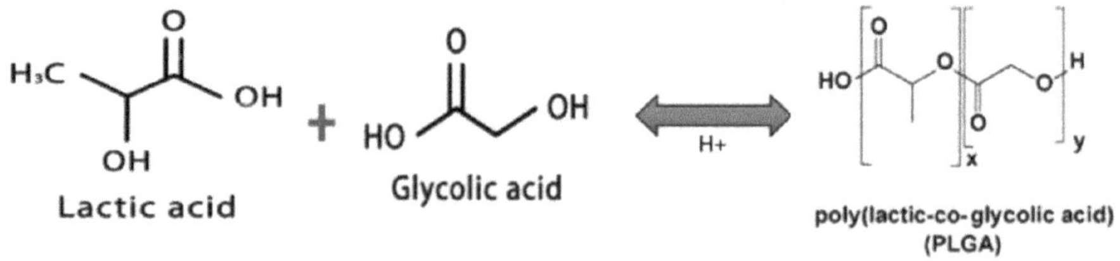

FIGURE 13.2 Poly(lactic-co-glycolic) acid-based bioresorbable polymers.

13.3.4 POLY(LACTIC ACID) (PLA)-BASED BIORESORBABLE POLYMERS

PLA is another biodegradable polymer widely applied in orthopedic and dental services [55, 56]. Yet, using PLA polymer alone has resulted in certain negative medical consequences [74]. Supplementary biocompatible ingredients, like tricalcium phosphate or hydroxyapatite, can be incorporated into the matrix to prevent or mitigate PLA-based inflammation or any other allergic reactions [58–60]. Regenerative medicine research on PLA-based composite materials, especially the blends of PLA and TCP, is extensive. Yanoso-Scholl et al. using a fast volumetric phase separation approach, examined the physical strength and microstructure characteristics of native and composite blends of PLA. It was shown that the native PLA had a porosity between 30 and 40%, which was dramatically reduced by the incorporation of TCP particles to 20.1%. Still, the torsional and compressive characteristics were markedly improved. The specific attributes of scaffolds as carriers were examined to achieve an optimally regulated release profile of osteogenic and angiogenic agents. The outcomes demonstrated the possible application of these as a delivery system for medicinal products to be delivered locally [61]. In a related study, Dong and colleagues used a melt combining technique to create PLA/tetra calcium phosphate (TTCP) that showed great mechanical stiffness. N-(2-aminoethyl)-3-aminopropyltrimethoxysilane (AEAPS) is routinely employed to alter the topography. The matrix contained pyromellitic dianhydride (PMDA) to ameliorate interfacial binding capabilities. Studies showed that it augmented the physical characteristics and increased adhesion, specifically among TTCP and PLA. Tensile strength escalated nearly from 50 to 70 MPa by using AEAPS. Based on the dynamical mechanical analysis, inserting a small amount of PMDA into this structured composite resulted in a 51% increase in storage modulus. The PLA/TTCP-based biodegradable blends show enhanced physical qualities and can prevent any inflammation-based reaction brought on by the PLA's degradation by-products [62]. As a way to improve osseointegration and physical strength for bone restoration, hydroxyapatite (HA) has served as one of the major bioactive ingredients [63–65]. Mathieu and colleagues used supercritical foaming to create composite materials for bone regeneration, which were then compared to TCP-based composites. This work examined the impact of the foaming and the structure's cellular compatibility. The findings showed that TCP produced a more homogeneous scaffold than HA because the latter tended to aggregate when dispersed across a matrix. HA obtained from natural sources (e.g., animal bones) has recently gained popularity as a substance for bone transplants and fillings.

13.3.5 POLYCAPROLACTONE-BASED BIORESORBABLE POLYMERS

Polycaprolactone is considered a bioresorbable polyester mainly used as a basal matrix in various tissue regeneration techniques [66]. Even though the native PCL polymer has certain benefits, including superb cellular compatibility, stability to temperature variations, and chemical resistance, it also has some drawbacks, such as minimal cell attachment that hinders its growth due to its hydrophobicity. As a result, PCL's surface functionalization and the creation of composites could enhance its efficiency [67–70]. Park and colleagues described the application of 3D bioprinting to create a matrix structure of PCL and TCP for bone regeneration. Researchers examined how adding more TCP (0 to 30 wt%) affected the scaffold's rigidity and capacity to promote osteogenic differentiation. According to the findings, it increased the mechanical strength, and the platform with 30 weight percent proved to be an ideal condition for bone regeneration. PCL and HA-based composites have undergone research as a potential substrate for bone tissue engineering. Leborg and colleagues [71] used a biomimetic growth method through a combined porogen leaching/phase inversion procedure to create a hybrid PCL-HAp scaffold. An examination of the scaffolds' mineralization was conducted, regardless of whether a nucleation treatment was used [72]. The addition of HAp increased the bioactivity of this matrix, and the mechanical properties were enhanced by including a nucleation treatment. The PCL-HAp composite showed promise as a suitable substrate for bone regeneration based on the findings of the automated tests.

13.4 CONCLUSION

Bioresorbable polymers have been studied recently and used heavily in tissue regeneration. However, this strategy is just starting, and barely any of them are currently used in clinical settings. The advantage of using a biodegradable polymer for internal fixation is that it prevents the requirement of secondary surgery for removal once the healing process is complete. Due to their capacity to offer the requisite mechanical qualities for tissue repair and rapid cell growth and attachment, bioresorbable composites are receiving increasing attention. The optimized breakdown process for this biodegradable material must occur within a feasible environment that guides it to fulfill a particular role inside the organ. Poly-lactate can meet the above requirements for various purposes due to the presence of chirality and the capacity for copolymerization with other polymers. The absorption and potential diffusion of nano-sized particles into neighboring tissues are significant obstacles for nano-composites. Before bioresorbable polymers are broadly accessible as routine implants, a multidisciplinary perspective is also required for their thorough consideration. Additionally, for widespread application in tissue engineering, material composites should be produced cost-effectively and in large quantities.

KEYWORDS

- **bioabsorbable polymers**
- **biomaterials**
- **copolymerization**
- **diffusion**
- **polymeric biomaterials**
- **tissue engineering**

References

1. Ciclo, X. X. II. (2010). *Dottorato Di Ricerca In Chimica Industriale: Porous Polymeric Bioresorbable Scaffolds for Tissue Engineering.*
2. Mather, M. L., Brion, M., White, L. J., Shakesheff, K. M., Howdle, S. M., Morgan, S. P., & Crowe, J. A. (2009). Time-lapsed imaging for in-process evaluation of supercritical fluid processing of tissue engineering scaffolds. *Biotechnology Progress, 25*(4), 1176–1183. https://doi.org/10.1002/btpr.191.
3. Cima, L. G., Vacanti, J. P., Vacanti, C., Ingber, D., Mooney, D., & Langer, R. (1991). Tissue engineering by cell transplantation using degradable polymer substrates. *Journal of Biomechanical Engineering, 113*(2), 143–151. https://doi.org/10.1115/1.2891228.
4. O'Brien, F. J. (2011). Biomaterials & scaffolds for tissue engineering. *Materials Today, 14*(3), 88–95. https://doi.org/10.1016/S1369-7021(11)70058-X.
5. Barry, J. J. A., Gidda, H. S., Scotchford, C. A., & Howdle, S. M. (2004). Porous methacrylate scaffolds: Supercritical fluid fabrication and in vitro chondrocyte responses. *Biomaterials, 25*(16), 3559–3568. https://doi.org/10.1016/j.biomaterials.2003.10.023.
6. Kang, H. W., Tabata, Y., & Ikada, Y. (1999). Fabrication of porous gelatin scaffolds for tissue engineering. *Biomaterials, 20*(14), 1339–1344. https://doi.org/10.1016/S0142-9612(99)00036-8.
7. Wang, M. (2006). Composite scaffolds for bone tissue engineering. *American Journal of Biochemistry and Biotechnology, 2*(2), 80–84. https://doi.org/10.3844/ajbbsp.2006.80.84.
8. Suh, J. K., & Matthew, H. W. (2000). Application of chitosan-based polysaccharide biomaterials in cartilage tissue engineering: A review. *Biomaterials, 21*(25), 2589–2598. https://doi.org/10.1016/S0142-9612(00)00126-5.
9. He, W., Yong, T., Teo, W. E., Ma, Z., & Ramakrishna, S. (2005). Fabrication and endothelialization of collagen-blended biodegradable polymer nanofibers: Potential vascular graft for blood vessel tissue engineering. *Tissue Engineering, 11*(11–12), 1574–1588. https://doi.org/10.1089/ten.2005.11.1574.

10. Chaudhari, A. A. (2016). Future prospects for scaffolding methods and biomaterials in skin tissue engineering: A review. *International Journal of Molecular Sciences, 17*(12). https://doi.org/10.3390/ijms17122088.
11. Avti, P. K., Patel, S. C., Uppal, P., O'Malley, G., Garlow, J., & Sitharaman, B. (2012). Nano biomaterials for tissue engineering. In *Tissue Engineering: Principles and Practices* (pp. 235–260). CRC Press.
12. Naleway, S. E., Lear, W., Kruzic, J. J., & Maughan, C. B. (2015). Mechanical properties of suture materials in general and cutaneous surgery. *Journal of Biomedical Materials Research Part B: Applied Biomaterials, 103*(4), 735–742. https://doi.org/10.1002/jbm.b.33171.
13. Kronenthal, R. (1975). *Polymers in medicine and surgery*. Island Press.
14. Mukherjee, D. P., & Pietrzak, W. S. (2011). Bioabsorbable fixation: Scientific, technical, and clinical concepts. *Journal of Craniofacial Surgery, 22*(2), 679–689. https://doi.org/10.1097/SCS.0b013e318207432f.
15. Vert, M., Li, S. M., Spenlehauer, G., & Guerin, P. (1992). Bioresorbability and biocompatibility of aliphatic polyesters. *Journal of Materials Science: Materials in Medicine, 3*(5), 432–446. https://doi.org/10.1007/BF00701240.
16. Uhrich, K. E., & Abdelhamid, D. (2016). Biodegradable and bio erodible polymers for medical applications. In L. Poole-Warren, P. Martens, & R. Green (Eds.), *Biosynthetic Polymers for Medical Applications* (pp. 63–83). Woodhead Publishing.
17. Generali, M., & Hoerstrup, S. P. (2014). Bioresorbable scaffolds for cardiovascular tissue engineering. *EMJ–International Cardiology, 1*(2), 91–99.
18. Akinapelli, A., Chen, J. P., Roy, K., Donnelly, J., Dawkins, K., Huibregtse, B., & Hou, D. (2017). Current state of bioabsorbable polymer-coated drug-eluting stents. *Current Cardiology Reviews, 13*(2), 139–154. https://doi.org/10.2174/1573403X12666161222155230.
19. Dhaliwal, K., & Dosanjh, P. (2018). Biodegradable polymers and their role in drug delivery systems. *Biomedical Journal of Scientific & Technical Research, 11*(3), 8315–8320. https://doi.org/10.26717/BJSTR.2018.11.002056.
20. Sheridan, M. H., Shea, L. D., Peters, M. C., & Mooney, D. J. (2000). Bioabsorbable polymer scaffolds for tissue engineering capable of sustained growth factor delivery. *Journal of Controlled Release, 64*(1), 91–102. https://doi.org/10.1016/S0168-3659(99)00138-8.
21. Alexy, R. D., & Levi, D. S. (2013). Materials and manufacturing technologies available for production of a pediatric bioabsorbable stent. *Biomedical Research International, 2013*, 137985. https://doi.org/10.1155/2013/137985.
22. Shikinami, Y., & Okuno, M. (2001). Bioresorbable devices made of forged composites of hydroxyapatite (HA) particles and poly l-lactide (PLLA). Part II: Practical properties of minis crews and miniplates. *Biomaterials, 22*(14), 3197–3211. https://doi.org/10.1016/S0142-9612(01)00072-2.
23. Ramakrishna, S., Mayer, J., Wintermantel, E., & Leong, K. W. (2001). Biomedical applications of polymer-composite materials: A review. *Composites Science and Technology, 61*(8), 1189–1224. https://doi.org/10.1016/S0266-3538(00)00241-4.
24. Eberhart, R. C., Su, S. H., Nguyen, K. T., Zilberman, M., Tang, L., Nelson, K. D., & Frenkel, P. (2003). Bioresorbable polymeric stents: Current status and future promise. *Journal of Biomaterials Science, Polymer Edition, 14*(3), 299–312. https://doi.org/10.1163/156856203321478838.

25. Ignjatovic, N., Wu, V., Ajduković, Z., Mihajilov-Krstev, T., Uskoković, V., & Uskoković, D. (2016). Chitosan-PLGA polymer blends as coatings for hydroxyapatite nanoparticles and their effect on antimicrobial properties, osteoconductivity, and regeneration of osseous tissues. *Materials Science and Engineering: C, Materials for Biological Applications, 60*, 357–364. https://doi.org/10.1016/j.msec.2015.11.061.
26. Santos, A. R. (2011). Bioresorbable polymers for tissue engineering. *Tissue Engineering, 18*(2), 225–246.
27. Loan, S., & Buruiana, L. I. (2017). Biodegradable polymers in tissue engineering. In V. K. Thakur, M. K. Thakur, & M. R. Kessler (Eds.), *Handbook of Composites from Renewable Materials* (pp. 145–182). John Wiley & Sons.
28. Shikinami, Y., Okazaki, K., Saito, M., Okuno, M., Hasegawa, S., Tamura, J., Fujibayashi, S., & Nakamura, T. (2006). Bioactive and bioresorbable cellular cubic-composite scaffolds for use in bone reconstruction. *Journal of the Royal Society Interface, 3*(9), 805–821. https://doi.org/10.1098/rsif.2006.0144.
29. Wuisman, P. I. J. M., & Smit, T. H. (2006). Bioresorbable polymers: Heading for a new generation of spinal cages. *European Spine Journal, 15*(2), 133–148. https://doi.org/10.1007/s00586-005-1003-6.
30. Ulery, B. D., Nair, L. S., & Laurencin, C. T. (2011). Biomedical applications of biodegradable polymers. *Journal of Polymer Science Part B: Polymer Physics, 49*(9), 832–864. https://doi.org/10.1002/polb.22259.
31. Buchanan, F. (2008). *Degradation Rate of Bioresorbable Materials*. Woodhead Publishing.
32. von Burkersroda, F., Schedl, L., & Gopferich, A. (2002). Why degradable polymers undergo surface erosion or bulk erosion. *Biomaterials, 23*(21), 4221–4231. https://doi.org/10.1016/S0142-9612(02)00170-9.
33. Tamada, J. A., & Langer, R. (1993). Erosion kinetics of hydrolytically degradable polymers. *Proceedings of the National Academy of Sciences USA, 90*(2), 552–556. https://doi.org/10.1073/pnas.90.2.552.
34. Li, S. M., Garreau, H., & Vert, M. (1990). Structure-property relationships in the case of the degradation of massive aliphatic poly- (α-hydroxy acids) in aqueous media. *Journal of Materials Science: Materials in Medicine, 1*(2), 123–130. https://doi.org/10.1007/BF00700871.
35. Alexis, F. (2005). Factors affecting the degradation and drug-release mechanism of poly (lactic acid) and poly [(lactic acid)-co- (glycolic acid)]. *Polymer International, 54*(1), 36–46. https://doi.org/10.1002/pi.1697.
36. Wang, J., Wang, L., Zhou, Z., Lai, H., Xu, P., Liao, L., & Wei, J. (2016). Biodegradable polymer membranes applied in guided bone/tissue regeneration: A review. *Polymers, 8*(4), 115. https://doi.org/10.3390/polym8040115.
37. Gupta, P., & Nayak, K. K. (2015). Characteristics of protein-based biopolymer and its application. *Polymer Engineering & Science, 55*(2), 485–498. https://doi.org/10.1002/pen.23928.
38. Crini, G. (2005). Recent developments in polysaccharide-based materials used as adsorbents in wastewater treatment. *Progress in Polymer Science, 30*(1), 38–70. https://doi.org/10.1016/j.progpolymsci.2004.11.002.
39. Lenz, R. W., & Marchessault, R. H. (2005). Bacterial polyesters: Biosynthesis, biodegradable plastics, and biotechnology. *Biomacromolecules, 6*(1), 1–8. https://doi.org/10.1021/bm049700c.

40. Paul, W., & Sharma, C. P. (2008). Natural bioresorbable polymers. In F. Buchanan (Ed.), *Degradation Rate of Bioresorbable Materials* (pp. 67–94). Woodhead Publishing.
41. Sampath, U., Ching, Y., Chuah, C., Sabariah, J., & Lin, P. C. (2016). Fabrication of porous materials from natural/synthetic biopolymers and their composites. *Materials, 9*(12), 991. https://doi.org/10.3390/ma9120991.
42. Chen, G. Q., & Wu, Q. (2005). The application of polyhydroxyalkanoates as tissue engineering materials. *Biomaterials, 26*(33), 6565–6578. https://doi.org/10.1016/j.biomaterials.2005.04.036.
43. Shavandi, A., Bekhit, A. E. D. A., Sun, Z., Ali, A., & Gould, M. (2015). A novel squid pen chitosan/hydroxyapatite/β-tricalcium phosphate composite for bone tissue engineering. *Materials Science and Engineering: C, Materials for Biological Applications, 55*, 373–383. https://doi.org/10.1016/j.msec.2015.05.029.
44. Guan, J., Sacks, M. S., Beckman, E. J., & Wagner, W. R. (2004). Biodegradable poly (ether ester urethane) urea elastomers based on poly (ether ester) triblock copolymers and putrescine: Synthesis, characterization, and cytocompatibility. *Biomaterials, 25*(1), 85–96. https://doi.org/10.1016/S0142-9612(03)00476-9.
45. Cameron, R. E., & Kamvari-Moghaddam, A. (2012). Synthetic bioresorbable polymers. In M. Jenkins & A. Stamboulis (Eds.), *Durability and Reliability of Medical Polymers* (pp. 96–118). Woodhead Publishing.
46. Albertsson, A. C., & Varma, I. K. (2002). Aliphatic polyesters: Synthesis, properties and applications. In *Degradable Aliphatic Polyesters* (pp. 1–40). Springer Berlin Heidelberg.
47. Nair, L. S., & Laurencin, C. T. (2007). Biodegradable polymers as biomaterials. *Progress in Polymer Science, 32*(8–9), 762–798. https://doi.org/10.1016/j.progpolymsci.2007.05.017.
48. Xiao, L., Wang, B., Yang, G., & Gauthier, M. (2012). Poly (lactic acid)-based biomaterials: Synthesis, modification and applications. In D. N. Ghista (Ed.), *Biomedical Science, Engineering and Technology*. IntechOpen. https://doi.org/10.5772/23927.
49. Cheng, Y., Deng, S., Chen, P., & Ruan, R. (2009). Polylactic acid (PLA) synthesis and modifications: A review. *Frontiers in Chemistry, 4*, 259–264. https://doi.org/10.1007/s11458-009-0092-x.
50. Makadia, H. K., & Siegel, S. J. (2011). Poly lactic-co-glycolic acid (PLGA) as biodegradable controlled drug delivery carrier. *Polymers, 3*(3), 1377–1397. https://doi.org/10.3390/polym3031377.
51. Baoyong, L., Jian, Z., Denglong, C., & Min, L. (2010). Evaluation of a new type of wound dressing made from recombinant spider silk protein using rat models. *Burns, 36*(6), 891–896. https://doi.org/10.1016/j.burns.2009.12.001.
52. Hollinger, J. (1993). Strategies for regenerating bone of the craniofacial complex. *Bone, 14*(6), 575–580. https://doi.org/10.1016/8756-3282(93)90196-H.
53. Zhang, R., & Ma, P. X. (1999). Poly (alpha-hydroxyl acids)/hydroxyapatite porous composites for bone-tissue engineering. I. Preparation and morphology. *Journal of Biomedical Materials Research, 44*(4), 446–455. https://doi.org/10.1002/(SICI)1097-4636(19990315)44:4<446:AID-JBM11>3.0.CO;2-F.
54. Cieślik, M., Mertas, A., Morawska-Chochół, A., Sabat, D., Orlicki, R., Owczarek, A., Król, W., & Cieślik, T. (2009). The evaluation of the possibilities of using PLGA co-polymer and its composites with carbon fibers or hydroxyapatite in the bone tissue

regeneration process–In vitro and in vivo examinations. *International Journal of Molecular Sciences, 10*(7), 3224–3234. https://doi.org/10.3390/ijms10073224.
55. Persson, M., Lorite, G. S., Kokkonen, H. E., Cho, S. W., Lehenkari, P. P., Skrifvars, M., & Tuukkanen, J. (2014). Effect of bioactive extruded PLA/HA composite films on focal adhesion formation of preosteoblastic cells. *Colloids and Surfaces B: Biointerfaces, 121*, 409–416. https://doi.org/10.1016/j.colsurfb.2014.06.029.
56. Kutikov, A. B., & Song, J. (2013). An amphiphilic degradable polymer/hydroxyapatite composite with enhanced handling characteristics promotes osteogenic gene expression in bone marrow stromal cells. *Acta Biomaterialia, 9*(8), 8354–8364. https://doi.org/10.1016/j.actbio.2013.06.013.
57. Hong, Z., Zhang, P., He, C., Qiu, X., Liu, A., Chen, L., Chen, X., & Jing, X. (2005). Nano-composite of poly(l-lactide) and surface grafted hydroxyapatite: Mechanical properties and biocompatibility. *Biomaterials, 26*(29), 6296–6304. https://doi.org/10.1016/j.biomaterials.2005.04.018.
58. Mathieu, L. M., Montjovent, M. O., Bourban, P. E., Pioletti, D. P., & Månson, J. A. E. (2005). Bioresorbable composites prepared by supercritical fluid foaming. *Journal of Biomedical Materials Research Part A, 75*(1), 89–97.
59. Lee, M. R., Lee, G. W., Kim, J. E., Yun, W. B., Choi, J. Y., Park, J. J., Kim, H. R., Song, B. R., Park, J. W., Kang, M. J., et al. (2019). Biocompatibility of a PLA-based composite containing hydroxyapatite derived from waste bones of dolphin *Neophocaena asiaeorientalis*. *Journal of the Australian Ceramic Society, 55*(3), 269–279. https://doi.org/10.1007/s41779-018-0232-1.
60. Rakmae, S., Ruksakulpiwat, Y., Sutapun, W., & Suppakarn, N. (2011). Physical properties and cytotoxicity of surface-modified bovine bone-based hydroxyapatite/poly (lactic acid) composites. *Journal of Composite Materials, 45*(12), 1259–1269. https://doi.org/10.1177/0021998310377934.
61. Kothapalli, C. R., Shaw, M. T., & Wei, M. (2005). Biodegradable HAPLA 3-D porous scaffolds: Effect of nano-sized filler content on scaffold properties. *Acta Biomaterialia, 1*(6), 653–662. https://doi.org/10.1016/j.actbio.2005.06.005.
62. Montjovent, M. O., Mathieu, L., Hinz, B., Applegate, L. L., Bourban, P. E., Zambelli, P. Y., Månson, J. A., & Pioletti, D. P. (2005). Biocompatibility of bioresorbable poly (L-lactic acid) composite scaffolds obtained by supercritical gas foaming with human fetal bone cells. *Tissue Engineering, 11*(11–12), 1640–1649. https://doi.org/10.1089/ten.2005.11.1640.
63. Sanchez-Arevalo, F. M., Munoz-Ramírez, L. D., Alvarez-Camacho, M., Rivera-Torres, F., Maciel-Cerda, A., Montiel-Campos, R., & Vera-Graziano, R. (2017). Macro- and micromechanical behaviors of poly (lactic acid)–hydroxyapatite electrospun composite scaffolds. *Journal of Materials Science, 52*(7), 3353–3367. https://doi.org/10.1007/s10853-016-0624-y.
64. McManus, A. J., Doremus, R. H., Siegel, R. W., & Bizios, R. (2005). Evaluation of cytocompatibility and bending modulus of nanoceramic/polymer composites. *Journal of Biomedical Materials Research, 72A* (1), 98–106. https://doi.org/10.1002/jbm.a.30204.
65. Akindoyo, J. O., Beg, M. D. H., Ghazali, S., Heim, H. P., & Feldmann, M. (2017). Effects of surface modification on dispersion, mechanical, thermal and dynamic mechanical properties of injection molded PLA-hydroxyapatite composites. *Composites Part A: Applied Science and Manufacturing, 103*, 96–105. https://doi.org/10.1016/j.compositesa.2017.09.013.

66. Oh, S. H., Park, I. K., Kim, J. M., & Lee, J. H. (2007). In vitro and in vivo characteristics of PCL scaffolds with pore size gradient fabricated by a centrifugation method. *Biomaterials, 28*(10), 1664–1671. https://doi.org/10.1016/j.biomaterials.2006.11.024.
67. Sousa, I. S., Mendes, A., & Bartolo, P. J. (2013). PCL scaffolds with collagen bio activator for applications in tissue engineering. *Procedia Engineering, 59*, 279–284. https://doi.org/10.1016/j.proeng.2013.05.122.
68. Dell'Erba, R., Groeninckx, G., Maglio, G., Malinconico, M., & Migliozzi, A. (2001). Immiscible polymer blends of semicrystalline biocompatible components: Thermal properties and phase morphology analysis of PLLA/PCL blends. *Polymer, 42*(16), 7831–7840. https://doi.org/10.1016/S0032-3861(01)00269-5.
69. Coombes, A. G. A., Rizzi, S. C., Williamson, M., Barralet, J. E., Downes, S., & Wallace, W. A. (2004). Precipitation casting of polycaprolactone for applications in tissue engineering and drug delivery. *Biomaterials, 25*(2), 315–325. https://doi.org/10.1016/S0142-9612(03)00535-0.
70. Averous, L. (2000). Properties of thermoplastic blends: Starch–polycaprolactone. *Polymer, 41*(11), 4157–4167. https://doi.org/10.1016/S0032-3861(99)00636-9.
71. Lebourg, M., Suay Anton, J., & Gomez Ribelles, J. L. (2010). Hybrid structure in PCL-HAp scaffold resulting from biomimetic apatite growth. *Journal of Materials Science: Materials in Medicine, 21*(1), 33–44. https://doi.org/10.1007/s10856-009-3838-6.
72. Park, S. H., Park, S. A., Kang, Y. G., Shin, J. W., Park, Y. S., Gu, S. R., Wu, Y. R., Wei, J., & Shin, J. W. (2017). PCL/β-TCP composite scaffolds exhibit positive osteogenic differentiation with mechanical stimulation. *Tissue Engineering and Regenerative Medicine, 14*(3), 349–358. https://doi.org/10.1007/s13770-017-0022-9.
73. Iqbal, N., Khan, A. S., Asif, A., Yar, M., Haycock, J. W., & Rehman, I. U. (2019). Recent concepts in biodegradable polymers for tissue engineering paradigms: A critical review. *International Materials Reviews, 64*(2), 91–126. https://doi.org/10.1080/09506608.2018.1460943.
74. Vert, M. (1989). Bioresorbable polymers for temporary therapeutic applications. *Angewandte Makromolekulare Chemie, 166*, 155–168. https://doi.org/10.1002/apmc.1989.051660111.
75. Vert, M., Li, S. M., Spenlehauer, G., & Guerin, P. (1992). Bioresorbability and biocompatibility of aliphatic polyesters. *Journal of Materials Science: Materials in Medicine, 3*(5), 432–446. https://doi.org/10.1007/BF00701240.

Index

α

α-amino acids, 9
α-chymotrypsin, 36

β

β-linked polysaccharide, 36
β-oxidation, 37
β-tricalcium phosphate (β-TCP), 137, 139, 140, 185, 254, 255

γ

γ-radiation, 22, 23

A

Abiotic deterioration, 119
Acetonitrile, 9
Acetylation, 7, 83
Acidic environments, 116
Acrylic acid grafting, 134
Actin filament organization, 137
Additive manufacturing (AM), 243, 245–247, 250, 251, 257, 259
Adenosine triphosphate (ATP), 14
Adhesion
  barriers, 249, 272
  prone tissues, 20
Adhesive, 212, 232, 234, 249, 272
Adipose-derived stem cells (ADSCs), 253
Agricultural waste, 113
Alginate, 34, 35, 41, 44–46, 49, 132, 153–155, 158, 165, 185, 231, 247–249, 252, 269, 272
  bio-nanocomposite, 153–155
    scaffolds, 35, 49
Aliphatic
  poly(amino acids), 248
  polyester, 34, 37, 250, 256
Alkaline treatment, 121, 122
Allergic reactions, 253, 275
Allogeneic grafts, 184
Allograft, 184, 185, 188, 194, 268
Alloplastic grafts, 184, 185
Allylamine, 66
Alternating magnetic field (AMF), 49, 51
Alumina, 191
Alveolar
  bone grafts, 184
  processes, 185
Alzheimer's disease (AD), 47
Amide functional groups, 5
Amikacin-loaded hydrogels, 223
Amino glucose macromolecule clustering process, 141
Aminopropyltrimethoxysilane (AEAPS), 275
Amoxicillin (AMX), 49, 223
Anaerobic composting environments, 24
Anatomical
  abnormality, 173
  regions, 183
  repair, 183
Angiogenesis, 182, 223, 226, 228, 230–232
  properties, 232
Angular stability, 172
Angulation, 172
Anisotropic, 130, 133, 165, 246
  features, 133
Anisotropy, 16, 41, 43, 163, 165
Anterior compression, 167
Antibacterial, 46, 81–83, 89, 91, 99, 119, 182, 203, 204, 206–209, 211, 212, 222, 223, 226–229, 232, 249
  activity, 46, 82, 91, 99, 204, 208, 209, 211, 222, 226, 227, 232, 249
  additives, 83, 206
  characteristics, 119
  films, 91
  properties, 82, 203, 207–209, 211, 212, 222, 223, 228
Antibiotics, 223
Anti-collagenase activity, 223
Antidiabetic treatments, 154

Antifungal
agents, 114
drugs, 229
Antiinflammatory, 182, 220, 224, 229, 230, 233
compounds, 233
Antimicrobial, 38, 44–46, 82, 89, 106, 114, 139, 149, 156, 159, 204, 206, 210, 220, 222, 223, 232, 233, 235, 249, 272
activity, 38, 89, 106, 149, 159, 206
agents, 156
amalgamation, 220
concentrations, 139
fillers, 210
hydrogels, 220, 222, 229, 235
medicines, 223
properties, 220, 272
Antioxidant, 114, 223
capacity, 223
Anti-oxidation effects, 220
Anti-swelling, 228
Anti-tumor activity, 156
Apatite formation ability, 255
Apical periodontitis, 203
Arbitrary chain scission, 112
Arrhythmogenic features, 136
Artificial
biodegradable polymers, 273
devices, 24
materials, 166, 182, 185
Aseptic loosening, 184
Atrophy, 181, 184
Autograft, 185, 194, 268
Autologous
bone transplant, 184
grafts, 184
Axial
compression, 167
stability, 165

B

Bacillus cereus, 156
Bacterial cellulose (BC), 38
Balloon kyphoplasty, 136
Benzoyl peroxide, 136
Betamethasone sodium phosphate (BSP), 48
Binder jetting (BJ), 246, 257
Bioabsorbable, 3, 5, 6, 9–11, 19–22, 32, 49, 50, 105–111, 116, 117, 122, 123, 192, 193, 245, 253, 258, 267, 270, 273, 277
bone fixation devices, 6
composites, 107, 122, 123
implants, 6, 11, 23
materials, 23, 105, 106, 111, 192
osteosynthetic material, 108
polymer (BAP), 1–3, 5, 6, 8, 10, 12, 13, 19, 22, 31, 32, 34, 41, 49, 50, 61, 81, 105, 109, 110, 129, 149, 163, 181, 203, 219, 243, 267, 269, 270, 277
plates, 111
polymer-based scaffolds, 49
polymeric composites, 106, 107, 109, 110, 122
Bio-absorption, 50, 51
Bioactive
capability, 210
ceramic, 197, 245
powders, 182
chitosan composites, 141
glass (BG), 137, 182, 184, 186, 191, 193, 253
ceramics, 137
fibers, 182
polyester composites, 182
shaping, 184
materials, 182, 192, 193
properties, 186, 192
Bioactivity, 81, 206
Bioadhesion capacity, 232
Bioadhesive, 154
hydrogels, 231, 232
Bio-anchors, 20
Bio-based
packaging methods, 82
polymeric materials, 91
resorbable composites, 164
Bioceramic, 129, 143, 191, 197
materials, 191
Biocompatibility, 1, 2, 31, 33, 35–38, 44, 49, 67, 71, 81, 82, 89, 91, 99, 108, 123, 129, 132, 134, 149, 153, 154, 185, 187, 190, 196, 203, 206, 207, 209, 210, 212, 220, 228, 229, 244, 248–250, 252, 254, 256, 258, 259, 271–274
Biocompatible
ceramics, 194

implant devices, 1
medicines, 159
nanocomposite hydrogels, 221
Biocomposite, 4, 81, 82, 163, 175, 181, 203–205, 207, 211, 212
materials, 203
Biodegradability, 24, 35–37, 73, 81, 82, 89, 118, 121, 122, 138, 139, 153, 154, 185, 193, 206, 229–231, 244, 248, 249, 255, 258, 272, 274
Biodegradable
material, 3, 5, 23, 120, 137, 138, 141, 149, 150, 231, 244, 276
metals, 183, 187
polyesters, 5
polymer, 2, 22, 24, 31, 47, 73, 81, 106, 114, 140, 192, 244, 258, 269, 273
processing, 257
polymeric materials, 32, 248, 249
scaffolds, 32
Biodegradation, 5, 7, 8, 13, 38, 50, 51, 63, 74, 109, 117, 138–140, 231, 270
Bioelectronic devices, 229
Bioengineering, 193, 194
Bio-erodible, 245
polymers, 269
Biofabrication method, 221
Bioglass, 190
Bioimplants, 23, 107
Bioinert
alloys, 182
ceramics, 197
Bio-inspired materials, 182
Biological
characteristics, 6, 184
compatibility, 63, 204, 274
materials, 182, 184, 185, 187
processes, 85, 183, 220, 268
reactions, 184, 186, 192
sciences, 184, 268
Biology, 64, 182
Biomarkers, 63
Biomaterials, 7, 8, 38, 72, 83, 89, 105, 111, 129–131, 149, 150, 164, 175, 182, 184–187, 191–194, 196, 197, 204, 205, 220, 221, 227, 231, 244, 246–248, 253, 258, 268–271, 277
Biomechanical
characteristics, 164, 165
findings, 163
force, 168
investigation, 169, 171
processes, 183
properties, 274
study, 166
testing, 168
Biomedical
3D applications, 243
applications, 5, 6, 21, 31, 32, 61, 62, 66, 105–107, 117, 118, 122, 123, 131, 149, 158, 227, 243, 250, 258, 259
devices, 1, 149, 268
implants, 105, 190
industry, 67, 69, 105, 106, 210
materials, 122, 184
science, 210
sectors, 123
Biomedicine, 61, 62, 68, 149, 159
Biometals, 183
Biomimetic, 194
composites, 143, 196, 197
growth method, 276
matrices, 194, 196
Biomimicry, 193, 258
Biomolecular linkages, 63
Biomolecule-functionalized nanoparticles, 64
Bio-nanocomposite, 115, 149–159
antimicrobial characteristic, 156
healthcare applications, 154
thermal
degradation, 114
stability, 115
Biopharmaceutical analysis, 66
Bio-polymer, 82, 88, 90, 114, 115, 143, 150, 152, 154, 159, 185, 249
ceramic composites, 129
matrix, 115
Bioprinting, 49, 158, 159, 196, 244, 253, 256, 257, 276
Bio-resorbability, 50
Bioresorbable, 1, 3, 5, 24, 47, 186, 243–245, 247, 248, 250, 252, 259, 269–272, 274–276
composites, 243, 276
material, 1, 243, 248
polymeric
composites, 248
materials, 243, 247, 248, 252
polymers, 1, 3, 24, 224, 247, 250, 252, 269, 270, 272, 274, 276
Biotechnology, 1, 24, 193, 258

Blood
brain
barrier (BBB), 47
tumor barrier (BBTB), 47
cerebrospinal fluid barrier, 47
coagulation, 227
vessel, 8, 19, 143, 248, 268
formation, 273
Bone, 2–4, 6–9, 12, 13, 19–22, 24, 33, 36, 37, 44–46, 48, 71, 72, 105–107, 110, 111, 116, 120, 121, 129–143, 157, 158, 163–169, 171, 172, 175, 181–188, 190–194, 196, 206, 245, 247, 248, 250–256, 268–270, 272–276
augmentation, 129, 131, 143
degeneration, 184
disease, 33, 129, 137, 138
extracellular matrix, 46
fracture, 2, 6, 130, 183
healing, 21, 183
therapy, 183
graft, 182, 184, 185, 196
healing, 4, 121, 130, 137, 185, 255
implant, 106, 164, 175
contact, 245
load-bearing replacement, 245
marrow stem cells (BMSCs), 252, 253, 256
matrix's size, 164
mimic approach, 132
mineralization, 141
morphogenetic protein (BMP), 185, 194
2 (BMP-2), 8
plates, 9, 165, 182, 183, 268
quality, 141, 169, 172, 183
reconstruction applications, 134
regeneration, 3, 4, 8, 22, 36, 44, 46, 48, 71, 72, 120, 138, 139, 182, 185, 187, 196, 250, 255, 256, 269, 273–276
matrix, 185
repair, 45, 46, 120, 184, 193, 247, 250, 254, 270
replacement, 129, 165, 183
scaffold applications, 37
tissue, 116, 130–133, 138, 140, 143, 157, 158, 182, 184, 187, 192, 193, 196, 252, 256, 270, 274, 276
engineering, 116, 131, 138, 143, 158, 182, 184, 196, 252, 256, 270, 274, 276
transplants, 184, 185, 275
Boron nitride (BN), 209
nanotubes (BNNTs), 210
Botanical medications, 224
Bovine serum albumin (BSA), 46
Brittleness, 38, 206
Bungee jumping, 164
Butyric-2-butenoate, 112

C

Calcium
carbonate, 49
chloride, 232, 233
orthophosphates, 131
phosphate, 6–8, 129, 131, 137, 139, 141, 187, 188, 209, 275
cement (CPC), 139, 188
nano-crystals, 8
particles, 6
Calendula, 224
Callus, 183
Cancellous bone fractures, 6
Cancer
immunotherapy, 49
therapy, 61, 62, 73, 149
treatment, 35, 36, 44, 47, 48, 50, 66, 67, 72
Carbides, 191
Carbon
composites, 235
dioxide gas, 40, 108
fiber (CF), 255, 274
monoxide, 112
multifunctional nanostructures, 227
nanomaterials, 226
nanotubes (CNT), 66–68, 70, 71, 73, 114, 115, 151, 210, 226, 228
Carboxyl-functionalized SPIONs, 70
Carboxylic acid, 36, 112
Carboxymethyl cellulose, 82
Carcinogenic treatment, 61
Cardiovascular applications, 105
Cartilage, 24, 34, 36, 143, 182, 183, 185, 248, 249, 268, 272
engineering, 249
Cefazolin (CEF), 46
Cell
adhesion, 8, 32, 244, 249, 269
binding sites, 273

delivery agents, 272
interaction, 248
membranes, 165
migration, 233
proliferation, 22, 32, 46, 47, 67, 116, 193, 222, 231, 245, 256
Cellular
compatibility, 70, 73, 74, 275, 276
growth, 273
Cellulose
bio-nanocomposites, 153
fibers, 116, 151, 153
nanocrystal (CNC), 48
nanowhiskers, 114, 115
thermal degradation, 113
Centellae herba, 224
Central nervous system (CNS), 47, 50
Ceramic, 107, 129, 137, 143, 184, 190, 191, 193, 194, 197, 245, 246, 268, 270
bioglass composites, 131
biomaterials, 105, 190
Chemical
catalyzed hydrolysis reactions, 272
characteristics, 62, 248, 250
composition, 17, 62, 68, 257, 271
cross-linking strategies, 234
decomposition, 105
degradation, 109, 267
inertness, 210, 256
interactions, 134
vapor deposition (CVD), 66
Chemotherapy, 20, 47
Chirality, 276
Chitin, 7, 34, 36, 82–87, 99, 140, 141, 153, 207
deacetylase enzyme, 87
Chitosan, 7, 8, 32–36, 41, 47, 48, 71, 81–84, 86–92, 99, 132, 140–142, 149, 153–158, 185, 194, 204, 207, 208, 211, 212, 222, 223, 231, 232, 247–250, 269, 271, 272, 274
alginate-based nanocomposite, 155
antimicrobial properties, 91
bio-nanocomposites, 153–157
composites, 141
derivatives, 88, 91, 141
dressings, 222
drug carriers, 36
films, 88
hydrogel-based sealant, 208
nanocomposites, 158
nanoparticles, 207, 208
natural polymer, 249
silk fibroin (CS/SF), 250
Chronic
exposure, 74
inflammation, 223, 225
wound, 219, 223–225, 229–233, 235
healing, 229, 230
remodeling, 229
therapy methods, 229
treatment, 225, 229, 231
Ciprofloxacin, 48
Cis-elimination, 112
Citrate-hydroxyapatite nanoparticles (cHA), 46
Cleft
lips, 182, 184
palates, 182, 184
Coacervates, 82
Cobalt alloys, 189
Collagen (Col), 6–8, 32, 34–37, 45–47, 71, 130, 133, 153, 164, 165, 185, 188, 189, 196, 223, 231, 244, 247–249, 269, 271, 272
brushite cement paste, 7
Colloidal stability, 62
Commercially pure titanium (CP-Ti), 190
Complex tissue
regeneration & repair, 143
Composite, 6–8, 12, 35, 40, 71, 89, 105–107, 109, 110, 116–120, 122, 129–134, 137, 139–143, 150, 151, 164, 166, 175, 182, 185, 188, 196, 203–206, 209–211, 225, 228, 245, 251–257, 259, 267, 268, 270, 272, 274–276
architecture, 110
biodegradable polymers, 137
materials, 204, 270
Compound annual growth rate (CAGR), 82
Computer-aided
design (CAD), 246, 255
wet-spinning (CAWS), 251
Conducting polymer (CPs), 228
hydrogels (CPHs), 228
Confocal laser scanning microscopy (CLSM), 251

micrograph, 251
Connective tissue, 24
Conventional
composites, 154
materials, 186
treatment strategies, 130
Copolymerization, 108, 115, 258, 276, 277
Copper
fluoride nanoparticles, 209
oxide nanoparticles, 209
Co-precipitation technique, 120, 142
Core/shell electrospun fiber, 47
Cori cycle, 14
Cosmetic, 149
industry, 154, 159
Covalent interactions, 62, 68
Crack bridging, 157, 182
Cranial
bone
deficiencies, 184
malformations, 181
fractures, 182
implants, 182
materials, 182
Craniofacial
area, 183
augmentation, 196
bone, 182
implants, 182
procedures, 184
reconstruction, 181, 184, 196
surgery, 108
Craniomaxillofacial surgery, 182
Cranium, 182
Creep test, 19
Cross-sectional area, 41
Crotonic acid, 112
Cryogels, 48
Crystalline
materials, 16
nanoparticles, 22
polymers, 10
Crystallinity, 7, 10, 13, 18, 22, 24, 34, 68, 108, 110, 115, 141, 270
Crystallization, 16, 109, 120, 186
characteristics, 120
Curcumae longae rhizome, 224
Curcumin, 47, 155, 156, 223
Cutting-edge traumatology implants, 165
Cyclic oligomers, 112
Cytocompatible chemical crosslinking techniques, 231
Cytotoxic killing, 66
Cytotoxicity, 63, 68, 71, 91, 99, 139, 223, 226, 227, 243

D

De Broglie wavelengths, 43
Deacetylated (DD), 7, 86
Deacetylation process, 86
Debye-Scherrer equation, 17
Decellularization, 185
Decolorization, 85
Deep tissue penetration, 223
Degradation
behavior, 106, 107, 110, 117, 118, 122, 231
kinetics, 250
mechanisms, 109
Degree of deacetylation (DD), 86, 90, 207
Demineralization, 85, 207, 208
Dental
applications, 149, 157, 159, 193, 203, 253
restoration, 204, 205
sealants, 204–207, 209–212
Dentistry, 182, 184, 194, 203–205, 212
Deproteinization, 85
Dextran, 70, 231, 248
Diabetic
foot ulcers, 230
wound, 35, 220, 235
healing, 35
Diagnostic imaging, 61
Dicalcium phosphate dehydrate (DCPD), 7
Dicarboxylic acid, 9
Differential
deterioration rates, 142
scanning calorimetry (DSC), 16, 18, 44, 113
thermal analysis (DTA), 113
Diffusion, 22, 36, 42, 62, 110, 116, 276, 277
erosion process, 250
Dilute solution viscometry, 19
Dimensional stability, 139, 142, 203
Dimethyl formamide (DMF), 19
Dissolution, 62, 136

Distal
radial fractures, 172
radius, 172, 175
Divinyl silicone rubber, 221
Dopamine, 232
Double
crosslinked hydrogel, 49
network hydrogels, 228
Doxorubicin (DOX), 36, 38, 46, 72
Drug
delivery system, 2–4, 9, 20, 23, 31–36, 38, 41, 44, 46–50, 61, 63, 71, 73, 105, 122, 149, 153, 154, 159, 222, 234, 247, 249, 252, 274
doxorubicin (DOX), 46
encapsulation, 64
loaded
mats, 46
microsphere, 49
scaffolds, 32, 33, 45, 50
loading
capacity, 154
system configuration, 251
releasing
carriers, 38
fiber system applications, 32
Dual
network, 227
responsive hydrogels, 221
Ductility, 12, 140
Dynamic compression plate (DCP), 168, 175

E

Eco-friendly medical utilization, 159
Elastic modulus, 12, 13, 44, 106, 191, 210
Electric arc discharge, 66
Electrochemistry, 64
Electrohydrodynamic jet (EHD-jet), 256
Electroporation (EP), 49
Electrospinning, 31, 35–37, 40, 45
Electrospraying, 35
Electrospun
nanofibers, 225
scaffolds, 37, 46
bioactivity, 22
Electrostatic attraction, 62
Ellagic acid, 47
Elongation (EB), 12, 40, 44, 90, 106, 119, 254
Endochondral ossification, 183, 187
Endocytosis, 68
Engineering thermoplastics, 2
Enhances the permeability and retention (EPR), 64, 72
Environmental
conditions, 110
variables, 107
Enzymatic
biodegradation, 231
catalysis, 247
concentration, 13
Epoxy resin sealer, 209
Ethylene
glycol dimethacrylate, 136
oxide (EtO), 22, 23
Exothermic temperatures, 136
External
compression, 167
torsion, 167
Extracellular matrix (ECM), 35, 46, 141, 193, 194, 219, 220, 231–233, 248, 253, 268, 272
Extrusion
3D printing, 246
bioprinter, 257
printing, 48

F

Fabricated implants, 164
Fabrication, 3, 24, 31–36, 38, 39, 41, 46, 49–51, 62, 110, 133, 134, 164, 190, 233, 246, 252, 254, 256, 258
processes, 133
Fatigue fracture, 184
Femoral head
circulation problems, 169
osteonecrosis, 139
Fiber orientation, 110
Fibrin, 182, 249, 272
Fibrinogen-mediated platelet adhesion, 132
Fibronectinmimetic peptide, 70
Finite element analysis (FEA), 247
Fluid shear stress (FSS), 164, 165
Fluorohectorite (FH), 115
Food
FDA (Food and Drug Administration), 2, 3, 5, 74

medical sectors, 153
packaging, 81–84, 88–90, 92, 96, 99, 119, 149, 156
systems, 89
Fossil fuels, 81
Fourth-generation biomaterials, 193
Fracture, 2, 9, 21, 23, 34, 45, 108, 120, 130, 133, 136–138, 163, 166, 169–172, 174, 175, 182–186, 191, 255
deflection, 182
morphology, 120
pieces, 183
plates, 183, 186
reduction, 169
Framework, 84, 183, 249, 268
Freeze-drying method, 41
Functionalized
gold nanoparticles, 64, 70
nanoparticles (FNP), 62, 64, 70, 72, 73
Fused
deposition modeling (FDM), 46, 48, 135, 245, 246, 249–251, 254, 255, 259
filament fabrication (FFF), 246

G

Gallic acid (GA), 113, 223, 232
Gas pycnometry, 41
Gastrointestinal environment, 252
Gel, 231
Gelatin, 41, 48, 67, 153, 157, 231, 232, 249, 251, 252, 272
methacrylate (GelMA), 67, 231, 251
Gemcitabine, 70
Gene therapy, 34, 47, 63
Glands, 182, 183
Glass
ceramics, 193
ionomer cement (GIC), 204
transition temperature, 10, 12, 24, 37, 41
Gliding nail (GN), 165, 169, 170, 175
technology, 170
Glycerophosphate pentahydrate (G-P), 208
Glycosaminoglycans, 141
Glyoxylate, 11, 14
Goldner trichrome (G/T), 254
Goniometer, 44
Granulation, 229, 231
Graphene oxide (GO), 209, 226, 227
Graphitic carbon nitride, 227
Grazing incidence X-ray diffraction (GIXRD), 17
Guar-gum-based thermoresponsive hydrogel, 48
Guided bone regeneration (GBR), 185, 254

H

Hair follicle maturation, 223
Healing properties, 182, 224
Health problems, 184
Healthcare, 1, 2, 68, 149, 150, 154, 156, 158, 159
applications, 149, 150, 154, 158, 159
expenses, 2
industry, 150
payers, 183
Hemicellulose thermal decomposition, 113
Hemostasis, 220, 222, 232
Hemostatic, 222, 227, 228, 232
Heterogeneous structures, 130
Heterologous bone, 185
High
density polyethylene (HDPE), 132, 133
intensity electric fields, 40
load-bearing skeleton-related applications, 141
Histological examination, 139, 254
Homogeneous mixtures, 134
Hot-melt extrusion, 250
Human
bone marrow-derived mesenchymal stem cells (hBMSCs), 250
clinical trials, 3, 5
mesenchymal stem cells, 117
serum albumin (HSA), 71
Humidity, 23, 90, 107
Hyaluronanmethylcellulose gel systems, 47
Hyaluronic acid (HA), 6, 8, 33–36, 48, 49, 72, 112, 116, 131–134, 137, 139–142, 185–189, 193, 223, 231, 245, 247, 248, 252–256, 273, 275, 276
bio-streptavidin-alginate (HBSA), 49
drug-eluting systems, 49
sintered powder, 134
sponge-type scaffolds, 48
Hybrid nanosheets' photocatalytic activity, 227
Hydrochloric acid, 88

Hydrogel, 1, 36, 45, 47–49, 67, 89, 141, 142, 208, 219–235, 245, 250, 252, 267, 269
conductive materials, 228
delivery vehicle, 234
dressings, 229, 232
drug delivery, 234
matrix, 233
precursor solution, 223
wound dressings, 230
Hydrolysis, 3, 7, 10, 12–14, 108, 109, 116–118, 138, 247, 252, 267, 270–273
Hydrolytic degradation, 13
Hydrophilic
molecule encapsulation, 47
nature, 152, 220
Hydrophilicity, 31, 44, 46, 116, 118, 132, 155, 206, 248, 270
Hydrophobic
nature, 108
particles, 235
Hydrophobicity, 210, 248, 270, 276
Hydrostatic extrusion, 133
Hydroxy
acids, 8, 245, 250, 252, 267, 269
carbonate apatite (HCA), 186
Hydroxyapatite (HAp), 6, 46, 71, 116, 130–133, 137–140, 157, 158, 164, 186, 188, 189, 196, 209, 245, 249, 251, 253–255, 272, 275, 276
poly(hydroxybutyrate) (HA-PHB), 140
Hydroxypropyl guar (HPG), 48

I

Ibuprofen, 155, 250
drug, 154
Immobilization, 172, 183
Immune cells, 73, 74
Immunocytochemistry, 257
Immunogenicity, 62, 250
Impact-resistant, 182
Implantable scaffolds, 48, 49
Implantology, 61
In situ, 140, 231
In vitro, 42, 254
In vivo, 7, 8, 22, 32, 36, 44, 45, 51, 62, 106, 108, 118, 122, 131, 134, 137–140, 165, 184, 190, 193, 197, 204, 227, 232, 244, 247, 252–256, 268, 269, 274
Inert biomaterials, 187
Inflammation, 11, 20, 70, 136, 139, 142, 220, 223–225, 233, 235, 273–275
Injectable
material technologies, 196
platelet-rich fibrin (I-PRF), 182
polymeric platforms, 32
Injection molding, 2, 115, 122, 190
Inorganic
ceramic composites, 130
materials, 184
nanoparticles, 73, 74, 114, 115
species, 154
Interlocked nails, 166, 174
Intermolecular transesterification, 12
Internal
compression, 167
fixation
devices, 3, 164, 204
implants, 2
techniques, 185
fracture, 182, 183
torsion, 167
Intestinal inflammation, 224
Intramedullary
implant, 169
nails, 185
static locked, 168
Intramembranous, 183
Intramolecular transesterification, 3, 112
Intraocular lenses, 268
Intricate multistage structure, 165
Intrinsic
birefringence, 17
viscosity, 19

J

Jaw-and-mouth, 181, 184
reconstruction, 181

K

Keratinocytes, 274
Kinetics, 107, 250
Kirschner wire, 171

L

Lactide monomer, 112

Lactobacillus species, 207, 209
Laponite nanosheets, 227
Large-scale availability, 249
Laser ablation, 66
Ligaments, 24, 182, 183, 248, 272
Lightweight green nanocomposite materials, 82
Lignocellulosic
fibers, 113
materials, 113
Limbrelated injuries, 167
Liquid
bonding agents, 246
photopolymers, 246
Load bearing
applications, 107, 131
capacity, 44
properties, 167
Local vascularization, 169
Locked compression plate (LCP), 168, 175
Longterm
degradation research, 122
durability, 184, 229
Low-density polyethylene (LDPE), 132
L-polylactic acid, 254
Lymphatic system, 73

M

M1 macrophage polarization, 250
Macro
microporous structure, 255
scale, 164
Macromolecular
adsorption, 91
systems, 64
Macron-sized ranges, 245
Macrophage-derived conditioned medium (M-CM), 250
Magnesium aluminate ($MgAl_2O_4$), 182
Magnetic
hybrid nanomaterials (MHNs), 69
nanoparticles, 49, 69
resonance imaging (MRI), 63, 69, 70, 158
Malarial drug quinine, 64
Mandibular bone, 181, 184
Marine brown algae, 153
Material
characterization, 254
stiffness, 134
Maxillary, 181, 184
Maxillofacial, 108, 111, 182, 185, 196
injuries, 185
osteo fixation, 108
osteosynthesis operations, 185
surgery, 108, 196
trauma surgery, 111
Mechanical
characteristics, 5, 13, 24, 71, 90, 108, 117, 120, 132, 133, 137–141, 163–165, 183, 223, 227, 228, 245, 247, 248, 250, 270, 272, 273
performance, 107, 134, 184, 190
property, 3, 11, 21, 23, 31, 38, 44, 64, 73, 82, 89, 106, 107, 109, 117–120, 122, 129–132, 138, 191, 206, 252, 254, 255, 257, 258, 276
qualities, 5, 7, 12, 24, 82, 137, 139, 165, 244, 268, 276
stability, 5, 33, 36, 111
stiffness, 275
stimulation, 130, 164
stimuli, 130, 164
strength, 6, 8, 12, 39, 41, 42, 91, 106, 108, 111, 132, 139, 141, 143, 156, 164, 182, 196, 204, 219, 234, 235, 254–257, 276
Medical
applications, 3, 35, 38, 63, 153, 184
sensors, 191
technological advancements, 243
textiles, 149
Medications, 65, 193, 210, 220, 223, 224, 230, 234
Medullary pins, 174
Melt
flow index, 19
molding, 141
spinning, 14
Melting temperature, 3, 12, 37, 191
Membrane lamination, 41
Meniscal
repair devices, 23
stingers, 20
Mercury volume readings, 43
Mesenchymal stromal cell cultures, 46
Mesh, 20, 40, 182
Metabiomaterials, 182

Metabolization, 244, 269
Metal, 182
ceramic-based biomaterials, 105
composites, 235
Metallic
implantable scaffolds, 49
implants, 130
materials, 189
oxidization, 130
scaffolds, 182
Metaphyseal fractures, 172
Methacrylate
cement, 139
chitosan (ChMA), 231
groups, 231
Methane, 112
Methotrexate, 70, 252
Methyl methacrylate (MMA), 136, 137, 139, 251
monomer, 136
Microbial
fermentation, 114, 115
perforations, 219
synthesis, 37
Micro-computed tomography tests, 255
Microcracking, 182
Microfractures, 12
Micro-granules, 8
Microleakage, 208
Micromechanical modeling, 247
Micrometric interfragmentary strain, 183
Micromotion, 183
Microscopic studies, 141
Microstructural organization, 10
Microstructure, 13, 275
Milliliters (mL), 19
Mimic, 184, 194, 252
bone structures, 182
Mineralization, 141, 192, 257, 276
Miniplates, 182
Minocycline hydrochloride (MH), 45, 46
Molar mass products, 12
Molecular
reinforcement, 142
weight (MW), 3, 6–9, 11, 22, 24, 65, 90, 107–109, 116–118, 132, 138–140, 245, 248, 269, 270, 272
Molten polymer, 14
Monoliths, 184
Monomer-associated liquids, 136
Montmorillonite (MMT), 115, 227
Mucor rouxii, 87
Multidisciplinary plates, 172
Multifaceted angle stability plates, 173
Multifunctional
bionanocomposites, 150
nanocomposites, 149
nanoparticles, 72
Multiscale modeling, 122
Muscles, 171, 182, 183
Musculoskeletal implants, 190

N

N-(2-aminoethyl)- 3-aminopropyltrimethoxysilane (AEAPS), 275
N-acetyl
D-glucosamine, 86, 140
glucosamine, 7
Nail insertion, 174, 175
Nano amorphous, 209
Nano drug delivery systems, 32
Nanoalginate materials, 153
Nano-carriers (NCs), 48
Nanoclays, 114, 115, 227
Nanocomposite, 92, 150–152, 276
applications, 150
materials, 82, 258
Nanocrystalline rod-like structure, 130
Nanodimensional fillers, 149
Nano-fiber, 40, 71, 107, 117, 222, 224, 225
hydrogel composites, 225
matrices, 6
multifunctional hydrogels, 225
Nano-fillers, 150
Nanogels, 64
Nanohydroxyapatite (nHA), 72, 140, 204, 209, 249, 254, 255, 257
Nanomaterial, 38, 50, 61, 62, 64, 69, 71–74, 82, 204, 210, 222, 226, 227
nanomedicines, 74
Nanomedicines, 74
Nanoparticle (NP), 22, 46, 49, 62–74, 107, 114, 115, 117, 139, 149, 151, 154, 159, 204, 207–211, 222, 223, 225–228, 234, 250, 252, 258
cytotoxicity, 68

Nano-reinforced composite hydrogels, 225
Nano-scaled fillers, 149
Nanosheets, 227, 228
Nanosilver, 204
Nanostructures, 61, 220, 225, 227, 270
Nanotechnology, 62, 64, 68, 70, 143, 149, 150
Nanowires, 228
Natural
  biopolymers, 114
  fibers, 114, 121
  hemostasis process, 232
  metabolites, 250, 273
  organic materials, 185
  polymers, 32, 35, 248, 272
  tissues, 184
N-dimethylacetamide, 9
Near-infrared (NIR), 49, 223
Neotissue formation, 42
Neovascularization, 223, 229
Nerve
  guide tubes, 9
  root radiculopathy, 136
Neural stem cells (NSCs), 45
Neurodegenerative diseases, 47
Neurosurgery, 182
Neurovascular network, 182, 183
New Jersey (NJ), 11
Nickel-titanium shape, 189
Nimodipine, 36
N-isopropyl acrylamide (NIPAM), 221
Nitrides, 191
Nitrobenzene, 9
Non-biodegradable medicines, 159
Noncariogenic plaque, 207
Non-immunogenic organic materials, 185
Non-interconnected pores, 42
Non-metallic bond fixation, 130
Nontoxic properties, 82
Nonvolatile solvent, 15
Novel polyesteramide copolymers, 5
Nozzle-based fused deposition modeling, 245
Nucleic acid transport, 71

O

Olecranon fractures, 171, 172
Oligomers, 112, 136, 137, 247, 271
One-pot synthesis, 65
Optical characterization, 18
Orbital floor procedures, 134
Organ
  acids, 88, 142, 207
  biomaterials, 184, 185
  materials, 130
  mimic implants, 62
Organs, 24, 38, 71–73, 184, 244, 258, 268, 272, 273
Orthognathic surgery, 111
Orthopedic, 2, 32, 105, 182, 189, 191, 204, 241
  applications, 117, 129, 130
  bone plates, 183
  implant, 2, 21, 106, 130, 138, 142, 184, 186, 241
  procedures, 23
  prostheses, 131
  remedies, 138
  surgeons, 166
  surgery, 20, 108, 130, 137
Orthosorb pins, 20
Osseointegration, 182, 194, 245, 254, 275
Osteoblast, 138, 187
  colonization, 186
Osteocalcin, 254
Osteoclasts, 138
Osteoconduction, 7
Osteoconductive, 6, 138, 182, 186, 187, 192
  materials, 182
Osteoconductivity, 132, 157, 196, 253, 257
Osteogenesis, 70, 253
Osteogenic
  activity, 252
  differentiation, 253, 256, 276
  performance, 252
Osteoinduction, 187
Osteoinductivity, 253
Osteointegratability, 157
Osteointegration, 7, 132, 186, 192
Osteoporosis, 6, 130, 149, 157, 159, 169
  treatment, 157
Osteo-related gene expression, 256
Osteostimulation, 183
Osteosynthesis, 2, 21, 138, 170–174, 185, 189, 255
  treatments, 138
Osteosynthetic state progression, 174
Osteotomy, 171
Oxidation responsiveness, 225

P

Paclitaxel (PTX), 36, 45–48, 70, 71
Palates, 182, 184
Parkinson's disease (PD), 47
Passive hydrolysis, 272
Patella fractures, 165, 171, 175
Patient health hazards, 183
Pediatric surgery, 111
Penetrometer, 43
Percutaneous insertion, 165
Periosteum, 183
Perivertebral veins, 136
Perkin Elmer diamond DMA, 19
Permeability, 38, 41, 42, 64, 89, 91, 220
Pertrochanteric
  fractures, 169
  injury, 169, 170
Phagocytic processes, 5
Phantom soft-thread, 20
Pharmaceutical
  applications, 64
  domains, 1
  treatments, 64
Pharmacokinetic properties, 62
pH, 72
Phloroglucinol triglycidyl methacrylate, 137
Phosphate-buffered saline (PBS), 32, 46, 48, 49, 115, 166
Photoacoustic imaging (PAI), 69
Photodynamic therapy, 47, 69
Photothermal
  conversion, 67
  therapy (PTT), 47, 65–67, 222, 223
  treatment, 66
Physical
  degradation, 109
  functionalization, 68
Physicochemical
  factors, 232
  properties, 61, 62, 211
  requirements, 182
Physicomechanical properties, 153
Pilon
  fractures, 173
  injuries, 175
Pinocytosis, 68
Piriformis fossa, 169
Plasma etching, 22
Plasmid DNA (pDNA), 70
Plasticization, 116
Plate osteosynthesis, 171, 173
Platelet-rich fibrin (PRF), 182, 196
P-nitrophenol, 9
Poly lactic-co-glycolic acid (PLGA), 182
Poly(2-hydroxyethyl methacrylate), 220
Poly(3- hydroxy octanoate), 249, 272
Poly-(3-hydroxybutyrate-co-3-hydroxyvalerate) (PHBV), 37, 249
Poly(3-hydroxybutyrate-co3-hydroxyvalerate-co-3-hydroxyhexanoate) (PHBVHHx), 37
Poly(4-hydroxybutyrate), 249
Poly(amides), 248
Poly(amino acid), 3, 5, 8
Poly(anhydrides), 248
Poly(butylene succinate) (PBS), 32, 115
Poly(caprolactone) (PCL), 32–34, 38, 44–47, 71, 110, 113, 114, 117, 152, 182, 251, 253–257, 276
Poly(D,L-lactide) (PDLLA), 111, 115, 251
Poly(dioxanone), 3, 5
Poly(ester amide), 3, 5
Poly(esters), 248, 271
Poly(glycolic acid) (PGA), 3, 5, 9, 37, 110, 248
Poly(hydroxybutyrate) (PHB), 140
Poly(hydroxyvalerate) (PHV), 140
Poly(lactic acid) (PLA), 3, 5, 9, 37, 110, 112, 252, 253, 255, 256, 258
  bioresorbable polymers, 274
Poly(lactic-coglycolic acid) (PLGA), 20, 22, 37, 41, 45, 48, 49, 71, 108, 109, 116, 120, 121, 182, 245, 248, 252, 253, 273, 274
  bioresorbable polymers, 273
Poly(methyl methacrylate) (PMMA), 134, 136–138, 182, 251
  bone cements, 136, 137
  cement extravasation, 136
Poly(ortho ester), 3, 5, 245, 248, 267, 269
Poly(phosphazenes), 248
Poly(propylene fumarate) (PPF), 138
Poly(trimethylene carbonate) (PTMC), 120, 121
Poly(ε-caprolactone) (PCL), 117
Poly-3-hydroxybutyrate (PHB), 37
Polyacid-modified monomer, 210
Polyallylamine, 64

Polyamide, 5, 271
  structure, 5
Polyamidoamine (PAMAM), 48
Polyamino acids, 271
Polyanhydrides, 3, 5, 38, 245, 267, 269
Polycaprolactone (PCL), 3, 5, 32, 38, 113, 152, 182, 250, 253, 275
  bioresorbable polymers, 275
  tricalcium phosphate (PCL/TCP), 253, 254
Polycationic properties, 91
Polydioxanone (PDO), 2, 9–14, 20–22, 38, 117, 118
Poly-D-lactic acid (PDLA), 108, 112, 273
Polydopamine (PDA), 223
Polyester, 5, 34, 37, 113, 119, 138, 139, 182, 245, 250, 256, 267, 269, 271, 272, 275
Polyesteramides (PEAs), 8
Polyethylene (PE), 47, 48, 64, 68, 70–72, 119, 132–134, 245, 267, 270
  glycol (PEG), 64, 68, 245, 267, 270
Polyethyleneimine (PEI), 68, 72
Polyglycolic acid (PGA), 2, 9–14, 20–22, 24, 34, 37, 40, 41, 107–112, 186, 188, 248, 252
Polyheterocycles, 22
Poly-hydroxy
  aliphatic esters, 1
  valerate, 3
Polyhydroxyalkanoate (PHA), 32, 37, 247–249, 272
Polyhydroxybutyrate (PHB), 3, 5, 37, 112–114, 140
  thermal degradation, 112
Polyhydroxyvalerate, 5
Poly-lactate, 276
Polylactic
  acid (PLA), 2, 3, 6, 9–14, 20–24, 32, 34, 37, 38, 40, 44–49, 108–110, 112–116, 152, 157, 186, 188, 245, 252–255, 273–275
    cellulose acetate-based nanofibrous mats, 46
    silica-based nanocomposite, 157
  coglycolic acid (PLGA), 245
Poly-L-CO-DL-Lactide (PLDLA), 108, 109
Poly-L-Lactic Acid (PLLA), 12, 20, 21, 40, 41, 108, 111, 112, 252, 254, 255, 273
Polymer, 1–3, 5–12, 14–24, 31–35, 37, 38, 40, 41, 44, 47–51, 61, 64–66, 70, 71, 73, 81–84, 88, 90, 91, 105–113, 115–119, 121, 123, 129, 131, 132, 134, 136, 138–140, 142, 143, 149, 150, 152, 153, 163, 181, 185, 188, 191–193, 203, 219–222, 227–229, 231, 232, 243–250, 252–259, 267–274, 276, 277
  composition, 110–112
  functionalization groups, 64
  linkages, 3
  matrix, 22, 38, 106, 109, 116–119, 134, 142, 271
    reaction, 134
  thermal degradation, 18
Polymerase chain reaction (PCR), 254, 257
Polymerceramic
  biomaterials, 105
  composite materials, 130
  interfaces, 134
Polymeric
  bioabsorbable
    composites, 137, 138
    substances, 245
  biomaterials, 130, 269, 270, 277
  coatings, 68
  composites, 12, 24, 105–107, 109, 110, 122, 123, 138, 139, 243, 248, 267
  fibers, 40, 111
  foam, 41, 255
  fragments, 65
  materials, 32, 91, 138, 243, 247–249, 252
  matrix, 106, 227
  membrane, 39
  solution, 39
  substances, 71, 107, 244, 270
Polymerization, 9, 16, 24, 37, 65, 108, 136, 204
Polymethyl methacrylate, 132
  resin, 209
Polyphasic composite, 182
Polyphenol-derived moieties, 232
Polyphosphazenes, 271
Polypropylene matrix, 121–123
Polypyrrole (PPy), 72, 222, 227
Polysaccharide, 32, 34, 82, 88, 152, 153, 221, 231, 272
  bio-nanocomposites, 152
  nanocomposites, 152

natural polymers, 248
polymeric compounds, 272
polymers, 248
Polyurethane, 244, 267, 269
Polyvinyl alcohol (PVA), 40, 45, 46, 152, 220
Porogens, 39
Porosity, 13, 38–43, 49, 50, 67, 109, 116, 132, 140–143, 190, 244, 275
Porous
iron oxide nano agents (PIONs), 69
tantalum, 182
Posterior compression, 167
Post
curing temperature, 259
implantation, 134, 139
modification strategy, 65
thrombotic sequelae, 173
Postoperative infection, 184
Potassium aluminum sulfate, 232, 233
Potential cytotoxicity, 63
Povidoneiodine (PVP-I), 208
Powder
bed fusion, 182, 196
metallurgy, 182
Power densities, 67
Preliminary clinical studies, 73
Pre-reacted glass ionomer (PRG), 211
Printability, 244, 249, 250, 257, 258
Proangiogenic
capabilities, 229
hydrogels, 230
Prodigiosin (PG), 48
Proliferation, 7, 8, 22, 32, 42, 46, 47, 67, 71, 116, 117, 143, 186, 193, 220, 222, 229, 231, 245, 248, 252–257
Propenyl-2-butenoate, 112
Propylene glycol, 138
Prosthetic
design, 169
transplant, 166
Protein
adsorption, 8, 64, 132
natural polymers, 249
polymers, 231, 248, 272
Proximal femoral nail (PFN), 169
Proximal humerus, 172, 173, 175
Psychological
effects, 184
impact, 182
Pulmonary embolism, 136
Pulp-dentin complex, 157
Pulverized injuries, 173
Puncture deformation, 90
Pure chitosan films, 88
Pyridine, 9
Pyromellitic dianhydride (PMDA), 275

R

Rabbit intramuscular implantation, 139
Radiation therapy, 47
Radiological images, 174
Rapid prototyping (RP), 41
Reactive oxygen species (ROS), 68, 72, 208, 223, 232
Reduced GO (rGO), 211, 227, 256, 257
Re-epithelialization, 226, 229
Refractory fractures, 183
Regenerative
medicine, 62, 72, 73, 149, 194, 227, 244, 268, 271, 273
therapy, 71
tissues, 154
Reinforcement, 110
Relative humidity (RH), 90
Resin, 204, 210
Resorbable
implants, 164
polymer systems, 193
Restorations, 205
Robust, 10, 12, 111, 121, 182, 206
Root canal sealant, 208
Rutin, 223

S

Salmon, 88
Sawbones, 255
Scaffold, 1, 2, 7, 8, 13, 20–22, 31, 32–51, 67, 71, 106, 117, 132, 134, 139–143, 149, 164, 165, 182, 184, 194, 196, 225, 228, 243, 244, 246–250, 252–257, 268–270, 272, 273, 275, 276
applications, 36
fabrication techniques, 32, 33
morphology, 257
Scanning electron microscopy (SEM), 41–43, 116–118, 156, 158, 256

Schiff base, 72
Screw osteotomies, 174
Sealant, 203, 204, 208, 209, 211, 212
Secondary
healing, 183
osteoporotic individuals, 136
Second-generation biomaterials, 186, 192
Segmental imperfections, 140
Selective
degradation behavior, 117
laser sintering (SLS), 134, 245–247, 251, 257
Self/non-self-recognition, 221
Selfassembled scaffolds, 225
Self-healing, 48, 220, 228
Self-reinforcement, 111
technique, 111
Self-reinforcing (SR), 10, 12, 13, 20, 21, 109, 111
Semicrystalline, 10, 23, 37
Semi-synthetic biopolymers, 152
Sensory abilities, 183
Septic encephalopathy, 69
Shear
orientation molding injection, 133
rate, 3
strength, 12, 13
Silk fibroin-based scaffolds, 41
Silver nanoparticle, 208, 209
Simonkolleite (SKT), 211
Simplex radiopaque, 136
Single
network hydrogels, 228
photon emission computed tomography, 69
Skin
diseases, 219
lesion disorders, 20
Small
angle X-ray scattering (SAXS), 17
nano-sized particles, 73
Smart screws, 20
Sodium alginate (SA), 44
Soft tissue, 20, 110, 165, 169, 172–174, 183, 191
Sol-gel transformation temperature, 47
Solvent
spinning, 2
sublimation, 142
Split skin grafting, 174
Sponge-shaped bio-nanocomposite, 155
Spray-dried
HA (sd HA), 48
materials, 134
Stainless steel bone screws, 138
Staphylococcus aureus, 156
Starch, 149, 151, 153, 248, 272
bio-nanocomposites, 153
Static magnetic field (SMF), 49, 51
Stereochemistry, 23
Stereolithography (SLA), 245–247, 257
Sterilization, 22
processes, 2
Stimuli-responsive
materials, 33
nanomaterials, 72
scaffold system, 49
Streptococcus sobrinus, 208
Stress shielding, 120, 130, 131, 139, 164, 183, 184, 187
Stretchability, 231
Subcutaneous tissues, 183
Sulfides, 191
Super toughness, 228
Supercritical foaming, 275
Superparamagnetic iron oxide nanoparticles (SPIONs), 69, 70
Superparamagnetism, 69
Supplementary
biocompatible ingredients, 274
remodeled infusions, 173
Supramolecular hydrogel, 225
Surface
adherent dependent cells, 141
area-to-volume ratio, 41, 42
erosion, 271
functionalization, 61, 66, 68, 276
roughness, 116, 209
sealants, 210
texture, 39
to-volume ratio, 210
water wettability, 120
Surgical
incisions, 233
meshes, 9
Sustainability, 89, 174
Synergistic interaction, 89, 222

Synthetic
bioabsorbable polymers, 267
biomaterials, 182, 186, 192
material, 164, 184–187, 203
molecules, 41
polymer, 32, 40, 90, 131, 269
bioresorbable composites, 273
films, 88

T

Tannic acid, 223, 232
Targeted
agent delivery, 63
delivery of pharmaceutical agents, 62
medicine delivery, 270
Temperature, 3, 10, 14–16, 18, 19, 24, 37, 41, 47, 48, 86, 107–110, 112, 113, 115, 119, 131, 136, 139, 191, 206, 220, 221, 231, 241, 259, 276
induced depolymerization, 3
variations, 276
Temporary prosthetic skin, 9
Tendons, 24, 171, 174, 185, 272
Tensile
modulus, 12, 120–122
strength, 12, 40, 44, 90, 106, 116–121, 133, 134, 137, 156, 157, 250, 254, 255, 275
Tension band
compression nail (TCN), 171
synthesis method, 171
Tetra calcium phosphate (TTCP), 275
Tetracycline hydrochloride, 38
Therapeutic properties, 156, 205
Thermal
deterioration, 8
distortion, 24
expansion coefficients, 210
gravimetric analysis (TGA), 18, 44, 113–115
history, 23, 24
properties, 112, 120
stability, 89, 106, 115, 118, 121, 154, 255, 256
Thermodynamic
analysis, 113
characteristics, 120
properties, 120
Thermogravimetric, 44, 113
analyzer (TGA), 18, 44
Thermogravimetry, 113
analysis (TGA), 113
Thermoplastic polymer filament, 246
Thermoresponsive
gel, 48
hydrogels, 47
Thin skin transplants, 173
Third-generation biomaterials, 193
Three-dimensional (3D)
bioprinting, 158, 159, 196, 244, 256, 276
medical scanned data, 258
porous structures, 193
printer-friendly software, 246
printing applications, 31, 32, 41, 46, 49, 189, 196, 228, 243, 244, 246, 249, 256, 258, 259
structures, 246
tissue modeling human pancreatic cancer cell spheroids, 251
Thymoquinone (TQ), 45, 46
loaded electrospun mats, 46
Tissue, 11, 20, 24, 38, 62–64, 69, 71, 72, 105, 143, 154, 165, 171, 181, 183, 184, 186, 187, 191–193, 196, 197, 219–221, 229, 231, 243, 244, 248, 258, 268, 270, 276
degeneration, 267
development, 184
engineering (TE), 1, 13, 21, 22, 24, 32, 34, 37–39, 44, 46, 61, 63, 67, 71, 72, 106, 116, 117, 122, 129, 131, 138, 141–143, 149, 154, 158, 159, 165, 182, 184, 188, 194, 196, 197, 220, 221, 226, 244, 247–249, 252, 253, 256, 258, 267–274, 276, 277
applications, 37, 39, 44, 117, 141, 221, 253, 256, 258
techniques, 196
growth, 49, 131, 132, 196, 197, 270
regeneration, 21, 116, 141, 143, 157, 184, 185, 219, 225, 229, 233, 248, 249, 270, 273, 275, 276
remodeling, 231
restoration process, 155
stability preservation, 268
Titania, 137, 191
Titanium alloys (Ti), 130, 182, 183, 189, 190
Tooth-sealant interface, 204
Torsional stiffness, 134
Toxicology, 99
Traditional
antibiotics, 226
Chinese medicine (TCM), 220, 222, 224
Transdermal drug delivery, 41

Transducer movement, 167
Transmission electron microscopy (TEM), 43, 140
Trauma, 71, 111, 129, 130, 163, 171, 182, 185, 222
Traumatic injuries, 183
Traumatologic procedures, 21
Triboelectric nanogenerators, 229
Tricalcium phosphate (TCP), 131, 137–140, 142, 182, 185, 188, 196, 253–256, 272–276
  composite structure, 272
Tri-dimensional anatomy accuracy, 196
Trimethoprim (TMP), 49
Triple
  helix type 1 collagen, 130
  negative breast cancer (TNBC), 48
Trochanteric
  area, 169
  fractures stabilization, 169
  injuries, 165, 170
Tumor
  clearance, 66
  excision, 182

U

Ubbelohde viscometer, 19
Ultimate tensile strength (UTS), 44
Ultrafine layered titanate, 114, 115
Ultra-high molecular weight polyethylene (UHMWPE), 132, 133, 241
Ultrasound-sensitive (US), 49, 130, 185
Ultraviolet (UV), 44, 68, 234, 246, 259
Unsaturated polyester resin, 119
Uronic acid residues, 153

V

Vaccinations, 68
Vascular endothelial growth factor (VEGF), 46, 73, 228
  laponite gels accelerated tubulogenesis, 228
Vascularization potential, 229
Violence, 181, 184
Volatile organic compounds (VOCs), 259

W

Warping, 142
Washburn equation, 43
Water-soluble nature, 49
Wear, 184, 187, 190, 206, 241
Wide-angle X-ray
  diffraction (WAXD), 17
  scattering (WAXS), 17
Wolfberries, 88
Wood flour (WF), 118, 119
Wound
  contraction, 229
  dressing, 21, 36, 46, 47, 149, 220, 222, 224, 225, 227, 230, 232, 234, 235, 249
  healing applications, 20, 32, 33, 35, 44, 105, 149, 154–156, 159, 219–227, 229, 230, 232–234, 249, 272

X

Xenogenic transplants, 184
Xenograft, 70, 185, 268
X-ray
  diffraction (XRD), 17, 18, 44
  spectroscopy, 42

Z

Zinc oxide (ZnO), 44, 73, 208, 209, 222, 226
  nanocomposite hydrogels, 226
  nanoparticle (ZnO NP), 44, 208, 209, 222, 226
Zirconia, 191
Zygomatic
  bones, 185
  fracture fixation, 108